IMPACT OF CARDIAC SURGERY ON THE QUALITY OF LIFE

Neurological and Psychological Aspects

IMPACT OF CARDIAC SURGERY ON THE QUALITY OF LIFE
Neurological and Psychological Aspects

Edited by

Allen E. Willner

Long Island Jewish Medical Center, Hillside Hospital
Glen Oaks, New York

and

Georg Rodewald

University Hospital Hamburg-Eppendorf
Hamburg, Federal Republic of Germany

PLENUM PRESS • NEW YORK AND LONDON

Library of Congress Cataloging-in-Publication Data

International Symposium on the Impact of Cardiac Surgery on the
  Quality of Life: Neurological and Psychological Aspects (3rd : 1989
  : New York, N.Y.)
    Impact of cardiac surgery on the quality of life : neurological
  and psychological aspects / edited by Allen E. Willner and Georg
  Rodewald.
      p.   cm.
    "Proceedings of the Third International Symposium on the Impact of
  Cardiac Surgery on the Quality of Life: Neurological and
  Psychological Aspects, held March 28-30, 1989, in New York, New
  York"--T.p. verso.
    Includes bibliographical references.
    Includes index.

    ISBN-13: 978-1-4612-7908-2   e-ISBN-13: 978-1-4613-0647-4
    DOI: 10.1007/978-1-4613-0647-4

    1. Heart--Surgery--Psychological aspects--Congresses. 2. Heart-
  -Surgery--Patients--Mental health--Congresses. 3. Heart--Surgery-
  -Patients--Psychological testing--Congresses. 4. Quality of life-
  -Evaluation--Congresses.   I. Willner, Allen E.   II. Rodewald,
  Georg.   III. Title.
    [DNLM: 1. Heart Surgery--adverse effects--congresses. 2. Heart
  Surgery--psychology--congresses. 3. Mental Disorders--etiology-
  -congresses. 4. Nervous System Diseases--etiology--congresses.
  5. Prognosis--congresses. 6. Psychological Tests--congresses.
  7. Quality of Life--congresses.   WG 169 I606i 1989]
  RD598.I537 1989
  617.4'12'0019--dc20
  DNLM/DLC
  for Library of Congress   90-14215
                                                           CIP

Proceedings of the Third International Symposium on the Impact of
Cardiac Surgery on the Quality of Life: Neurological and Psychological Aspects,
held March 28–30, 1989, in New York, New York

© 1990 Plenum Press, New York
Softcover reprint of the hardcover 1st edition 1990

A Division of Plenum Publishing Corporation
233 Spring Street, New York, N.Y. 10013

ACKNOWLEDGEMENTS

On behalf of our Consortium we would all like to thank several people who helped to make possible the International Symposium and this book:

1. All our colleagues without whose efforts this International study could never have been carried out.

2. Three intelligent and diligent young women: Sharon Windwer, Carol Ritter, and Janet Sendar, who did the essential but tedious work of scoring, checking and entering the data into the computer.

3. Ms. Ann Boehme and her co-workers from the LIJ Department of Continuing Education, Debbie Mohr and Mindy Gordon, who helped us accomplish the almost impossible task of organizing an International Symposium within two months rather than the customary two years.

4. Carol Ritter, who was unflaggingly cheerful, intelligent and thorough in carrying out the seemingly interminable tasks required in turning a collection of manuscripts into a book.

5. Ginny Fay, for her tireless efforts in typing the manuscript.

6. Plenum Publishing Corp. for its help in quickly putting this book into print and especially Melanie Yelity and Greg Safford for their thoughtfulness and direction.

7. Ken Moeller, Ph.D., for his many years of work in the earlier stages of this research.

8. And finally, Dr. Robert Flemma for his enthusiasm and guidance during the long planning stages of the International Study.

CONTENTS

NEUROLOGICAL ISSUES

PSYCHOMETRIC ISSUES

MEDICAL/SURGICAL DATA

CORRELATIONS BETWEEN MEDICAL/SURGICAL DATA AND POSTOPERATIVE PSYCHIATRIC, NEUROLOGICAL AND PSYCHOMETRIC CONDITION

CORRELATIONS BETWEEN PSYCHIATRIC, NEUROLOGICAL AND PSYCHOMETRIC VARIABLES

PREDICTION AND POSTOPERATIVE OUTCOME

QUALITY OF LIFE

INTRODUCTION

Georg Rodewald
University of Hamburg
Hamburg, Federal Republic of Germany

Allen E. Willner
Hillside Hospital
Glen Oaks, NY

In contrast to the initial years of cardiac surgery (37 years ago), there is now increasing interest in cerebral protection. Rodewald [1] in 1978 was among the first to point out the surgeon's concern with "psychopathological problems" and Taylor [2] in 1989 stressed that " . . . the awareness of the cerebral consequences of open heart surgery has risen considerably in recent years . . . " This book reviews the evidence for neurological, psychological, and neuropsychological reactions to cardiac surgery.

In previous studies one problem is that small samples of patients were studied with different measuring instruments so that it was difficult to make sense of inconsistent findings. Considerable controversy resulted with little ability to sort out discrepant findings. It appeared that a large multi-center study using uniform measures might help clarify the picture.

FORMATION AND DEVELOPMENT OF THE INTERNATIONAL CONSORTIUM AND INTERNATIONAL STUDY

With support from the Deutsche Forschungsgemeinschaft (German Research Society), between 1974 and 1982, eight institutions of the University of Hamburg conducted a project devoted to: "An analysis of the factors causing postoperative psychopathological and neurological dysfunctions in patients who had undergone cardiac surgery involving extracorporeal circulation."

Impact of Cardiac Surgery on the Quality of Life
Edited by A. E. Willner and G. Rodewald
Plenum Press, New York, 1990

In this connection, the first International Symposium took place in Hamburg in 1978 followed by a second in Milwaukee in 1980 [3, 4]. During these meetings it was agreed that neurological and psychiatric-psychological reactions to open heart surgery constitute a very serious problem. However, it was noticed that results of corresponding investigations often differed considerably as regards to severity as well as frequency of findings.

There were several possible reasons for these discrepant results: retrospective versus prospective examinations; type and severity of heart disease; actual conduct of anesthesia, surgery, and especially extracorporeal circulation; post-operative treatment in the I.C.U.; methods used in specific examinations, and qualification and training of those conducting these examinations.

In order to cope with these problems an International Forum was created during the Milwaukee Meeting in 1980. Sub-sequently, the International Consortium was founded in 1982 in order to carry out an international study. All participants would use the same protocol as well as identical methods for neurological and psychiatric-psychological investigation, the "common yardstick" in this study. In order to meet this requirement a basic protocol was developed at two workshops in Milwaukee in May and October 1982.

The entire documentation (i.e. all the data compiled for each patient) was very extensive. It covers 69 pages and contains 12 questionnaires and 12 test procedures. The considerable degree of resources required dictated that in any one center it would be difficult to examine more than two patients a week.

Since the total number of patients for one center alone was too small to allow extensive statistical conclusions to be drawn, it was essential that the study be conducted on a multicenter basis. Eventually 9 centers entered the study, although initially more institutions were interested in participating. For the latter, the main difficulty was problems of interdisciplinary cooperation and lack of finan-cial support, because each center was required to provide its own financial resources for the study. Table 1 shows the 9 centers participating in the study.

In contrast to typical studies with different measuring instruments and small samples, the International Study is a multicenter study with a final sample of 900 to 1000 patients, in which exactly the same protocol is used across 9 centers in

Europe, South America and the United States. Our intention was to partial out and identify the effects associated with centers having widely differing geographical locations and social systems in order to specify the common factors associated with neurological, psychological, and neuro-psychological impairment in the patient after the surgery.

Table 1. List of the 9 Centers Participating in the Study

Institution	City	Language
Long Island Jewish Medical Center	New York	English
St. Francis Hospital	Evanston, Illinois, USA	English
Clinica Shaio	Bogota, Colombia	Spanish
Univ. of Milan Med. School	Milan, Italy	Italian
Heart Institute Hospital das Clinicas	Sao Paulo, Brazil	Portuguese
Medical School, Univ. of Oulu	Oulu, Finland	Finnish, Swedish
University Hosp., Eppendorf	Hamburg, FRG	German
CAU Univ. Hospital	Kiel, FRG	German
Rehabilitation Center	Bad Krozingen, FRG	German

The International Study is a polyglot enterprise as illustrated here by the seven different languages involved. It was therefore necessary to translate some tests and instructions from English. In order to guarantee sufficient reliability for the administration of psychological tests and clinical interviews, three training sessions were held, one at Cambridge, England, and two at New York.

The first patient entered the study in New York in April 1985. To date our central data registry at the Long Island Jewish Medical Center has received data from more than 700 patients.

Preliminiary results were presented at the 3rd International Symposium "The Impact of Cardiac Surgery Upon Quality of Life: Psychological and Neurological Aspects" in New York, March 28-30, 1989. The results presented there and reported in this Proceedings volume are based upon the data of 498 patients which were available in October 1988. We intend to report the results of the planned total of 900 patients in May 1992 in a 4th International Symposium in Hamburg, Germany. The proceedings of that meeting also will be published.

One may well ask why these preliminary results are being published now, rather than waiting for the final volume in 1993 or 1994. We have several reasons for this:

The first and simplest is to provide some feedback after the many years that we have been studying these issues. The second and more important motive is to report our preliminary results to a broader audience. Despite the fact that these are preliminary and incomplete, we thought it would be valuable for the further progress of our study to have the criticism and comments of a wider audience. The third reason is to invite colleagues who are not Consortium members but who have made major contributions to the field to participate in this volume. We are very pleased that so many have done so.

This book contains papers describing the International Study variables and the preliminary results of the study. The study has both the advantages and the disadvantages of size. The sample is large enough that one can control for many background variables while examining the main effects of the study. However, because of the size and scope of the study, variations may creep in despite the aim of using a uniform method. For example, because of the different social systems in the cities in which the study took place, there were differences in the social supports available to the patients. Although both Bogota, Colombia and Hamburg, Germany have Social Security benefits available for at least some patients, the nature of these benefits is very different in the two cities. Furthermore, even within one center there can be wide differences. As Meffert points out in his chapter, "Comparison of In-Hospital Conditions for "International Study" and "Non-Study" Patients," the mechanisms for carrying out the study in Hamburg transformed the experience of the study patients into something different (fortunately better) than that of the non-study patients.

We intend to use the advantage of the large number of subjects in the final sample to aid in partialling out such effects, and to weigh their influence upon the final results.

This book includes 19 contributions presenting analyses of the combined consortium data. We would like to emphasize that each of these authors is representing the efforts of all our colleagues at the various centers who contributed to these findings. A complete list of the participants in this Study and their institutions may be found in the Appendix. The remaining 38 contributions are a sampling of papers reporting important findings in the field.

On behalf of our Consortium we would above all like to thank several people who helped make possible the International Symposium and this book:

1.   All our colleagues without whose efforts this International Study could never have been carried out.

2.   Three intelligent and diligent young women: Sharon Windwer, Carol Ritter, and Janet Sendar, who did the essential but tedious work of scoring, checking and entering the data into the computer.

3.   Ms. Ann Boehme and her co-workers from the LIJ Department of Continuing Education, Debbie Mohr and Mindy Gordon, who helped us accomplish the almost impossible task of organizing an International Symposium within two months rather than the customary two years.

4.   Carol Ritter, who was unflaggingly cheerful, intelligent and thorough in carrying out the seemingly interminable tasks required in turning a collection of manuscripts into a book.

5.   Ginny Fay, for her tireless efforts in typing the manuscript.

6.   Plenum Publishing Corp. for its help in quickly putting this book into print and especially Melanie Yelity and Greg Stafford for their thoughtfulness and direction.

7.   Ken Moeller, Ph.D., for his many years of work in the earlier stages of this research.

8.   And finally, the late Dr. Robert Flemma for his leadership, enthusiasm and guidance during the long planning stages of the International Study.

REFERENCES

1.   G. Rodewald, Introduction to the Subject, in: "Psychic and
        Neurological Dysfunctions After Open Heart Surgery,"
        H. Speidel and G. Rodewald, eds., Georg Thieme Verlag,
        Stuttgart, New York (1980).
2.   K. Taylor, Editorial: The cerebral consequences of
        cardiac surgery. Perfusion, 4:81-82 (1989).
3.   H. Speidel and G. Rodewald, Eds., "Psychic and
        Neurological Dysfunctions after Open-Heart Surgery,
        First International Symposium in Hamburg," Georg Thieme
        Verlag, Stuttgart, New York (1980).
4.   Becker, J. Katz, Polonius, H. Speidel, eds.,
        "Psychopathological & Neurological Dysfunctions
        Following Open-Heart Surgery, Second International
        Symposium," Springer Verlag, Berlin (1982).

PSYCHIATRIC ISSUES

METHODS - CONSTRUCTION AND CLINICAL APPLICATION OF THE

HAMBURG RATING SCALE FOR PSYCHIC DISTURBANCES (HRPD)

Paul Gotze, Bernhard Dahme, Ulrich Lamparter,
Sabine Falck

University of Hamburg
Hamburg, W. Germany

INTRODUCTION

In our review of the research on psychic disorders
after open heart surgery published 10 years ago [1], we
pointed out the heterogeneity in description, assessment
and classification of these disorders. One of the major
consequences of the heterogeneity was a great variation
in data on the prevalence of postoperative psychic
disturbances; frequencies ranged from about 5 to more
than 40 per cent.

By constructing the Hamburg Rating Scale for Psychic
Disorders (HRPD), we hoped to contribute to a more standardized assessment, description and classification of
psychopathological disorders after open heart surgery.
This seems to us the most important prerequisite for
comparing data about postoperative psychic disorders
coming from different cardio-surgical centers.

Since we have rather explicitly described the
psychometric construction and evaluation of the HRPD in
an English version [2, 3], and in a somewhat more
extensive and refined German version [4], we can
concentrate here on the major principles and some new
developments.

Impact of Cardiac Surgery on the Quality of Life
Edited by A. E. Willner and G. Rodewald
Plenum Press, New York, 1990

METHODS AND RESULTS OF THE ORIGINAL HRPD CONSTRUCTION AND
EVALUATION

Sample

The original construction of the HRPD was founded on
a sample of 100 patients undergoing open heart surgery
for: congenital heart disease (n = 12; 6 m, 6 f), valve
replacement (n = 57; 33 m, 24 f), coronary heart disease
(n = 26; 22 m, 4 f) and 5 patients for combined heart
diseases. One patient died immediately after surgery.

Symptom Assessment

By means of a much larger symptom list - a modified
version of the Arbeitsgemeinschaft Fur Dokumentation und
Methodik in der Psychiatrie (AMPD) inventory of psychopathological status with a list of 90 symptom items -
each patient was rated by an experienced psychiatrist at
3 periods:

- preoperative assessment: once during the last week
  before surgery;
- early postoperative assessment; once at each of the
  first 4 days after surgery at the intensive care unit
  (ICU);
- late postoperative assessment: once during the 4th
  week after surgery at the normal ward.

Psychometric Methods of HRPD Construction and Analysis

The psychometric scale construction was achieved by
methods of classical test theory (CTT), by item and
factor analysis of the 90 symptom items. This resulted
in a list of 36 items, which were judged to be sufficient
for symptom assessment of postoperative psychic disorders
both from a psychometric and also a clinical viewpoint.
All psychometric analyses were based exclusively upon the
early postoperative assessments. Only those symptoms
were taken into account in HRPD construction that occurred
at least once during the first four postoperative days in
at least five per cent of patients, except for some rare
symptoms of great clinical relevance (e.g. visual hallucinations, suicidal ideas). The resulting list of 36
items constitutes the Hamburg Rating Scale of Psychic
Disorders (HRPD).

In a further step of test construction these 36 items were condensed to 8 symptom scales by factor analysis (principle components and Varimax rotation). These were: (1) Disorientation, (2) Impaired thinking/ concentration, (3) Paranoid-hallucinatory symptoms, (4) Anxiety, (5) Depression, (6) Hostility, (7) Loss of control, (8) Resignation [2, 4].

These 8 HRPD scales are formed by summing up the item ratings with substantial loadings (.40 or more) in the respective factors.

Statistical Classification of Patients into Symptomatic or Syndrome Groups

In order to obtain objective, homogeneous symptomatic subgroups, we applied methods of cluster analysis (especially K means algorithm 5), based upon the symptom profiles of each of the 99 remaining patients during the first 4 postoperative days. Each daily symptom profile was composed of the summed raw scores in the above mentioned 8 symptom scales. (So cluster analysis was based upon 99 x 32 raw values.) By the K means algorithm we tried to get subgroups (clusters) with maximal symptom homogeneity within groups and maximal symptom variance between groups. Six subgroups resulted from this analysis. For comparison with the new results of the current international study, we concentrate upon the symptom profiles (mean raw scores) of the 2nd (Fig. 1) postoperative day (for more details [4]).

(1)   About 1/4 of all patients had no signs of psycho-pathological symptoms at all (n = 28);
(2)   about 1/3 of patients had distinct, but clinically unremarkable, signs of anxious and depressive mood (n = 32);
(3)   a further 1/4 of patients suffered from a psycho-organic syndrome with disturbances in orientation, concentration, memory and reasoning, associated with depressive mood (n = 23);
(4)   4 patients manifested a severe psycho-organic syndrome;
(5)   8 patients manifested aggressive hostility and paranoid-hallucinatory symptoms mainly at the 2nd post-operative day after a rather symptom free first post-operative day;
(6)   4 patients suffered from a severe, generalized delirious syndrome with maximum severity at the 3rd and 4th post-operative day.

HRPD:78, HH, N = 99: 6 Clusters of Postoperative Psychic Status (2 nd day)

Cluster 1: "Unnoticeable"

        (n = 28)   m: 17 f: 11   mean age: 45.9

Disorientation	0.32
Impaired thinking/conc.	2.64
Paranoid-Halluc. Sympt.	0.00
Anxiety	3.25
Depression	1.04
Hostility	0.93
Loss of control	0.46
Given up	0.04

Cluster 2: "Rather unnoticeable"

        (n = 32)   m: 20 f: 12   mean age: 45.7

Disorientation	1.09
Impaired thinking/conc.	5.25
Paranoid-Halluc. Sympt.	1.31
Anxiety	7.72
Depression	3.09
Hostility	0.63
Loss of control	0.44
Given up	0.28

Cluster 3: "Slight psycho-organic syndrom"

        (n = 23)   m: 16 f: 7   mean age: 47.3

Disorientation	2.78
Impaired thinking/conc.	11.17
Paranoid-Halluc. Sympt.	0.25
Anxiety	12.74
Depression	8.26
Hostility	0.74
Loss of control	0.78
Given up	1.26

-> 2 ->

Figure 1.   Clusters of postoperative psychic status at
2nd day after surgery: Original sample of
HRPD construction from 1978 (N=99)

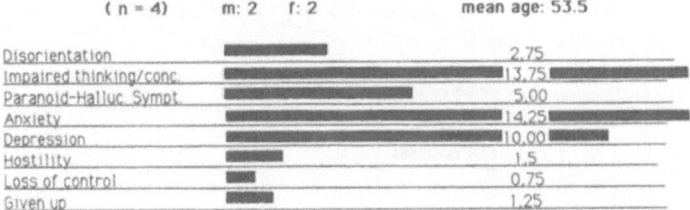

Cluster 4: "Severe psycho-organic syndrom"

| (n = 4) | m: 3   f: 1 | mean age: 56.0 |

Disorientation	12.25
Impaired thinking/conc.	12.50
Paranoid-Halluc. Sympt.	1.75
Anxiety	6.50
Depression	1.50
Hostility	1.25
Loss of control	8.50
Given up	0.0

Cluster 5: "Hostility"

| (n = 8) | m: 6   f: 2 | mean age: 53.5 |

Disorientation	3.38
Impaired thinking/conc.	7.63
Paranoid-Halluc. Sympt.	4.25
Anxiety	14.63
Depression	6.13
Hostility	7.50
Loss of control	0.87
Given up	1.88

Cluster 6: "Delirous Syndrome"

| (n = 4) | m: 2   f: 2 | mean age: 53.5 |

Disorientation	2.75
Impaired thinking/conc.	13.75
Paranoid-Halluc. Sympt.	5.00
Anxiety	14.25
Depression	10.00
Hostility	1.5
Loss of control	0.75
Given up	1.25

Figure 1 (continued).   Clusters of postoperative psychic
status at 2nd day after surgery:
Original sample of HRPD
construction from 1978 (N=99)

RESULTS OF HRPD ASSESSMENT AND CLUSTER ANALYSIS IN A NEW SAMPLE

We are able to present results of a new but <u>small</u>
sample of 58 patients who underwent open heart surgery in
Hamburg University Hospital during the last 2 years and
who participated in the current international
multi-center study. All patients had been rated on the
36 HRPD symptom items, again by an experienced psychiatrist (1) preoperatively, (2) at 2nd or 3rd day, and
(3) about 10 to 12 days after surgery. For further data

HRPD:88, HH, N = 58: 6 Clusters of Postoperative Psychic Status (2 nd or 3rd day)

Cluster 1: "Unremarkable"

(n = 22)   m: 20   f: 2   mean age: 50.5

Disorientation	I	0.05
Impaired thinking/conc.	▪	0.46
Paranoid-Halluc. Sympt.		0.00
Anxiety	▪	0.77
Depression	▪	0.64
Hostility	I	0.05
Loss of control	I	0.09
Given up		0.00

Pt.no: 1 3 6 8 9 12 13 14 15 22 26 27 28 31 32 35 43 45 46 49 51 59

Cluster 2: "Impaired Thinking / Concentration, Depression, Anxiety"

(n = 23)   m: 18   f: 5   mean age: 58.65

Disorientation	▪	0.65
Impaired thinking/conc.	▬▬▬▬	3.70
Paranoid-Halluc. Sympt.	I	0.09
Anxiety	▬▬	1.78
Depression	▬▬▬	3.61
Hostility	▪	0.48
Loss of control	▪	0.35
Given up		0.00

Pt.no.: 2 4 5 7 16 17 19 20 23 24 29 30 33 36 37 40 48 52 53 54 56 57 58

Cluster 3: "Anxiety, Depression, Impaired Thinking / Concentration"

(n = 8)   m: 8   mean age: 54.75

Disorientation	▪	0.25
Impaired thinking/conc.	▬▬▬	2.75
Paranoid-Halluc. Sympt.	I	0.13
Anxiety	▬▬▬	4.25
Depression	▬▬▬	3.75
Hostility	▪	0.25
Loss of control	▪	0.38
Given up		0.00

Pt.no: 25 34 39 41 42 44 47 50

-> 2 ->

Figure 2. Clusters of postoperative psychic status at 2nd or 3rd day after surgery: Sample from the international multicenter study in 1988 (N=58)

analysis, the 36 severity ratings of the early postoperative assessment were summed up into the respective 8 symptom scales mentioned above for each patient. These data were submitted to a cluster analysis performed by the Clustan program package [5] (especially by the subroutine Relocate). Again, 6 clusters or homogeneous subgroups came out of this analysis (Fig. 2):

Cluster 4: "Anxiety, Depression, Hostility"

(n = 2)   m: 2   age: 45, 55

Disorientation	▬	1.0
Impaired thinking/conc.	▬▬▬	2.5
Paranoid-Halluc. Sympt.		0.0
Anxiety	▬▬▬▬▬▬	6.0
Depression	▬▬▬▬▬▬	6.0
Hostility	▬▬▬▬	3.5
Loss of control		0.0
Given up		0.0

Pt.no: 10 11

Cluster 5: "Psycho-organic Syndrome"

(n = 2)   m: 1   f: 1   age: 65, 53

Disorientation	▬▬▬▬▬	5.5
Impaired thinking/conc.	▬▬▬▬▬▬	6.0
Paranoid-Halluc. Sympt.	▬▬	2.0
Anxiety	▬▬▬	3.5
Depression	▬▬▬	3.5
Hostility	▬	1.5
Loss of control	▬	1.5
Given up	▬	1.0

Pt.no: 55 60

Cluster 6: "Severe Psycho-organic (delirious) Syndrome"

(n = 1)   m: 1   age: 60

Disorientation	▬▬▬▬▬▬▬	10.0
Impaired thinking/conc.	▬▬▬▬▬▬▬▬▬	15.0
Paranoid-Halluc. Sympt.	▬▬▬▬▬	7.0
Anxiety	▬▬	2.0
Depression	▬▬▬▬	5.0
Hostility	▬▬	3.0
Loss of control	▬▬▬▬	5.0
Given up	▬	1.0

Pt.no: 38

Figure 2 (continued).   Clusters of postoperative psychic status at 2nd or 3rd day after surgery: Sample from the international multicenter study in 1988 (N=58).

(1) Nearly half of the patients had no clinical signs of psychic disturbances (n = 22).
(2) About the same number of patients had slight cognitive impairments accompanied by depression and anxiety (n = 23).
(3) 8 patients showed symptoms of mild anxiety, depression and impaired concentration/reasoning.
(4) 2 patients manifested remarkable anxiety, depression and hostility accompanied by mild disturbances in concentration and orientation.

(5) 2 patients suffered from a psycho-organic syndrome
     with more severe disorientation and disorders in
     concentration, anxiety and depression.
(6) 1 patient suffered from a severe delirious syndrome,
     even with the experience of loss of self-control.

DISCUSSION

HRPD Construction and Evaluation

     We think that psychometric construction and evalua-
tion of the HRPD was an important step toward realizing a
more objective and unequivocal diagnosis of postoperative
psychic disorders. Consequently, we obtained more differentiated statements about the frequency and intensity
of various symptom or syndrome manifestations, and
generally came to a more complex but even more transparent
symptomatology. But the real proof of the quality of the
HRPD in regard to the classical test criteria, i.e.,
objectivity, reliability and validity lies ahead, when we
begin to analyze the HRPD data that have been assembled
in the multicenter study.

Comparison of the Subgrouping in the Old and the New
Sample

     Generally, it is a good proof of validity of a given
scientific instrument if you come to approximately the
same results with the aid of this instrument in 2 different samples. Unfortunately, things are not so easy in
the present matter. There are some relevant, distinct
differences between the two samples that have to be
carefully considered in evaluating the HRPD results:

(1) The former sample was nearly a random sample. The
     new sample is not at all random. Only patients
     motivated for this study were selected, 2 patients a
     week who knew each other. So we can suppose higher
     motivation and mutual interactive psychological
     support ("tandem effect");
(2) there is a 10 year interval between both samplings
     with great progress in some techniques of open heart
     surgery;
(3) only a quarter of the patients of the first sample
     suffered from coronary heart disease. Now, on the
     contrary, all patients of the new sample had bypass
     surgery because of coronary heart disease;
(4) there are differences in age and sex distribution
     between both samples (old sample: 48 males, 47

females, mean age: 48 years; new sample: 50 males, 8 females, mean age: 55 years). In the new sample there are many more males and the mean age is higher than in the first sample 10 years ago;

(5) the absolute symptom frequency and intensity have been diminished; both are less severe in the new sample, but this can be due to systematic interrater differences in symptom assessment;

(6) Mood disturbances seem to prevail over cognitive deficits in the new sample;

(7) there is an important methodological difference: The new clusters are based only on a single one-day symptom assessment (2nd or 3rd postoperative day), whereas the former ones were made over the complete symptom profiles of the first 4 days after surgery. In other words, the new clusters represent the psychic status of patients at the 2nd or 3rd post-operative day, whereas the former clusters represent the status and development of symptoms during the first 4 postoperative days, i.e. they represent "symptom dynamics." Consequently, the psychic status of the 2nd or 3rd day is not necessarily comparable between the former and the new clusters.

CONCLUSIONS

In constructing and analyzing the Hamburg Rating Scale of Psychic Disturbances (HRPD) we offered a psycho-metric and diagnostic tool for research about psychic disturbances after open heart surgery. The scientific usefulness of this tool still has to be further evaluated.

REFERENCES

1. H. Speidel, B. Dahme, B. Flemming, P. Goetze, G. Huse-Kleinstoll, N. J. Meffert, G. Rodewald, Probleme der Klassifizierung psychopathologischer Auffalligkeiten nach Herzoperationen mit extrakorporaler Zirkulation, Psychiatria Clinica, 12:57 (1979).

2. B. Dahme, P. Goetze, M. Wessel, Brief psychiatric inventory for assessment of psychopathological disorders after open heart surgery, in: "Psycho-pathological and neurological dysfunctions following open heart surgery," R. Becker, J. Katz, M. J. Polonius, H. Speidel, eds., Springer, Berlin, Heidelberg, New York, 68 (1982).

3. P. Goetze, B. Dahme, Hamburg Rating Scale for Psychic
    Disturbances - HRPD, in: "Psychopathological and
    neurological dysfunctions following open heart
    surgery," R. Becker, J. Katz, M. J. Polonius, H.
    Speidel, eds., Springer, Berlin, Heidelberg, New
    York, 77 (1982).
4. P. Goetze, B. Dahme, M. Wessel, Die Hamburger
    Schatzskala fur psychische Storungen nach
    Herzoperationen, European Archives of Psychiatry
    and Neurological Sciences, 234: 308 (1985).
5. J. MacQueen, "Some methods for classification and
    analysis of multivariate observations,"
    Proceedings of the 5th Berkeley Symposium on
    Mathematical Statistics and Probability, 1:281
    (1967).

PSYCHIATRIC METHODS OF THE INTERNATIONAL STUDY:

HAMILTON DEPRESSION AND ANXIETY SCALES

Bernhard Strauss, Gunnar Paulsen

Depts. Psychotherapy & Psychosomatics and
Psychiatry, Kiel University
Kiel, Fed. Republic of Germany

The Hamilton Scales for the rating of clinical
anxiety and depression are well established instruments
for psychiatric research, and have been used in numerous
studies, mainly in the field of psychopharmacology.
Within the International Study, the scales are one of the
constituents of the psychiatric part of the investigation,
in conjunction with the HRPD [1] and a psychosocial
interview.

Both scales are derived from clinical experience,
summarize the important symptoms of anxiety and depression, and are designed to measure anxiety and depressive
states, rather than stable personality traits. Originally,
they were intended to be used on patients already diagnosed as suffering from neurotic anxiety or depression,
and not for assessing anxiety and depression in patients
suffering from other disorders [2]. However, numerous
studies in the field of psychosomatic research have
demonstrated that the scales are suitable for measuring
depressive and anxious symptoms in several other groups,
including patients suffering from somatic diseases.

The Hamilton Anxiety Scale [3] covers symptoms of
anxiety, culled from clinical experience, summarized in a
total of 14 groups of symptoms, together with a rating of
the patient's behavior at the interview (Table I). The
symptoms are judged on the basis of a clinical interview (with no time limit), on 5 point-scales by one or
more psychiatrists or clinical psychologists. Normally
the ratings refer not only to the time of the interview
but also to the days before.

Impact of Cardiac Surgery on the Quality of Life
Edited by A. E. Willner and G. Rodewald
Plenum Press, New York, 1990

Several studies have shown that the groups of
symptoms can be factorially divided into two subgroups:
symptoms such as anxious mood, tension or fears as well
as behavior during the interview constitute the factor
"psychic anxiety"; those items describing different
somatic symptoms constitute a second factor named
"somatic anxiety."

Similarly, the Hamilton Depression Scale [4]
provides an instrument for rating depressive symptomatology in adults, likewise based upon an interview
(Table II). The usual form of the scale comprises 21
symptoms or symptom-complexes. In contrast to the
anxiety scale, the degree of the symptoms is operation-
ally defined and judged on 3- or 5-point scales. Thus, a
rating of "0" would be given for the item "retardation"
if the patient's thought and speech appears normal during
the interview. A "1" could be given if the activity of
the patient is minimally decreased, a "2" if the patient's
activity is diminished substantially. A rating of "3"
means that the exploration of the patient is difficult
and a rating of "4" means that the patient is in a marked
stupor. Usually, the scale is analysed on the basis of a
total score derived from the sum of the 21 ratings. Some
authors have suggested dividing the scales on the basis
of factor analyses into two subscales covering "retarded
depression" and "somatic depression aspects" [5].

Table 1. Hamilton Anxiety Scale - Items/Subscales

Anxious Mood	Somatic (muscular) Symptoms
Tension	Somatic (sensory) Symptoms
Fears	Cardiovascular Symptoms
Insomnia	Respiratory Symptoms
Intellectual (cognitive) Impairment	Gastrointestinal Symptoms
Depressed Mood	Genitourinary Symptoms
Behavior at Interview	Autonomic Symptoms
Psychic Anxiety	Somatic Anxiety

As far as psychometric properties are concerned,
interrator reliability has been shown to be high for both
scales, provided that the interviewers are clinically
experienced. The scales have been validated in several
studies and found to be sensitive to change. Especially

in psychopharmacological investigations it has been demonstrated that total scores decrease significantly during treatment, which suggests that they cover aspects of anxiety and depression that can be influenced by anxiolytic or antidepressive drugs.

Table 2. Hamilton Depression Scale - Items

Depressed Mood	Feelings of Guilt
Suicide	Insomnia -early -middle -late
Impaired Work and Activities	
Retardation	Agitation
Anxiety -psychic -somatic	Hypochondriasis
Somatic symptoms: -gastrointestinal -general -genital	Loss of weight Insight (Denial)
Diurnal variation	Depersonalization and Derealization
Paranoid Symptoms	Obsessional and Compulsive Symptoms

The following results are based on the preliminary analysis of the Hamilton data at our center, collected by one of the authors (G.P.), who carried out the interviews with the patients prior to surgery, postoperatively and prior to the patient's discharge. The preoperative interview lasted about 60 minutes, with the latter interviews lasting about 30 to 45 minutes. The analyses cover the data of a maximum of 79 patients investigated within the International Study at Kiel.

Table III shows some correlational results. The correlations indicate that the interrelationship between the two aspects, anxiety and depression, is fairly high on each of the three occasions (i.e. pre-, postoperative as well as at discharge) with correlation coefficients between .90 and .92. The intercorrelations between the single measurements on one scale on the three occasions are higher on the anxiety scale than the depression scale, which indicates that changes in anxiety are less extensive than changes in depression.

Within the psychometric part of the International Study, self-ratings on anxiety were obtained pre-operatively and at discharge by using the State-Trait-Anxiety Inventory (STAI) [6]. These self reports should be related to the clinical ratings of anxiety in the Hamilton Scale. As the table shows, this was not the case: neither the preoperative nor the postoperative State-Anxiety Scores correlated significantly with the total scores in the Hamilton Scale. The same proved true for the trait anxiety score, a result which was to be expected since the Hamilton test covers anxious states rather than traits.

There are several possible explanations for the unexpected result concerning the State Anxiety Scores: it could be that the STAI covers aspects of anxiety distinguishable from those rated in the Hamilton Scale. Another explanation would be that the ratings made by clinically experienced psychiatrists may be more reliable for determining the degree of the patients' anxiety, whereas the self-ratings may be confounded by the patients' denial. The lack of a correlation could also be explained by the fact that the self-ratings have to be related to the present state (at any time during the psychometric testing) while the interviews cover a longer period of time prior to or following cardiac surgery.

Of special interest within the International Study were the changes in the psychiatric measurements pre-and postoperatively.

Figure 1 shows the mean total scores of the Hamilton Scales on the three occasions, again these figures are based on the data collected in Kiel. The figure shows that changes in both scales are highly significant, characterized by an increase of anxiety and depression immediately following surgery. While the depression scores return to the preoperative level prior to the discharge, the anxiety scores at this time are consider-ably decreased compared to the preoperative values.

Table 3.   Intercorrelations between the Hamilton Scores
and between Anxiety ratings and patient's
self-reports (STAI)

STAI Trait		Hamilton Anxiety			Hamilton Depression			STAI State	
		II	III	I	II	III	I	III	I
Hamilton Anxiety	I	.44	.43	.92	.33	.42	.01	.02	-.01
	II		.61		.90	.49	-.31	-.23	-.03
	III				.92	-.18	-.01	-.03
Hamilton Depression	I					.34	.41		
	II						.43		

I: preoperative   II: postoperative   III: discharge

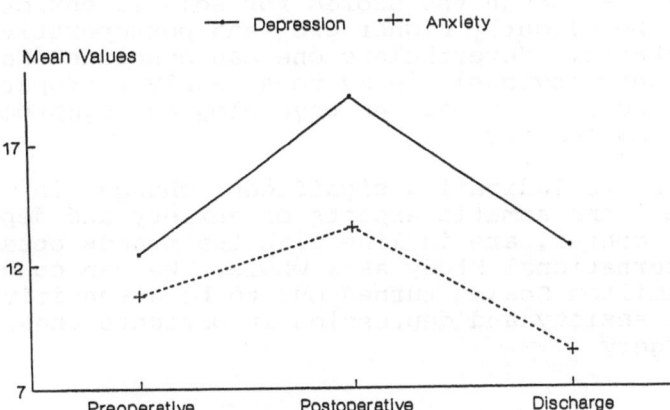

Fig. 1.   Hamilton Anxiety and Depression Scores (Mean
values); changes are statistically significant
(p<.001; ANOVA).

There is one specific aspect which could be important when determining the usefulness of such scales for
studying psychiatric complications following cardiac
surgery: both scales cover several items which describe
somatic symptoms of anxiety and depression.   One could
argue that a postoperative increase in the total scores
could be explained by an increase of somatic complaints.
These complaints, such as abdominal pain, autonomic
symptoms, insomnia or respiratory symptoms, could equally
be the consequence of surgery rather than the expression
of an altered psychological state in the patient.   To
test this assumption we looked into the amount and type
of changes in the single symptoms covered by each scale.

Starting with the symptoms of the Hamilton Depression Scale (Figure 2) it can be shown that two of the
symptoms, agitation and psychic anxiety, decrease significantly from the preoperative to the third interview.
The remaining seven items showing significant change
cover several somatic symptoms such as gastrointestinal
or genital symptoms, as well as psychological symptoms
such as insight (or denial) and retardation.   The changes
for all these seven items can be described as an increase
from the preoperative to the postoperative level followed
by a further decrease until the time of the patients'
discharge.

A similar pattern was found (Figure 3) for the
anxiety scale in a more differentiated analysis of the
scores by dividing them into the two subscales "psychic
anxiety" and "somatic anxiety."   Changes in both scales
run parallel, although the scores for somatic anxiety
turn out to be slightly higher pre- and postoperatively
and at discharge.   Nevertheless one can conclude that
cardiac surgery obviously leads to an early postoperative
increase of somatic as well as psychological symptoms of
depression and anxiety.

The results indicating significant changes in
psychological and somatic aspects of anxiety and depression at one center, are in line with the trends obtained
for the International Study as a whole.   We can conclude
that the Hamilton Scales turned out to be a sensitive
measure for anxiety and depression in patients undergoing
cardiac surgery.

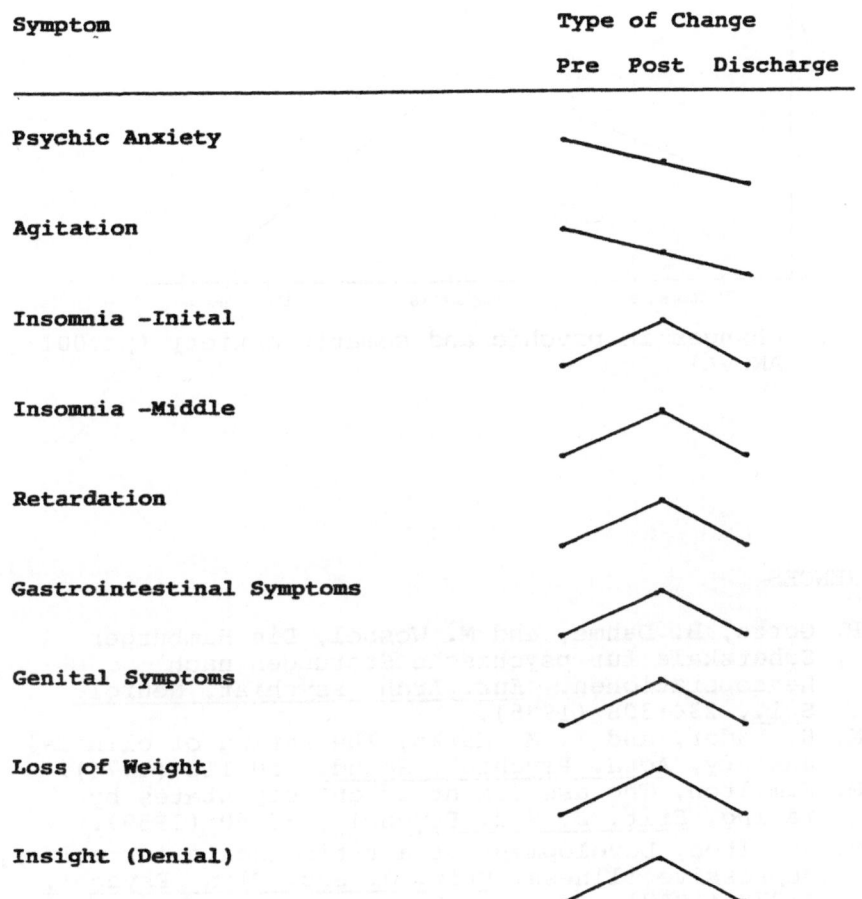

Fig. 2. Items of the Hamilton Depression Scale showing significant changes (p<.01; Cochran's Q)

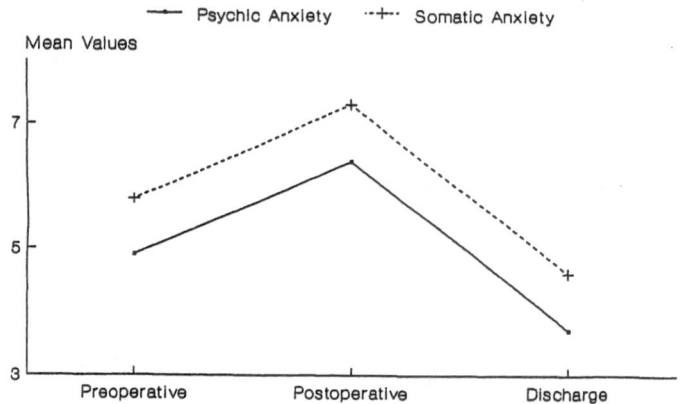

Fig. 3.   Changes in psychic and somatic anxiety (p<.001; ANOVA)

REFERENCES

1.   P. Gotze, B. Dahme, and M. Wessel, Die Hamburger Schatzkala fur psychische Storungen nach Herzoperationen. Eur. Arch. Psychiat. Neurol. Sci., 234:308 (1985).
2.   M. H. Lader, and I. M. Marks, The rating of clinical anxiety, Acta. Psychiat. Scand., 50:112 (1974).
3.   M. Hamilton, The assessment of anxiety states by rating, Brit. J. Med. Psychol., 32:50 (1959).
4.   M. Hamilton, Development of a rating scale for primary depressive illness, Brit. J. Soc. Clin. Psychol., 6:278 (1967).
5.   U. Baumann, Methodische untersuchungen zur Hamilton-Depressionsskala, Arch. Psychiatr. Nervenkr., 222:359 (1976).
6.   C. Spielberger, R. Gorsuch, R. Lushene, P. Vagg, and G. Jacobs, "Manual for the State Trait Anxiety Inventory," Consulting Psychologist Press, Palo Alto (1983).

PSYCHIATRIC ISSUES: SIMPLE FREQUENCIES PRE- AND POSTOPERATIVELY

H. Speidel

Dept. Psychotherapy & Psychosomatics
Kiel, Federal Republic of Germany

The paper of Rodewald and Willner has informed us about the history, aims, design and the state of the art of the International Study. Dahme & Goetze as well as Strauss & Paulsen have introduced three of the standardized psychiatric instruments used in the study and the latter have presented results obtained with two of these instruments, the Hamilton Scales, in one of the centers (Kiel, FRG). The purpose of this paper will be the presentation of global results (i.e. pre- and postoperative frequencies) based upon the Hamilton Depression Scale, the Hamilton Anxiety Scale and the Hamburg Rating Scale for Psychic Disturbances (HRPD) [1]. These results are based upon the preliminary analysis of the data obtained within the different centers which participate in the International Study.

Hamilton Depression Scale

Fig. 1 shows that the depression scores increase from the preoperative (1 or 2 days prior to surgery) to the postoperative measurement (1 or 2 days postop.) and decline at the time of discharge (approximately 8 days following surgery). The discharge measure appears higher than the preoperative score. This is interesting in comparison to the results of Strauss & Paulsen. In the Kiel population the preoperative and discharge scores did not differ, whereas the preoperative measure is the same in the Kiel population as in the total sample. In addition, the postoperative measure is higher in Kiel than in the overall sample which indicates that the increase as well as the decline of the depression scores are more distinct in the Kiel sample than in the total sample of the study.

Impact of Cardiac Surgery on the Quality of Life
Edited by A. E. Willner and G. Rodewald
Plenum Press, New York, 1990

27

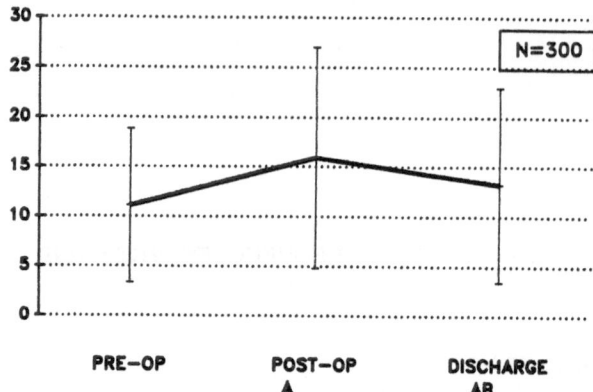

Fig. 1. Hamilton Depression Scale.

This might be important for further evaluations,
especially in light of the different conditions within
the participating centers. The difference could result
from different rating styles of the researchers. Another
possible explanation might be the following: The postoperative measure could be related to the quality of
postoperative care, whereas the discharge measure could
reflect different "destinies" of the patients following
discharge in West Germany and other countries. In the
Federal Republic of Germany most patients are transferred
to rehabilitation clinics immediately following their
discharge from the surgical unit and therefore might have
a moratorium before restarting their normal life.

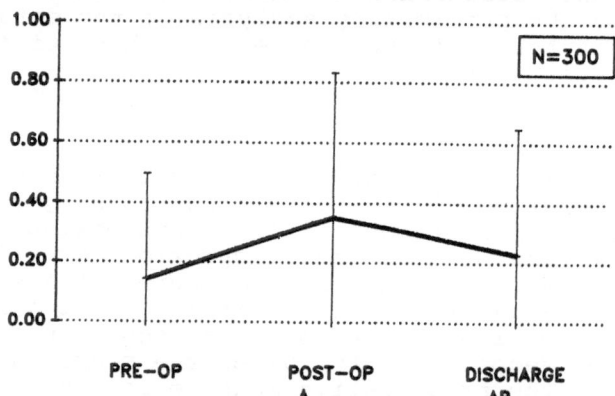

Fig. 2.   Hamilton Depression Scale: Proportion of cases
in the clinically depressed range.

Compared to the preceding figure, Figure 2 shows more distinct differences between the preoperative and discharge measure and the postoperative measure. The proportion of patients who are in the depressed range preoperatively increases in the first postoperative days. The proportion of patients having a problematic mood condition increases following surgery compared to the preoperative state. This is certainly an important result, related to preoperative and postoperative psychological care. Generally, the depressive as well as the non-depressive patients are described as more depressed at discharge than prior to surgery.

Hamilton Anxiety Scale

The results from Kiel indicate that patients are rated as more anxious in the first postoperative days than prior to surgery and at discharge. This result is rather surprising. We could well understand if patients were more anxious prior to surgery since they don't know if they will survive. As we learned from Blacher [2] the "inner statistic" of patients is not a 1%-mortality rate but a 50:50 rate. But why are they more anxious following surgery?

This question will be discussed in combination with the results of the anxiety scale of the HRPD. First, another interesting detail should be noted: the results obtained with the Hamilton Anxiety Scale (Fig. 3) in the whole sample and in the Kiel sample are the same. In both samples, a postoperative increase of anxiety can be

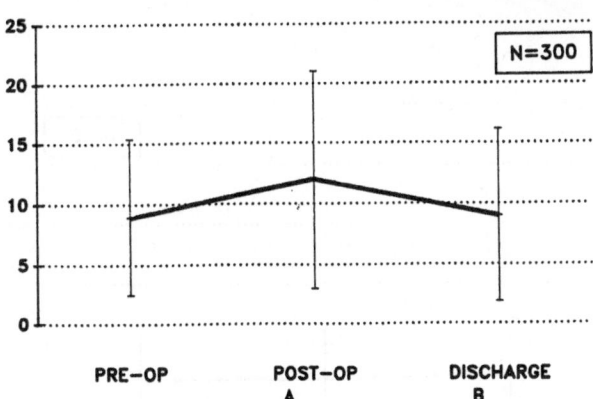

Fig. 3. Hamilton Anxiety Scale.

observed. But if we glance at the results prior to
discharge, we can see again a characteristic difference
between the total sample and the Kiel patients: in the
total sample, the anxiety score returns to the preoperative value. In the Kiel sample the score at
discharge is lower than prior to surgery.

Again, we can presume a researcher effect. Another
alternative hypothesis could relate to what follows in
the post-discharge phase: perhaps the patients in West
Germany have less reason to be anxious at the time of
discharge because they feel safer in view of the pending
treatment in a rehabilitation clinic.

HRPD-Factor 1: Disorientation

As Fig. 4 shows, disorientation, an alarming
symptom, is very uncommon postoperatively, but surprisingly there are no changes in the measures between the
three occasions. Based upon other studies and clinical
experience, we usually see this important symptom as one
of the typical early postoperative transitory signs of a
fugitive brain syndrome. Contrary to expectation, the
data from the International Study reveal continuity from
the preoperative to the discharge measurement. This
certanly might be a reference to preexisting brain disorders, as Willner & Rabiner [3] and Goetze, et al. [4]
have shown. Preoperatively disoriented people, on the
other hand, are rare. Questions caused by this result
provide a challenge for subsequent evaluations,
especially the study of subgroups.

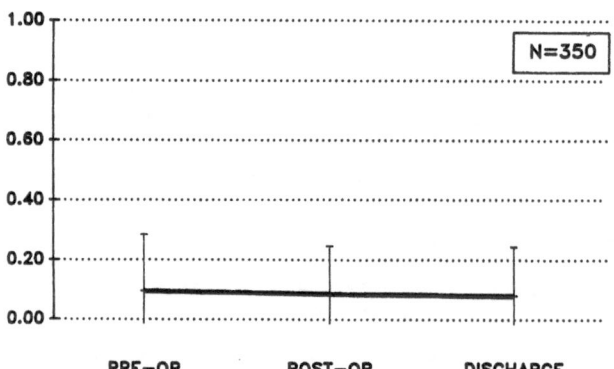

Fig. 4. HRPD Factor 1: Disorientation.

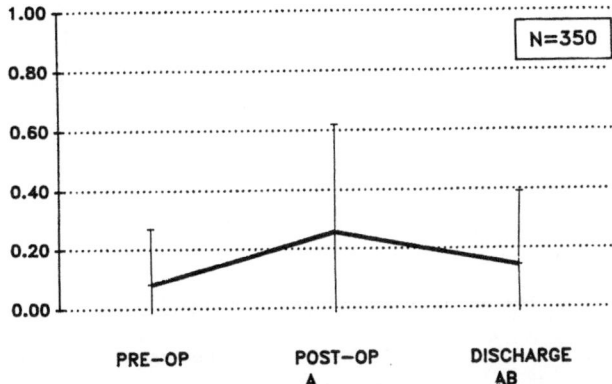

Fig. 5. HRPD Factor 2: Disturbed Concentration/Thinking.

HRPD-Factor 2:   Disturbed Concentration/Thinking

The results shown in Fig. 5 had to be expected. We know that many patients are slightly damaged in their higher intellectual functions when they come to heart surgery. This is a consequence of:

a) chronic circulatory problems,

b) the basic disease of the vessels manifested both in the heart and in the brain,

c) preoperative fatigue and diminished vitality,

d) masked or open depression,

e) preoperative anxiety.

As one of the consequences of the postoperative illness, where all physiological measures are in the pathological range, the higher intellectual functions are diminished, too.

The fact that the measures of disturbed concentration/thinking do not return to the preoperative level prior to the patients' discharge certainly might be caused by an amount of depression, resulting from the patients' awareness of their damage. Further analyses are necessary to isolate characteristics of patients with remaining deterioration of thinking. The investigations of Willner and Rabiner [3] have shown how important this factor can be for the further destiny of patients following heart surgery.

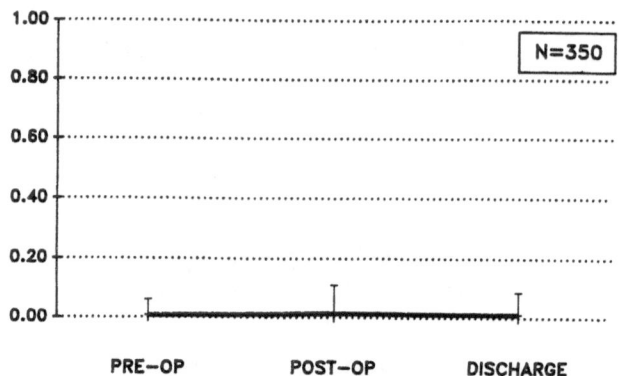

Fig. 6.   HRPD Factor 3:   Paranoid/Hallucinatory Symptoms.

HRPD-Factor 3:   Paranoid Hallucinatory Symptoms
_____

        In our overall sample, this syndrome is rare
(Fig. 6), and we therefore have no figures concerning
the postoperative development of this dramatic
psychopathology.

HRPD-Factor 4:   Anxiety
_____

        As expected, preoperative anxiety measured with the
HRPD is high and declines postoperatively (Fig. 7).   The
patient is still alive and is aware of that fact.   It is
surprising that the anxiety measures are higher at the
time of discharge: with concentration and thinking being
similarly impaired, it could be the patient doesn't know
how he will function in the future.

        The Hamilton Anxiety measures were inverse in the
total sample and in the Kiel sample as compared to the
results of the HRPD in the total sample.   There are
several possible interpretations for these contradictory
results:

a) The heart surgeons in Kiel support the patients'
   preoperative denial more than elsewhere, which breaks
   down during the first postoperative days and is
   restituted afterwards, when patients can feel safer.
   But this interpretation can not explain the results of
   the Hamilton Anxiety Scale.

b) The postoperative psychological care in Kiel could be worse than elsewhere and thus more anxiety provoking; but again, in this case the Hamilton Anxiety Scale should present a similar pattern.

c) The anxiety, measured by the Hamilton Anxiety Scale, is different from that anxiety measured by the HRPD. The results of Strauss & Paulsen indicate that within the subscales "psychic anxiety" and "agitation" of the Depression scale, there is a continuing diminution of the anxiety score, whereas the other subscales show a peak immediately following surgery.

If we assume that the Hamilton subscales "psychic anxiety" and "agitation" are associated with deadly peril and the other subscales like "insomnia," "retardation," "gastrointestinal" and "genital" symptoms, "loss of weight" and "insight" relate to postoperative somatic complaints, and if we further suppose that the HRPD covers psychic signs of anxiety, then the diminution of anxiety from the preoperative to the early postoperative measurement is similar to the results from Kiel, with the exception that discharge is not a source of anxiety for the patients at Kiel because of their transfer to the rehabilitation clinic.

HRPD-Factor 5:   Masked Depression Symptoms

The above figure (Fig. 8) shows the overall results of Factor 5 of the HRPD: we can observe an increase of the scores from the preoperative to the postoperative measure and a decline to the measure prior to discharge.

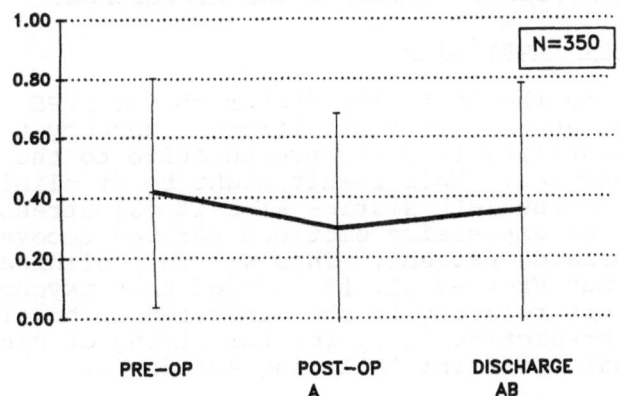

Fig. 7.   HRPD Factor 4:   Anxiety Symptoms.

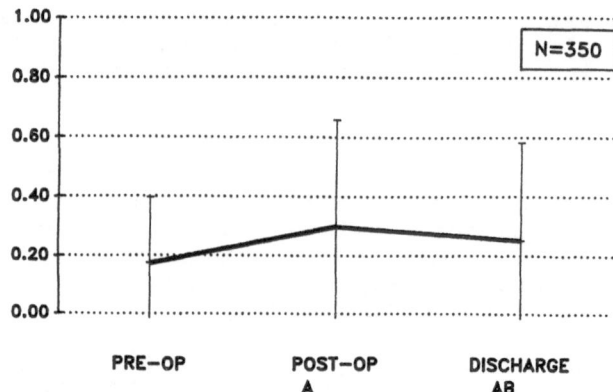

Fig. 8.   HRPD Factor 5:   Masked Depression Symptoms.

        This result is not surprising and similar to the
result with the Hamilton Depression Scale in Kiel.   But
there is a slight difference.   In the Kiel sample, the
Hamilton depression score returns to the preoperative
value, whereas the HRPD depression score at discharge is
higher than the preoperative score.   The overall results
of the Hamilton Depression Scale indicated the same
difference.   The depression scores of the total sample
have a corresponding course and are consequently both
different from the Hamilton depression score of the Kiel
sample.   In analogy to the interpretation of the differences in the Hamilton and HRPD anxiety scores between the
total sample and the Kiel subsample, we can assume that
the different course after discharge, home versus
rehabilitation clinic, explains the difference.

HRPD-Factor 6:   Hostility

        Concerning the hostility factor of the HRPD
(Fig. 9), we can observe a significant tendency towards
more overt hostility from the preoperative to the postoperative measures.   This result might be of clinical
relevance.   In the late sixties Kimball [5] stressed the
significance of expressing emotions for the recovery of
the heart-operated patient.   This was only clinical
experience, but Frey et al. [6] proved that psychological factors relating to the direction of hostility
are of high predictive value for the timing of discharge
after clinical treatment following accidents.

        Prior to surgery patients are totally dependent on
the relationship to the surgeon and the clinic, and this

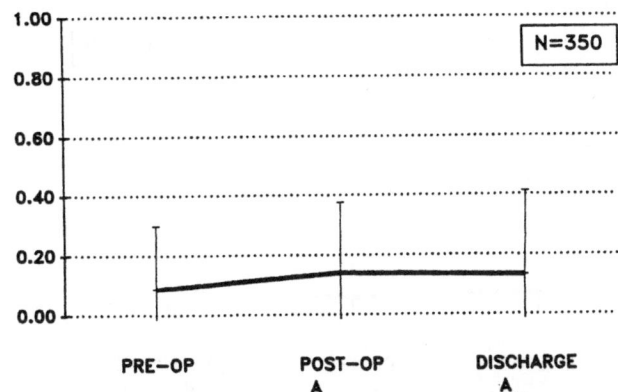

Fig. 9. HRDP Factor 6: Hostility.

is an "inner contraindication" for hostility. It is
certainly favorable for recovery if patients show more
hostility. In future evaluations, this item should be
controlled and subgroups with high and low scores should
be compared with respect to the recovery criteria and
time.

HRPD-Factor 7: Loss of Control

Concerning Factor 7 - Loss of Control - there is a
significant tendency towards a low level (Fig. 10).
Prior to surgery and to discharge, loss of control seems
to be more marked than at the postoperative time. This
tendency is hard to interpret. Possibly, the maximal
dependency on external factors, e.g., the surgeon before
operation, the uncertainty after discharge -- produces a
feeling of loss of control, whereas the feeling of having
mastered the operation reduces it. Further evaluation
with subgroups will produce more relevant results.
Generally, Factor 7 represents a difficult concept: it
includes very different items like perseverative and
fuzzy thinking, suicidal tendencies and so on.

HRPD-Factor 8: Self-Criticism

There are no significant differences within the
measures of this factor (Fig. 11). This is not surprising: preoperatively and in the first days following
surgery the patient's attention is focused mainly on his
body and his complaints. Prior to discharge, psychic
properties and the strength of the ego are challenged,
and therefore the patient is confronted with his
restrictions.

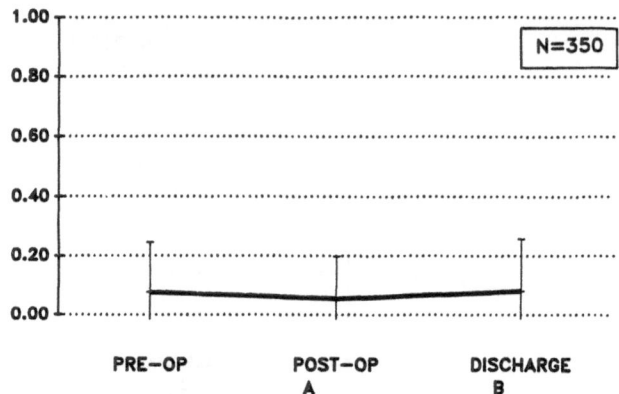

Fig. 10. HRPD Factor 7: Loss of Control.

SUMMARY

These results of the global evaluation of the three
instruments - Hamilton Depression Scale, Hamilton Anxiety
Scale and the Hamburg Rating Scale for Psychic Disorders
are preliminary. They provide us with more questions
than answers. What we can see is that there are many
psychological changes within a few days. These changes
may have an influence on the recovery process, but are in
turn influenced by the circumstances of postoperative
care. The comparison of the results of one center with
the global results of all centers showed interesting
differences. Further detailed evaluations and comparisons between the participating centers will give
interesting information which will be useful for the
surgical routine.

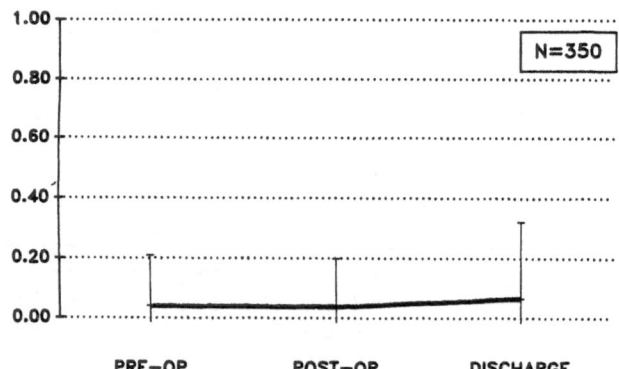

Fig. 11. HRPD Factor 8: Self Critical.

REFERENCES

1. P. Goetze, B. Dahme, B. Flemming, G. Huse-Kleinstoll, H. J. Meffert, H. Speidel, M. Wessel, Hamburg rating scale for psychic disturbances - HRPD, in: "Psychopathological and Neurological Dysfunctions Following Open Heart Surgery," R. Becker, J. Katz, M. J. Polonius, H. Speidel, eds., Springer, Berlin, Heidelberg, New York (1982).
2. R. Blacher, Discussion Part III, in: "Psychic and Neurological Dysfunction After Open Heart Surgery. First International Symposium, Hamburg," H. Speidel, G. Rodewald, eds., Georg Thieme Publ., Stuttgart, New York (1980).
3. A. E. Willner, C. J. Rabiner, The psychopathological and cognitive disorder syndrome (PCD) in open heart surgery patients, in: "Psychopathological and Neurological Dysfunctions Following Open Heart Surgery," Springer, Berlin, Heidelberg, New York (1982).
4. P. Götze, B. Flemming, G. Huse-Kleinstoll, H. J. Meffert, C. Reimer, H. Speidel, Relationship between psychopathological syndromes before and after open heart surgery, in: "Psychological and Neurological Dysfunctions Following Open Heart Surgery," R. Becker, J. Katz, M. J. Polonius, H. Speidel, eds., Springer, Berlin, Heidelberg, New York (1982).
5. C. P. Kimball, The experience of open heart surgery, VI: Research and consultation - liaison psychiatry, in: "Psychic and Neurological Dysfunctions After Open Heart Surgery, First International Symposium, Hamburg," H. Speidel, G. Rodewald, eds., Georg Thieme Publ., Stuttgart, New York (1980).
6. D. Frey, D. Havemann, O. Rogner, "Kognitive und Psychosoziale Determinaten des Genesungsprozesses von Unfallpatienten." Unpublished final report, Kiel, Germany (1983).

FANTASIES EVOKED BY CARDIAC SURGERY

Richard S. Blacher

Tufts University School of Medicine
New England Medical Center
750 Washington Street
Box 266
Boston, MA   02111

"When you have my heart in your hand, could you please take the bitterness out of it?" This remarkable request addressed to a cardiac surgeon epitomizes some of the problems facing the heart patient since his view of surgery can be so different from ours. The request was not a metaphor, and when I asked him about it he looked puzzled and asked, "Where else would my bitterness be?!"

While for surgeons, an operation is an everyday occurrence, for the cardiac patients, heart surgery may be the most dramatic event in their lives. They deal with it as a matter of life and death. Whatever the realistic risk stated by the surgeon, the anticipation of mortality that the patient brings to his operation is 50%, and I believe this represents not only the dramatic quality of the operation but also the way the heart works. The heart, after all, from the patient's point of view is the only binary organ in the body. It either functions and the person lives, or it doesn't and the person dies. Thus 50/50.

> A statistician was told that he had a
> 1% chance of dying with his coronary
> operation. He notified us that since
> he could die, that meant he could either
> live or die, "And so, statistically,
> that means that my risk is 50%."

Impact of Cardiac Surgery on the Quality of Life
Edited by A. E. Willner and G. Rodewald
Plenum Press, New York, 1990

How a patient views his medical condition or surgery often plays a significant role in whether he is comfortable or anxious, whether he complies with his medical regimen, and whether he is able to cooperate in the postoperative program. Heart surgery conjures up an array of frightening and even awesome thoughts and fantasies and since the focus for the patient of heart surgery is a struggle between life and death, these fantasies are often more powerful than those seen with other operations. Heart surgery might be viewed as a natural experiment in stress.

Although the surgeon may explain the procedure in great detail to the patient, the latter's anxiety may preclude his hearing what is said, and later distortion of what and how the material was presented is not at all uncommon. It is not unusual for me to hear patients ask, "When they take my heart out and put it on the heart-lung machine, will they keep it in the same room as my body?" At times the surgeons have been asked this question but more commonly, I believe, it is addressed to the primary physician, to the psychiatrist, or to the anesthesiologist.

In a series of patients who had valve replacements, I sat with a surgeon who explained the operation to the patient using a heart model. He would open the model, point to the valve, and say "This is the valve we are going to remove. We will then replace it and sew up your heart." Later, after the surgery, I asked the patients to describe how they thought the operation was done. Twenty percent of the patients said to me "They take your heart and lungs out and put them on a machine." When I then asked how they changed the valve, the patients became noticeably uncomfortable and would avoid the question. When finally asked whether the surgeon had opened their hearts, they turned pale and said, "Absolutely not!" These patients' view of surgery was much more traumatic than dictated by reality. More than half of the entire patient group felt that the heart was not opened for the valve repair. They believed the valves were located in the large vessels, so that touching the heart was unnecessary [1, 2].

Many of our patients have seen television programs on heart surgery, since public television has shown actual operations a number of times. Often they are most struck by the fact that during the procedure there is a stopping of the heart. After all, it was only in recent years that physicians decided that death should be measured by a flat

electroencephalogram; the <u>historical</u> measure of death has
been the stopping of the heart. Thus it should not
surprise us that our patients think that during the
surgery they will die and then will be brought back to
life. Patients facing any sort of surgery are most afraid
that their hearts will stop. <u>Our</u> patients have to accept
the fact that their hearts <u>will</u> stop and then worry about
whether they will start again. Certain patients, who are
religious, have an anticipation that during the time of
cardioplegia, when they are "dead," their souls will go to
heaven and visit members of their family who have died.
This becomes for some people a geographical problem. I
have seen a number of patients afraid of undergoing
surgery lest they be put into conflict when the surgeon
restarts their hearts at the termination of the procedure.
Should they stay in heaven with their long lost family
members or should they come back to their current lives?
While this may seem far-fetched to many people, to these
patients it is a realistic, logistical problem.

>A 60 year old woman was agitated before
>coronary surgery, following an upsetting
>dream. Her older sister, a nun, had died
>10 years before of heart disease. The
>entire dream consisted of her sister
>appearing, and in an uncharacteristically
>angry tone saying, "I'm very disappointed
>in you!" The patient had seen the operation
>on television and kept noting that during
>the surgery her heart would be dead. "Not
>me, mind you, but my heart," she said
>several times. I suggested that she was
>in conflict about staying in heaven when
>the surgeon restarted her heart, and she
>nodded vigorously and said, "I've already
>decided I want to come back to my husband."
>She then thought that since her sister was
>in heaven for eternity, that she'd be able
>to wait a while longer for the patient's
>company. With this, her anxiety abated.

Aside from these relatively common fantasies about
surgery, we sometimes see other worries. For instance,
patients who are chronic smokers will worry that during
the surgery, cancer of the lungs will be discovered. More
dramatic was the patient who asked the surgeon to remove
his bitterness. Such distortions should not surprise us,
since we are dealing with the organ that has been thought

of for millenia as the seat of emotions, the source of
love, and even the center of intellect.

Reality, as well as fantasies, can also be dealt with
in various ways. A sternal incision can be elaborated by
some patients into, "They cut open your chest and spread
you apart like a chicken." Plastic valve replacements can
be thought of by some patients as made of impervious,
tough material, or else of the kind of plastic seen in
inexpensive toys - a not too reassuring thought.

Postoperatively a historical danger for the patient
has been psychosis involving paranoia. The regressed
patient being treated in the intensive care unit feels
that he is being tortured. Forced to take deep breaths
against a sternal incision, moved around when he would
rather be left alone, and treated in other ways that cause
him pain and discomfort, he feels abused. To be angry at
those who hold life and death in their hands is not safe,
and yet the anger at his treatment must go somewhere.
What he does is project it, and then feels, "It is not I
who is angry but it is the nurses; they are trying to
hurt me or kill me, and this explains why they do these
painful things." It is interesting that it is the nurses
almost invariably who are the persecutors for the paranoid
patient, almost never the doctors - since the nurses are
the inflictors of the painful procedures. Paranoia, in
our intensive care unit, is a rare occurrence, ever since
we persuaded the nurses to give the patients permission to
be angry, and even to encourage them to resent the treatment. They will tell the patients, "It is a natural
reaction to dislike these treatments," and the theme
becomes one of, "You don't have to like what we do to you;
you just have to tolerate it." The patients can then be
resentful without danger, and have no need to project.

Our patients bring their own fantasies to their
surgical experience. These may affect the content, the
form, and at times even the question of whether they will
develop major psychological reactions. It behooves us to
bear in mind that patients probably do not have information about medical matters which we take for granted.
They all bring the information they do have, elaborated
and changed by personal and family experiences and by
societal and individual expectations. Whatever the
fantasies, we must recognize their importance to the
patient and the influence they can play in his care and
recovery.

REFERENCES

1. R. S. Blacher, Open Heart Surgery - The Patient's
    Point of View, <u>Mt. Sinai J. Med</u> 38:74 (1971).
2. R. S. Blacher, Heart Surgery: The Patient's
    Experience <u>in</u>: "The Psychological Experience of
    Surgery," R. S. Blacher, ed., John Wiley and Sons,
    New York (1987).

THE EVALUATION OF THE EMOTIONAL CLIMATE

IN THE FAMILIES OF CARDIAC SURGERY PATIENTS

G. Invernizzi, R. Basile, A. Passerini,
N. Calchi Novati, C. Bressi, A. Repossini,
P. Biglioli

Istituto Di Clinica Psichiatrica
Milano, Italy

FOREWORD

Some authors have particularly stressed that, in order
to obtain a good postoperative adaptation, in the short and
in the long run, you need a caretaker for the patient as
well as valid family relationships. The research on
EXPRESSED EMOTION [1] (E.E.) has tried to answer this
problem and provided an instrument of investigation, the
Camberwell Family Interview (C.F.I.) [2, 3]. The Expressed
Emotion (EE) methodology has until now been considered a
very useful tool to evaluate the "temperature" of families
with psychological problems. Actually, an important conceptual shift is now in progress. EE is being used more
and more with different pathologies. Here we consider the
usefulness of the EE measurement in evaluating families
of patients with severe coronary artery pathology,
surgically treated. Environmental pressures are, in fact,
distressing factors that can affect the course of such
pathology.

METHODOLOGY

Eight coronary bypass patients who underwent surgery
12 months before the start of the present research entered
the study. Their ages range from 40 to 65. Subjective and

Impact of Cardiac Surgery on the Quality of Life
Edited by A. E. Willner and G. Rodewald
Plenum Press, New York, 1990

objective (echocardiographic) evaluation of the course of cardiac symptoms in the postoperative phase was carried out. The evaluation of the family was carried out by means of the C.F.I. It was administered to the relatives living with the patient and spending at least 35 hours per week with him.

The evaluation of the interviews led to the measurement of 5 item scales:

- emotional overinvolvement (EOI)
- criticism (CR)
- hostility (H)
- warmth (W)
- positive remarks (PR)

According to the general Italian population the EE can be defined as high when EOI $\geq$ 4, criticism $\geq$ 6 and hostility is present. The EE can be defined as low when EOI < 4 and criticism < 6. These evaluations are administered one year after surgery.

RESULTS

The following table (Table 1) compares the characteristics of our sample with those of a larger one of Italian bypass patients.

Table 1

	General bypass population	Sample of this research
Total number of patients	94	8
Average age	57 $\pm$ 2.1	55 $\pm$ 4.5
Sex males	80 (85.1%)	7 (87.5%)
Sex females	14 (14.9%)	1 (12.5%)

The comparison of the average values of the EE scales in three diferent populations are presented in Table 2:

Table 2.   Average Values on EE Scales for 3 Different
            Populations

EE	Cardiac Surgery (n=8)	Renal haemodialisys (n=10)	Multiple sclerosis (n=6)
EOI	3.5	2.6	2.3
CR	0.75	5.0	5.0
H	0	0.6	1.0
W	4	3.8	3.0
PR	1.75	3.6	1.6
High EE	75%	60%	37%
Low EE	25%	40%	63%

The characteristics of the relatives of bypass
patients who underwent the C.F.I. can be summarized as
follows:

1. Evidence of a positive relationship with the patient,
   also present before the onset of the disease.

2. A high empathic level; immediate "emotional communication" between the patient and his relatives is common.

3. Virtual absence of criticism towards the patient.

4. "Relationship of service" towards the disease, i.e.,
   relatives report depressive reactions only after the
   patient overcomes the critical phase.

A very high level of EOI and W and a very low level
of C (with absence of H) characterize the cardiac surgery
sample. It seems possible to us to draw from these
characteristics, a few hypotheses:

a: The coupling of EOI/W is related mostly to the
    intrafamilial relationships predating the disease.

b: The absence of C., as well as the "relationships of
    service" are related to the peculiar situation of
    vulnerability and fragility of the patients, as
    experienced by their relatives.

As far as the patients' heart function is concerned,
none of them complained of relapses of angina, nor of a
reduction in tolerance to physical efforts. Echocardiog-
raphy never showed a worsening of signs of cardiac ischemic
suffering.

CONCLUSIONS

These conclusions may be regarded as preliminary impressions because of the small number of coronary bypass surgery patients (8) involved. Bearing this in mind, the following comments can be made: In the chronic organic diseases (as showed in a larger research study) a high level of C and H seems to be related to a bad outcome, while the high level of W and PR well relate to favorable outcomes. The EOI that, in psychic disturbances, is connected to a bad course of the disease, acquires in organic disease a positive influence. According to our preliminary data, therefore, these families seem to adequately support the patient during his postoperative recovery and to enhance a prompt return to the former psychosocial adaptation level. In contrast, the presence of a family climate characterised by C and H should require an intervention of psychosocial counselling.

REFERENCES

1. C. Maffei, G. Cereda, C. Bressi, P. Bertrando, S. Ciussani, C. Da Ponte, and C.L. Cazzullo, Expressed Emotion (EE): rassegna storica e prospettive teoriche. Rivista sperimentale di freniatria, Vol. CX, Fasc. 1, 1986.
2. J. P. Jeff, C. E. Vaughn, "EE in Families," The Jard. Press. NY (1985).
3. L. Knipers, EE: A review, Brit. J. Soc. Clin. Psychol., 18:237-243 (1979).

PSYCHOLOGIC SEQUELAE OF CARDIAC VALVE IMPLANTATION

James G. Peden, Jr.

Departments of Medicine and Psychiatry
East Carolina University School of Medicine
Greenville, NC 27858-4354

INTRODUCTION

Since the advent of cardiac surgery, there has been an increasing amount of research concerned with the psychological after-effects of these procedures. Numerous studies have examined the clinical features of post-cardiotomy delirium, which occurs in up to one-third of cases, as well as the factors which seem to predispose patients to this complication [1]. Other studies have investigated the adjustment of patients to artificial pacemaker implantation (both transthoracic and trans-venous), which typically results in few long-term psychiatric symptoms [2]. More recent papers have dealt with the psychological aspects of coronary artery bypass grafting, such as the persistent anxiety and depression seen in up to one-third of all patients [3, 4].

This research project examined the psychologic sequelae of a specific type of cardiac surgery, cardiac valve implantation. We investigated the prevalence of anxiety, depression, and cognitive dysfunction before and after valve replacement as reported by patients. We also examined the extent to which cardiac valve recipients were made aware of their prostheses in their daily lives.

METHOD

Names and addresses of appropriate patients were solicited from physicians in Greenville, N.C., and a

Impact of Cardiac Surgery on the Quality of Life
Edited by A. E. Willner and G. Rodewald
Plenum Press, New York, 1990

total of 101 individuals who had previously received
cardiac valve implantation were identified. Twenty-four
could not be contacted, and 11 patients had died since
their surgery. The remaining 66 potential subjects were
contacted over the telephone by a single researcher, and
after informed consent 59 (89%) agreed to participate in
a semi-structured interview.

Using an instrument designed for this project, demographic data provided by the referring physician were
confirmed and information on current medical status was
obtained. Participants were asked to retrospectively
describe their feelings and reactions to their valve
implantations. After spontaneous comments were recorded,
subjects were asked several overlapping and redundant
questions designed to elicit the presence of specific
psychiatric symptoms such as anxiety, depression, and
cognitive dysfunction. The history of symptoms was
obtained for 3 distinct periods: the time before surgery,
the immediate postoperative period, and the time of the
interview (which was anywhere from months to years
following surgery). Other questions concerned the
presence of vegetative signs, physiologic signs of
anxiety, disorders of thought, pre-operative psychiatric
diagnoses, and the prescription of medications for these
symptoms since valve implantation. Finally, patients
were questioned on their subjective awareness of the
implanted valves, and specifically on any sounds which
their artificial valves made.

RESULTS

There were 33 men and 26 women ranging in age from
26 to 85 years who participated in this survey. Cardiac
valve implantation had occurred from 2 to 50 months prior
to the interview, and in 7 (12%) this procedure had been
performed to replace a previously implanted prosthesis.
There was no significant difference in these demographic
variables between subjects and those potential subjects
who either declined participation or could not be located.

Almost half of the subjects (27, or 46%) recounted
that they were anxious prior to surgery, and that this
had resolved in all but 4 (7%) during the postoperative
period. However, one third of the subjects (20, or 34%)
related that they currently experienced feelings of
anxiety. The prevalence of depressive symptoms before
and after implantation was less frequently reported (by

6, or 10%, and 3, or 5% respectively), but one quarter (15) described such symptoms at the time of the interview and 21 (36%) stated that they had experienced suicidal ideation since their procedure. Nearly a third (18, or 31%) noted cognitive difficulties in the postoperative period, compared with 2 (3%) prior to surgery, and a substantial number of subjects reported persistent memory deficits (19, or 32%), impaired cognition (13, or 22%), and poor memory (11, or 19%).

A majority of subjects (33, or 56%) related an ongoing awareness of their prostheses which they ascribed to the sounds produced by the valves. Of these 33, 30 (91%) had received mechanical valves, which typically produce a distinct clicking noise as they open and close. The remaining 3 subjects (9%) who reported valve sound awareness had received animal tissue valves, which are generally silent in operation. In contrast, of the minority (26, or 44%) who denied perception of valve sounds, only 8 (31%) were mechanical valve recipients, while the remaining 18 (69%) had tissue valve implants.

There was no statistically significant correlation between the awareness of valve sounds and the prevalence of current anxious, depressive, or cognitive symptoms. However, 14 of 33 subjects (42%) who heard artificial valve sounds had suicidal ideation, compared to 7 of 26 (27%) who did not hear any valve sounds.

DISCUSSION

While the majority of patients who receive cardiac valve implantation report that they experience no long-term psychologic sequelae, a substantial minority do relate persistent difficulties with anxiety, depression, and cognitive impairment. This is similar in magnitude and type to the changes seen in many patients following coronary artery bypass grafting [4], and higher than that seen in the general population.

A situation unique to cardiac valve implantation is a subjective awareness of the prosthesis, usually engendered by the perception of sounds generated by the artificial valve. As could be expected from the physical characteristics of different valves, patients who received mechanical valves were more prone to notice sounds caused by their prostheses than were patients implanted with tissue valves. The finding that a subset

of patients with presumably silent tissue valves report
perception of valve sounds will require further investigation to uncover the etiological factors involved,
although increased somatic awareness and masked depression (which would probably not be detected by this
study's interview instrument) are possible explanations.

A surprising finding was the number of patients who
reported having suicidal ideation since their surgery.
While this data does not have statistical significance,
it suggests that an awareness of valve sounds may be
associated with an increased risk of suicidality. There
appears to be no correlation between the perception of
valve sounds and any other psychologic sequelae of valve
implantation.

An obvious limitation in the extent to which these
results can be generalized is that all data was obtained
through the subjective reports of patients, which may not
accurately describe their actual psychological and cognitive states. Prospective studies utilizing objective
clinical and psychometric assessment in addition to
subjective reports are required for a fuller understanding
of this intriguing phenomenon.

ACKNOWLEDGMENTS

The author wishes to thank C. Kenneth Mitchell, MS2,
for his efforts as research technician, as well as Dr. W.
R. Chitwood for his assistance and support.

REFERENCES

1. E. Vasquez, W. R. Chitwood, Postcardiotomy delirium:
    An overview, Int J. Psychiat in Med. 6:373-383
    (1975).
2. W. A. Greene, A. J. Moss, Psychosocial factors in the
    adjustment of patients with permanently implanted
    cardiac pacemakers, Ann Intern Med. 70:897-902
    (1969).
3. S. S. Heller, K. A. Frank, D. S. Kornfeld, J. R. Malm,
    F. O. Bowman, Psychological outcome following open
    heart surgery, Arch Intern Med. 135:908-914 (1974).
4. D. Hogan, B. Davies, D. Hunt, G. W. Westlake, and M.
    Mullerworth, Psychiatric aspects of coronary artery
    surgery, Med J. Aust. 141:587-590 (1984).

WHAT DO PATIENTS WITH INCOMPLETE POSTOPERATIVE DATA
TELL US? THE PROBLEM OF FATAL OUTCOME AND REFUSING
POSTOPERATIVE TESTING: PSYCHIATRIC ASPECTS

Gunnar Paulsen

Department of Psychiatry
Kiel University
Kiel, Federal Republic of Germany

The data presented here are part of the International Study and based upon the standard measuring
techniques of the study. One aim of our project was to
describe patients with missing data after coronary bypass
surgery. Drop-out of subjects from the time of the
pretest to posttest must be minimized and monitored to
identify sources of bias in the data. Incomplete data
due to subject fatigue, pain, death or refusal are common
sources of error. Our experience suggests that the
greatest amount of missing data occurs in the most
impaired subjects. According to Bashein et al. [1], one
approach to this problem is to set missing values in the
data to the worst possible score, so that the most
impaired patients are not dropped from statistical
analyses. Woidera et al. [2] describe 13 per cent of
their patients as having missing data after cardiac
surgery.

This study deals with patients who died of surgery
or were in the Intensive Care Unit (ICU) for longer than
three days, or refused our postoperative neuropsychological testing.

Eighty patients who received coronary artery bypass
grafts were prospectively studied by a standardized
psychiatric investigation and tested psychometrically to
determine the presence of brain dysfunction before and
after operation. At the onset of our study all patients

Impact of Cardiac Surgery on the Quality of Life
Edited by A. E. Willner and G. Rodewald
Plenum Press, New York, 1990

were informed about the aims and gave informed consent to
participate. The psychiatric evaluation (Hamburg Scale
HRPD, Hamilton Depression Scale HAMD, and Hamilton
Anxiety Scale HAMA, semistructured interview) was performed by the same interviewer 1 - 3 days before surgery
and 2 - 3 days, as well as 6 - 7 days after surgery. The
neuropsychological tests were administered by the
psychologist a few days before, and one week after, the
operation.

The study group consisted of 65 males and 15 females
aged 39 to 78 years (mean 59.5). Three patients (mean
age 65) died postoperatively because of severe arrhythmias
and cardiac arrest. For medical reasons 5 patients (3
males, 2 females) stayed longer than three days in the
ICU. Nine patients (6 males and 3 females) refused the
postoperative neuropsychological testing without comment.

Procedure

The whole sample was divided into three groups.

Group I: Patients who died after surgery or stayed in
              the ICU longer than 3 days. Both subgroups
              were combined for statistical reasons
              (n = 8).

Group II: Patients who refused the neuropsychological
              testing postoperatively (n = 9).

Group III: Remaining patients (n = 63).

The data were analysed statistically by correlational procedures, t-test and Friedman test (two-way)
with the criterion for statistical significance at 0.05
level. The means of the several groups and the significant differences between the means are shown in Tables 1
and 2.

The curves of the mean scores for all tests are
graphically shown in Figures 1, 2 and 3.

To specify the anxiety in more detail, the HAMA
scores were separately calculated for psychic anxiety
(item 1-6, 14) and somatic anxiety (item 7 - 13). The
results are presented in Table 3 and 4.

TABLE 1. Comparison of the means between Group I (> 3 days in ICU) and Group III (remaining patients)
** p < 0.01   * p < 0.05

Test	Time of testing	Means Group I	Group III	t	Significance
HAMA	pre op	11.66	9.95	ns	
	post op	22.50	12.54	3.22	* *
	discharge	16.33	7.77	3.32	* *
HAMD	pre op	12.77	11.76	ns	
	post op	25.50	17.56	2.50	*
	discharge	20.60	12.32	2.53	*
HRPD	pre op	8.44	6.56	ns	
	post op	20.40	10.32	2.96	* *
	discharge	17.00	6.62	3.64	* *

TABLE 2. Comparison of the means between Group II (refusing patients) and Group III (remaining patients)
** p < 0.01   * p < 0.05

Test	Time of testing	Means Group II	Group III	t	Significance
HAMA	pre op	15.44	9.95	2.66	* *
	post op	17.83	12.54	ns	
	discharge	7.87	7.77	ns	
HAMD	pre op	16.88	11.76	2.21	*
	post op	23.66	17.56	2.19	*
	discharge	11.87	12.32	ns	
HRPD	pre op	11.33	6.56	2.82	* *
	post op	14.22	10.32	ns	
	discharge	7.50	6.62	ns	

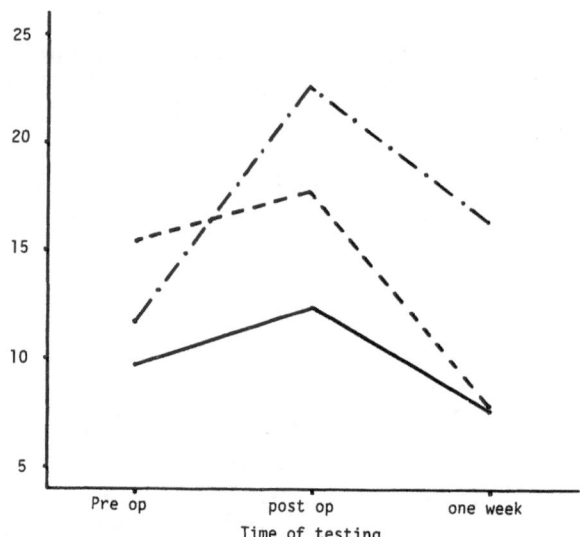

Fig. 1 Mean HAMA scores of the three groups
—·— = group I, longer than 3 days in ICU;
——— = group II, refusing patients;
——— = group III, remaining patients.

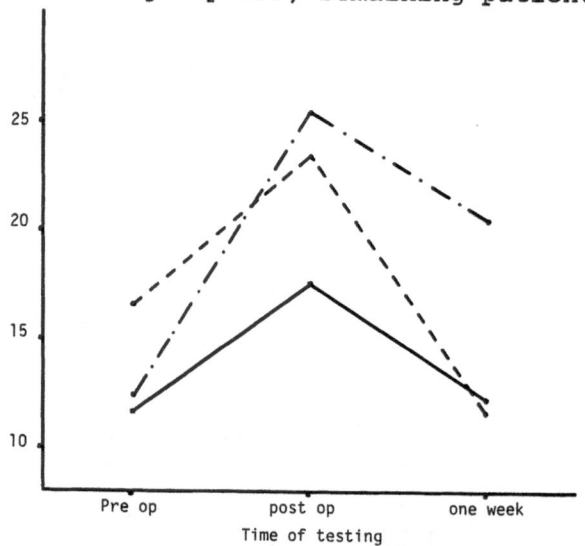

Fig. 2 Mean HAMD scores of the three groups
—·— = group I, longer than 3 days in ICU;
——— = group II, refusing patients;
——— = group III, remaining patients.

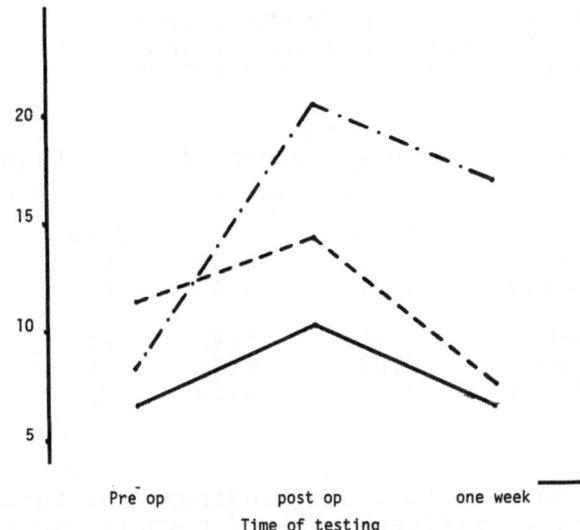

Fig. 3   Mean HRPD scores of the three groups
         - . - = group I, longer than 3 days in ICU;
         - . - = group II, refusing patients;
         - . - = group III, remaining patients.

TABLE 3.   Comparison of the means (psychic vs. somatic
           anxiety) between Group I and Group III
           * * p < 0.01   * p < 0.05

Test	Time of testing	Means Group I	Group III	t	Significance
HAMA psychic anxiety	pre op	5.11	4.53	ns	
	post op	10.50	6.00	2.60	*
	discharge	7.50	3.41	2.96	* *
HAMA somatic anxiety	pre op	6.55	5.42	ns	
	post op	12.00	6.54	3.34	* *
	discharge	8.83	4.36	3.19	* *

In the preoperative HAMA scale the correlations
between psychic and somatic anxiety for the Group II were
$r = 0.76$ and for the Group III $r = 0.67$. Using the
Friedman test we could find significant changes on all
psychiatric scales for Group III after coronary bypass

TABLE 4. Comparison of the means (psychic vs. somatic
          anxiety) between Group II and Group III
          * * p < 0.01   * p < 0.05

Test	Time of testing	Means Group II	Group III	t	Significance
HAMA psychic anxiety	pre op post op discharge	7.88 8.00 3.87	4.53 6.00 3.41	2.96 ns ns	* *ᵢ
HAMA somatic anxiety	pre op post op discharge	7.55 9.83 4.00	5.42 6.54 4.36	ns ns ns	

surgery. In contrast to these findings, the refusing
patients had no significant rise of psychiatric disturbances after surgery only. This suggests that these
patients have a high level of psychiatric symptoms prior
to surgery.

Comparing the three groups (Group I: patients who
stayed longer than 3 days in the ICU, Group II: patients
who refused the psychological testing postoperatively,
Group III: remaining patients) we could find significant
differences in the HRPD, HAMA and HAMD scales.

1. Patients categorized as "refusing the neuropsychological tests" showed evidence of higher anxiety
and higher emotional reactions, including depression on
the HAMD scale before coronary bypass surgery. In addition, we could demonstrate that in these patients only
the psychic anxiety was raised, whereas the signs of
somatic anxiety were less marked.

2. After surgery there is a significant rise of
psychiatric disturbances in Group I (patients who stayed
in ICU longer than 3 days) and Group III (remaining
patients) as well. Especially the patients who stayed in
the ICU for longer than three days displayed a high level
of psychiatric symptoms until the end of the hospitalization. Preoperative psychic complications were not found
more frequently in this group.

The finding that patients who refused postop testing
have more psychic symptoms and a higher level of psychic

anxiety preoperatively is surprising. Physical reasons could not be found as a causal factor for this. Also, we had no evidence of differences between the three groups in terms of results of their psychological pretests. Patients' time of testing was not longer than usual. In the psychological literature there are few explanations of why a subject leaves testing. This is a methodological problem as well.

In our study we can find some reasons for refusal of testing. It is known that patients with coronary heart disease suffer much bodily impairment, inactivity and loss of autonomy combined with the operation. Aggressive impulses against the medical staff treating them must be suppressed and denied preoperatively because they depend on them. Psychologists, being seen as supporters of the medical staff, were confronted with the patients' aggressive impulses as well. Patients impulses' are mobilized by disillusions after operation, e.g. they still feel the impaired body, realize a new scar, etc. On the other hand, for some patients, refusing our tests could well be a symptom of a newly acquired regulation of self confidence.

Until now patients refusing postoperative testing have not been taken into account. Our results show some interesting correlations. On the other hand, we are well aware that the number of patients is too small. We suggest further investigations to study this complex and multidetermined phenomenon.

REFERENCES

1. G. Bashein, S. W. Bledsoe, B. D. Townes, and
       D. B. Coppel, Tools for assessing central nervous
       system injury in the cardiac surgery patient, in:
       "Brain injury and protection during heart
       surgery," M. Hilberman, ed., Martinus Nijhoff
       Publishing, Boston (1988).
2. R. Woidera and A. Salm, Bedingungen psychischen
       Befindens nach Operationen am offenen Herzen, in:
       "Psychosoziale Kardiologie, Jahrbuch der
       medizinischen Psychologie Bd. 1," B. F. Klapp and
       B. Dahme, eds., Springer, Berlin, Heidelberg, New
       York (1988).

PSYCHOLOGICAL ADAPTATION OF PATIENTS 3 TO 5 YEARS AFTER

HEART SURGERY

A. Boll
Rehabilitationszentrum
Bad Segeberg, Fed. Republic of Germany

B. Dahme
Psychologisches Institut III
Universitat Hamburg
Hamburg, Fed. Republic of Germany

H.J. Meffert
Abt. fur Herz-und Gefabchirurgie,
Universitatskrankenhaus Hamburg-Eppendorf,
Fed. Republic of Germany

H. Speidel
Abt. Psychotherapie und Psychosomatik im
Zentrum Nervenheilkunde der Christian-
Albrecht-Universitat Kiel,
Fed. Republic of Germany

Psychosomatic research in the field of heart surgery started with the description and evaluation of psycho-pathological and emotional disturbances in the acute phases immediately before and after surgery [1, 2]. Currently our interest is also dedicated to the years afterward; problems the heart-operated patient must face in his private and public life are taken into consideration [3]. Since we regard the recovery process after surgery and its outcome as a multifaceted phenomenon, we have to include emotional and social aspects as well as the patient's physical condition. Follow-up studies in heart disease, as in other chronic illness, have shown that the extent of physical damage and the dysfunction resulting from it are not in them-selves sufficient to enable us to predict the subsequent psychological and social disadvantages for the patient.

Impact of Cardiac Surgery on the Quality of Life
Edited by A. E. Willner and G. Rodewald
Plenum Press, New York, 1990

This investigation primarily concentrates on
patients' psychological adaptation 3 to 5 years after
surgery. The questions in detail are:

1. How well adjusted are patients emotionally several
    years after heart surgery, and what differences are
    noticeable between them? Is it possible to identify
    subgroups of patients who show different psycho-
    logical adaptations at this point of time?

2. What correlations are there between the patients'
    long-term emotional adjustment and their medical,
    psychosocial and vocational rehabilitation?

3. What influence do preoperative psychological, social
    and somatic factors have on patients' long-term
    psychological adaptation?

Methods

Our sample consisted of 62 patients, 41 men (66%)
and 21 women (34%). These patients were part of a
bigger sample extensively scrutinized in an interdisciplinary research project carried out at the
Universitatskrankenhaus Hamburg-Eppendorf (Federal
Republic of Germany) from 1974 to 1981. The average age
of the patients when examined 3 - 5 years after the
operation was 51.5 years. Thirty-four patients (54%)
had valve replacements, in 9 patients (15%) a congenital
defect was corrected, and 19 patients (31%) had a CABS,
with an additional aneurysmectomy where necessary.

At the time of follow-up, 26 patients (42%) were
holding down jobs, 30 patients (48%) were drawing pensions, and 6 women were housewives without any supple-
mentary pension. Twelve patients retired after the
operation, and 18 patients had retired before it.

These patients were examined before surgery and
several times after it (1st - 4th postoperative day,
7th - 10th postoperative day, 3rd - 4th postoperative
week and 3rd - 5th postoperative year) by means of a
battery of customary personality tests and methods of
rating, such as the Freiburg Personality Inventory
(FPI), the Saarbruecken Anxiety List (SAL), the Giessen
Test (GT), the Complaint List (CL), and a personality
profile (PP). These were augmented by mood lists (ML),
questionnaires, and interviews designed by ourselves.
Psychopathological disturbances were established by

means of the Arbeitsgemeinschaft fur Methodik und
Dokumentation in der Psychiatrie (AMPD).

Results

 The variables which show how the patients adapted
3 - 5 years after the operation are those usually
examined when inquiring into the psychosomatic aspects
of chronic disease: the severity and frequency of
depressive moods and anxiety, the incidence of psychosomatic complaints, and the way the patient relates to
others. Patients' data in these variables were subjected
to cluster analysis with the intent to identify subgroups
which adapted psychologically in a similar manner, and
which may constitute the so-called 'criterion groups' of
the study. The 4-cluster solution (Figure 1) was
statistically adequate and psychologically plausible;
its validity was checked by comparing the 3- and
5-cluster solutions, and by random alteration in the
size of the sample.

 In line with the profile values the clusters were
named as follows:

Cluster I (Labile)   consists of 13 patients (21%)
                              who show a high degree of
                              depressive and anxious
                              feelings, who have many
                              psychosomatic complaints, and
                              negative resonance in social
                              contacts.

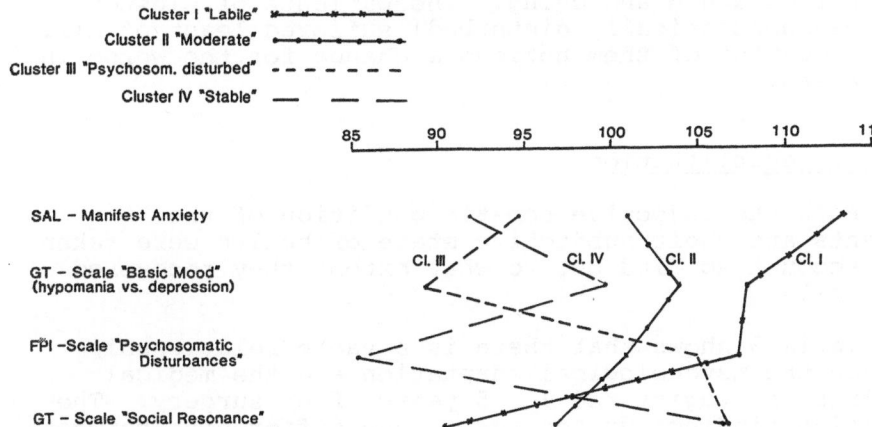

Fig. 1. Profiles of the 4 cluster solution.

Cluster II (Moderate)   consists of 20 patients (32%)
                             who have moderate levels in all
                             4 variables.

Cluster III (Psychosomatically disturbed)
                             consists of 16 patients (26%),
                             with few symptoms of manifest
                             anxiety, with emphasis on their
                             independence and assertiveness,
                             with many positive reinforce-
                             ments in social contacts, but
                             with an increased number of
                             psychosomatic complaints.

Cluster IV (Stable)   consists of ~13 patients (21%)
                             who have an extremely low level
                             of manifest anxiety, with
                             neither depressive nor hypo-
                             manic tendencies, relatively
                             few psychosomatic complaints,
                             and much positive reinforce-
                             ment in social contacts.

The validity of the grouping is underlined by
further differences in psychological parameters as they
were obtained by ratings after a psychoanalytically-
oriented interview.

As expected, patients from Cluster I (Labile) were
rated to have the highest increase of emotional problems
since the operation and to be troubled mostly by
thoughts of death and dying. The patients of Cluster
III (Psychosomatically disturbed) suffered least of all.
Only a quarter of them noticed a change for the worse in
both areas.

Medical Rehabilitation

Both the objective somatic condition of the
patients and their subjective state of health were taken
into account to find out to what extent they recovered
physically.

Table 3 shows that there is a vague relationship
between the psychological adaptation and the medical
findings, as registered 3 - 5 years after surgery. The
objective findings do not reveal any differences between
the criterion groups, except for cardiac arrhythmias.

Table 1.   Comparison between the 4 criterion groups:
           incidence of negative emotional changes

	Cl. I	Cl. II	Cl. III	Cl. IV	
No	4	8	13	7	32
Yes	8	11	3	5	27
Total	12	19	16	12	59

CHI^2 = 8.02;   df = 3;   p = .05

Table 2.   Comparison between the 4 criterion groups:
           incidence of problems connected with death and
           dying

	Cl. I	Cl. II	Cl. III	Cl. IV	
No	4	15	13	7	39
Yes	8	4	3	5	20
Total	12	19	16	12	59

CHI^2 = 9.11;   df = 3;   p = .03

It is worth noting that a relatively high proportion of patients (11 out of 16) in Cluster III (Psychosomatically disturbed) have occasional or frequent extrasystoli, and to some extent even multifocal extrasystoli. In comparison with Cluster I this holds only for 2 out of 16 patients. We found significant differences in the patients' subjective assessment of the severity of their stenocardias, their cardiac arrhythmias, and their psychosomatic symptoms. The patients in Cluster I, and to a lesser extent in Cluster II, judged their state of health to be worse than the patients in Clusters III and IV.

Table 3. Overview of results in comparing the 4 criterion groups in variables of their objective physical condition and their subjective state of health 3 to 5 years after surgery.

Variable		CHI^2	Significance
Heart failure	(obj.)	6.59	p = .36
Heart failure	(subj.)	9.39	p = .15
Stenocardias	(obj.)	3.2	p = .78
Stenocardias	(subj.)	16.08	p = .06
Arrhythmias	(obj.)	10.48	p = .1
Arrhythmias	(subj.)	12.67	p = .05
Other physical disorders		4.98	p = .5
Other physical complaints		9.16	p = .17
Psychosomatic complaints		15.55	p = .07

When we compared medical findings with subjective complaints, it became evident that patients tended to rate their symptoms more seriously than might be anticipated from the cardiac diagnosis. This discrepancy seems to be highest with the emotionally stressed patients of Cluster I.

Vocational and Psychosocial Rehabilitation

Patients who returned to work after surgery and those who did not (those who retired prematurely) are equally distributed among the 4 criterion groups. The financial situation, however, makes a difference; there is a clear link with psychological adjustment (CHI^2= 9.7, df = 3, p = .02). Of the 9 patients who reported having financial problems, 5 come from Cluster I. We did not find any statistically significant relationship

between the incidence of family or partnership problems
and our criterion of psychological adjustment.

Influence of Preoperative Psychological, Social, and Somatic Variables

Altogether we looked into about 20 different
variables, associated with the patient's state of mind
(AMDP), his actual emotional condition (Mood List), his
psychosocial situation, and his characteristic responses
to the operation (preoperative questionnaire and interview). Only 3 of these variables have a lasting effect
on patients' long-term psychological adaptation: negative emotional changes brought on by the illness,
annoyance, and depressive mood. No statistically significant influence could be found either for the
preoperative or for the immediate postoperative psychological disturbances as they were assessed by the AMDP
rating system.

When we studied psychological variables measured as
traits by use of personality tests and ratings, we found
more and clearer correlations. Emotional and vegetative
instability, depression, anxiety, and complaining, as
well as the preoperative diagnosis of a dominant
personality, are significantly linked with psychological
adjustment 3 to 5 years later.

The mean values listed in Table 4 demonstrate that
the patients of Cluster I (Labile) are preoperatively
noteworthy for their recurrent and powerful emotional
reactions under the stress of illness and surgery.
Prior to surgery, neurotic tendencies are more pronounced in this cluster than in the others. The
difference between the 4 clusters in the preoperative
rating of dominance means that the patients of Cluster
IV (Stable), who 3 to 5 years later show low anxiety and
depression with considerable positive resonance, were
assessed before the operation as more independent and
less symbiotic.

The comparison of the criterion groups in their
preoperative cardiac condition indicates that the
patients in Cluster III (Psychosomatically disturbed)
tend to be more seriously ill preoperatively. This also
applies to the patients with the least favorable psychological long-term adjustment in Cluster I. But the
differences are small and had diminished at the time of
follow-up. It is worth noting that the type and the
severity of the operation are not associated with the
prognosis of adjustment.

Table 4. Significant differences of the 4 criterion
          groups in preoperative psychological,
          psychosomatic and somatic variables - results
          of 1-way variance analysis.

Variable	$M_{Cl.I}$	$M_{Cl.II}$	$M_{Cl.III}$	$M_{Cl.IV}$	F	P
Negative emotional changes brought on by illness (Quest. A)	38.00	32.67	34.75	29.67	2.33	.09
Annoyance (ML)	10.52	8.35	7.60	9.53	3.31	.03
Depressive Mood (ML)	2.70	0.91	1.17	0.90	2.74	.05
Number of emotional and physical complaints (CL)	22.96	13.95	15.33	9.93	6.44	.00
Psychosomatic disturbances (FPI)	3.16	2.79	3.02	1.89	12.03	.00
Depression (FPI)	2.92	2.38	1.76	1.52	10.87	.00
Emotional instability (FPI)	2.95	1.77	1.69	1.36	14.48	.00
Manifest anxiety (SAL)	27.87	18.44	15.14	11.39	17.97	.00
Dominance (PP)	23.23	20.79	25.30	25.50	3.69	.02
Heart failure (NYHA)	2.95	2.68	3.13	2.62	2.34	.08

Discussion

While Brown & Rawlinson [4], Lutzenkirchen et al.
[5] and Heller et al. [6], in their follow-ups, could
detect general trends which were valid for the entire

sample when comparing them with either the preoperative level or the normal population, our results gained by cluster analysis answer the question: In which and in how many patients are distress reactions greater or smaller than expected? Twenty-one percent of our sample (Cluster I) show clear signs of above-average emotional, physical, and social distress. This proportion tallies with the findings of Heller et al. [7], Kimball [8], and Dahme et al. [9] who also identified at least 20% of the patients after heart surgery as having serious long-term psychological problems which call for psychiatric or psychotherapeutic help.

One central issue is the long-term correlation between the degree of medical rehabilitation and the psychological adjustment in chronically ill patients. Our results suggest there is little connection between the objective medical findings and the patient's emotional condition at the time of follow-up. This fits with the results already mentioned in the introduction: Cardiac findings constitute only one dimension of the ultimate outcome; they are not sufficient for determining the patients' quality of life after heart surgery. On the other hand, there are clearer correlations between psychological adjustment and the subjective cardiac complaints caused by cardiac arrhythmias and stenocardias. In Cluster I the severity of such complaints is more pronounced than might have been expected from the objective findings. One therefore gets the impression that these patients are hyperconscious of their hearts, and that their basically anxious and depressive attitudes have hypochondriacal elements. We found no justification whatsoever for the assumption that these labile patients are more severely or even fatally ill, as might have been concluded from the distress they experience subjectively.

One result, however, indicates that the patients' fears, their resignation and their numerous bodily complaints arise not only from a neurotic background. The patients in Cluster I also have to face more psychosocial problems caused by a lack of financial security.

The danger that a particular patient will have difficulties in adjusting to the operation and its consequences can partly be predicted before the operation. Considerable habitual, emotional, and vegetative instability before the operation, coupled with a great deal of strain arising from heart disease

which the patient can barely cope with, and a non-
dominant, passive and dependent attitude are all serious
risk factors for the patient's successful rehabilitation
3 - 5 years later. These results confirm the importance
of preoperatively intact ego functions, postulated by
Mohlen et al. [10], and the negative prognostic significance of regressive, symbiotic tendencies before the
operation. Unusually powerful emotional reactions to
stress before the operation, brought about by the
illness itself in combination with more pronounced
neurotic tendencies, as seen in the labile patients in
Group I, can be interpreted as a sign that this group
could not cope adequately with the burden and strains
inherent in this illness even before the operation.
This means that such patients undergo surgery in a state
when their defenses are already shaky and they do not
have the resources to protect themselves from the
anxiety and insecurity which the operation and the postoperative course induce in them. Huse-Kleinstoll et al.
[11] have already identified a high level of emotional
stress as a risk factor when the patient is confronted
with the pressures involved in a stay in the intensive
care unit.

Conclusions

Patients who were already emotionally at risk preoperatively have the highest number of emotional problems 3 - 5 years later. This comes as no surprise;
after all, one might say cardiac surgery is not intended
to cure neuroses. We could say, however, that the heart
is, to a large extent, incorporated into the neurotic
patterns, mainly via the hypochondriacal fixation of
some patients. The postoperative 'quality of life' of
these patients is lessened by dissatisfaction with the
result of the operation, as well as by an overcautious-
ness for which there is no objective need.

Aiming at improved care for patients at risk of
psychological maladjustment, we want to make the
following suggestions:

-   Early identification of the patient at risk of
    psychological maladjustment while the patient is
    in the hospital where the operation is carried
    out, if possible.

-   Improved cooperation between the psychological
    and psychiatric services in the surgical

hospital, the cardiologic rehabilitation center and - as far as possible - in out-patient care.
- Improvement of psychological services in heart surgery centers and in the cardiologic rehabilitation centers so that specific psychological and psychotherapeutic support can be given for immediate coping with the operation and heart disease as such.

- Improved utilization of opportunities which are available in the rehabilitation center and in the out-patient coronary training group to teach patients how to differentiate more accurately between 'dangerous' and 'innocuous' cardiac symptoms.

- Intensifying patient-centered information concerning cardiac symptoms.

- Providing more opportunities for out-patient psychotherapeutic treatment, especially for those patients whose emotional problems result from poor methods of coping with the illness and surgery which are interrelated with neurotic problems.

- Using the opportunities of social services to keep financial problems at a minimum.

References

1. H. Speidel and G. Rodewald, "Psychic and neurological dysfunctions after open-heart surgery," Thieme, Stuttgart, New York (1980).
2. R. Becker, J. Katz, M. J. Polonius and H. Speidel, "Psychological and neurological dysfunctions following open-heart surgery," Springer, Berlin, Heidelberg, New York (1982).
3. P. J. Walter, "Return to work after coronary artery bypass surgery - psychosocial and economic aspects," Springer, Berlin, Heidelberg, New York, Tokyo (1985).
4. J. S. Brown and M. Rawlinson, Relinquishing the sick role following open-heart surgery, J. Health and Soc Behav 16: 12-27 (1975).
5. N. J. Lutzenkirchen, K. Lamprecht, J. Walter and A. Dietz, The sociomedical situation and personality after heart surgery, in "Psychic and neurological dysfunctions after open-heart

surgery," H. Speidel and G. Rodewald, eds.,
Thieme, Stuttgart, New York (1980).

6. S. S. Heller, K. A. Frank, G. S. Kornfeld, S. N.
   Wilson and J. R. Malm, Psychological and
   behavioral responses following coronary artery
   bypass surgery, in "Psychopathological and
   neurological dysfunctions following open-heart
   surgery," R. Becker, J. Katz, M. J. Polonius
   and H. Speidel, eds., Springer, Berlin,
   Heidelberg, New York, Tokyo (1982).

7. S. S. Heller, K. A. Krank, D. S. Kornfeld, J. R.
   Malm and F. O. Bowman Jr., Psychological outcome
   followng open-heart surgery, Arch Int Med 134:
   908-914 (1974).

8. C. P. Kimball, The experience of cardiac surgery
   and cardiac transplant, in "Modern perspectives
   in the psychiatric aspects of surgery," J. G.
   Howells, ed., Brunner & Mazel, New York (1976).

9. G. Dahme, B. Dahme, A. Vollers and G.
   Huse-Kleinstoll, Fulfillment of patients'
   expectations concerning outcome of open-heart
   surgery, in: "Psychic and neurological
   dysfunctions after open-heart surgery," H.
   Speidel and G. Rodewald, eds., Thieme, Stuttgart,
   New York (1980).

10. K. Mohlen, S. Davies-Osterkamp, H. Muller, H.
    Scheld and G. Siefen, Relationship between pre-
    operative coping styles, immediate postoperative
    reactions and some aspects of the psychosocial
    situation of open-heart surgery patients one
    year after the operation, in "Psychopathological
    and neurological dysfunctions following open-
    heart surgery," R. Becker, J. Katz., M. J.
    Polonius and H. Speidel, eds., Springer, Berlin,
    Heidelberg, New York, Tokyo (1982).

11. G. Huse-Kleinstoll, A. Boll and P. Gotze, Angst und
    Angstbewaltigung vor und nach operativen
    Eingriffen, in "Leitsymptom Angst," P. Gotze,
    ed., Springer, Berlin, Heidelberg, New York,
    Tokyo (1984).

AN INTERPRETIVE STUDY OF THE METAPHORS MALE CORONARY
ARTERY SURGERY PATIENTS USE TO DESCRIBE THE SURGICAL
EXPERIENCE

Mary H. Hawthorne

Assistant Professor
School of Nursing
Duke University
Durham, North Carolina

BACKGROUND OF THE STUDY

Coronary artery disease remains the leading cause of
mortality and premature morbidity in the United States,
accounting for over 50% of the reported yearly deaths.
Approximately 560,000 Americans succumb each year from
myocardial infarctions, with another 4.6 million of the
population reporting either a history of angina or myocardial infarction [1]. In response to this major health
problem, myocardial revascularization via coronary artery
bypass grafting has emerged as one of the most dramatic,
invasive, as well as disputed, treatment modalities for
the management of coronary artery disease.

Since its popularization in 1967, the rate of revascularization procedures performed each year has increased dramatically. Unpublished data from the National
Center for Health Statistics of the Department of Health
and Human Services revealed that in 1987, 332,000 coronary
bypass operations were performed in the United States,
this figure representing an increase exceeding 60,000
procedures over the 1985 statistics [2]. Thus, coronary
artery surgery ranks as one of the most frequently performed, as well as the most costly procedures in the
United States [3].

Impact of Cardiac Surgery on the Quality of Life
Edited by A. E. Willner and G. Rodewald
Plenum Press, New York, 1990

The conclusions which emerged from the large, randomized trials have produced significant changes in the
decision tree utilized for the management of coronary
artery disease [4]. Once considered first-line defense
for significant coronary occlusive disease, this procedure
was most often utilized for the white male, expecting to
return post-operatively to full activity [5]. In contrast,
the procedure currently is viewed as appropriate for those
individuals who have failed medical management via an
impressive array of technologic and pharmacologic
armantaria, including coronary angioplasty, with some
noted exceptions such as in the instance of left main
coronary artery occlusion. Older patients (over 65),
often presenting with congestive heart failure, were once
excluded from surgical intervention. Currently, however,
it is thought that this subgroup of patients benefits not
only in terms of symptomatic relief, but especially
regarding the prolongation of life [6 - 10].

Empirical evidence expressed by both nurses and
physicians in the care of these patients indicates that
the cumulative effect of these changes in the selection of
surgical candidates has been a gradual and significant
shift in the client base. The traditional coronary bypass
population consisted of a group of individuals usually
anticipating full recovery post-operatively, and often
viewing the procedure as a cure versus palliation within a
chronic disease trajectory. The population of today still
includes a significant number of patients who will often
improve with surgery but may continue to suffer marked
infirmity and disability. Considering this evidence
within the context of an aging society, significant implications can be drawn regarding trends for the future care
of this patient population. It appears reasonable to
predict that the numbers of individuals experiencing
disability from their cardiac disease will rise as the
available technology reduces mortality and generates
illness chronicity [11].

The significance of this for nursing is the recognition of a growing population of patients for whom the
period of recovery after major surgery is likely to be
more complex, this group encountering surgery later in
life than previously and perhaps encountering greater
post-operative morbidity. The provision of appropriate
nursing care for this patient population, as with all
other patient groups, is contingent upon the authenticity

of the nurse-patient interaction [12], wherein patient needs and concerns are accurately and appropriately identified. Authenticity in interaction is dependent upon the nurse's existential awareness of illness as a reality experienced by the patient, rather than the presentation of objective signs and symptoms of disease. This ontologic approach to nursing care assumes that the understanding of the patient's illness reality is central, as well as essential, to the provision of humanistic care.

As the concern is to construct appropriate nursing care based upon an understanding of the illness reality of the patient, the approach to care becomes meaning-centered, as it is the meaning of experience which actually constitutes reality [13]. In other words, the individual constructs an illness reality by assigning meaning to this unique experience [14]. Patients' nursing needs are thus identified and constructed through the nurse's understanding of the meaning of the illness experience for the individual.

From a meaning-centered approach the provision of care for coronary artery surgical patients is thus contingent upon an understanding of the patient's illness reality as transformed by the experience of surgery. The overall concern of this study, therefore, was to enhance such understanding. As illness reality is thought to be constructed of a confluence of meanings, among the most prominent being those meanings associated with the symbols of medical science [15], the specific concern was an understanding of the symbolic meaning of the cardiac surgical experience as it shapes the patient's restructuring of life patterns during the period of post-operative recovery.

Discerning meaning and one's construction of reality cannot be achieved directly. From the perspective of hermeneutic philosophy as articulated by Ricouer [16], the sole route to achieving such understanding is obtained through the intepretation of language, specifically the metaphor, a language entity noted for its polysemic nature. The purpose of this qualitative study was therefore to investigate the language patients utilized to describe the coronary artery surgical experience. The intent in so doing was to obtain insight into the ideologic framework of the individual which is utilized to interpret and assign meaning to the surgical experience.

METHODOLOGY

    Participants in this study were recruited from the
sample of male coronary artery surgery patients at University Hospital, State University of New York at Stony
Brook. The investigator, using a semi-structured interview
technique, asked each participant to relate his story of
cardiac illness, describing the surgical experience.
Specific questions were utilized to elicit information
concerning the patient's perception of the effects of
the procedure upon his illness. Interviews were tape-
recorded and transcribed. The investigator also constructed fieldnotes throughout the interview process.
Using the rule of redundancy as a guide for sample size
[17], the investigator conducted a total of six interviews. The transcriptions and fieldnotes were coded and
analyzed employing the technique of thematic analysis.

RESULTS

    Analysis of this qualitative investigation resulted
in 13 major themes and 6 minor themes which provide
insight into the belief system the patients in this sample
utilized to interpret the surgical event.

Theme #1

    Cardiac illness and major cardiac events such as
heart attacks, surgery and angiography represent a frightening confrontation with one's mortality. Surgery, however,
as an intentional confrontation, is viewed as a necessary
exposure to life threat in order to escape the greater
risk posed by one's cardiac illness.

Theme #2

    Cardiac illness and the recognition of one's mor-
tality result in the "rude awakening" that one is not
indestructible. There is a dramatic shift in one's self
concept from that of strength and boundless energy to
vulnerability and fragility.

Theme #3

    Recognition of one's mortality and vulnerability
stimulates a life reassessment, not unlike a midlife

transition. Perspectives change and priorities shift.
Patients feel significantly altered, not only regarding
their physical health, but in terms of their thoughts and
emotions.

Theme #4

Coronary revascularization is perceived by patients
to be a resounding success as a treatment for significant
coronary artery disease. Surgery, exceptionally successful in relieving symptoms, transforms an uncertain, risk-
laden situation into a more predictable, risk-free
appearing disease trajectory.

Theme #5

The experience of cardiac surgery can be empowering.
Some patients report that successful recovery leaves them
feeling enhanced rather than diminished by the experience.
The patient, like the mythical heroes of American culture
who face adversity, feels renewed vigor, having survived
the life or death challenge of cardiac surgery. Surgery,
as such, may be a more desirable treatment option than
more conservative measures as it is consistent with the
desired male image within American society.

Theme #6

The widespread availability and frequent performance
of coronary artery surgery have resulted in the view of
the procedure as being an ordinary, rather mundane
experience.

Theme #7

The participants' descriptions of cardiac illness and
surgery reflect a belief system dominated by the Received
View of sciences, a perspective espoused and promulgated
by the logical positivists of the Vienna Circle. This
worldview supports the illusion of a surgical cure.

Theme #8

Patients' descriptions of illness reflect a world
constructed with discrete numbers and facts. Describing
illness in terms of numerical parameters generates the
illusion that disease is a tangible, hence manageable
phenomenon.

Theme #9

Cardiac surgery as a treatment choice is consistent
with the American spirit of mastery over illness and
adversity, approaching a difficult problem with definitive
action.

Theme #10

There is an element of consumerism apparent in
cardiac surgical care, wherein the process of selecting
care can be likened to purchasing a product. Such an
atmosphere of capitalist mass production generates fears
of depersonalization and dehumanization.

Theme #11

The experience of cardiac surgery generates a unique
type of intimacy. Central to this phenomenon is a bond of
trust that develops between the patient and the surgeon,
which makes legitimate for the patient both the intimacy
and extreme vulnerability associated with the surgery.

Theme #12

Patients' descriptions of cardiac illness and the
appraisal of threat posed by the illness contain classic
illustrations of the use of denial as a psychological
defense mechanism. The primary expression of this
phenomenon lies within the realm of unrealistic expecta-
tions/benefits anticipated from the surgical intervention.

Theme #13

Patients in the aftermath of cardiac surgery, like
other patients after minor cardiac events, search for
causative factors to explain their illnesses. Linked with
this search is an element of self-blame for the cardiac
illness.

Minor Themes

1. Myths about cardiac surgery abound despite the fact
    that there has been extensive information available to
    the public and the procedure is widespread in
    application.

2. Hallucinations and nightmares are a common experience
    following cardiac surgery.

3. Stress in the workplace is connected or contributes to
    cardiac disease.

4. Networking with other patients after surgery is an
    important component of recovery.

5. The experience of surgery and anesthesia is perceived
    as a loss of self.

6. Participants acknowledged the importance in care of
    expert communication; the ability to interpret and
    communicate clinical events.

CONCLUSIONS

The first conclusion which emerges from an examination
of the themes from this study is that the Received View of
science, espoused by the logical positivists of the Vienna
Circle [18], perseveres as a significant component of the
contemporary American scientific worldview. Views of
illness and surgery of the participants were dominated by
the tenets of reductionism, empiricism and disease causa-
tion. Views of health and medicine, as illustrated in
Themes #7 and #8, appear to be dominated by an approach
which values cure over prevention, views which also fuel
the incessant quest for a magic bullet for each medical
problem or imperfection that emerges [19].

The study findings also indicate that the procedure
of coronary artery surgery is consistent with the preferred manner of approach this society has defined for
problem solving. Cultures define primary modes for
approaching problems [20, 21], and in American society the
primary mode is taking direct action and employing instru-
mentation. Taking action is also part of the American
approach to dealing with or, as Ernst Becker [22] articu-
lates, the avoidance of the recognition of one's own
mortality through constant activity and risk taking.

The preferred model of male behavior in this culture
thus embodies this activist approach to the issue of
death, as men in this society are primarily socialized to
be solitary, independent risk-takers [23]. Cardiac
surgery perceived as a confrontation with death is consistent with the preferred image of the male American hero,
who will face any or all odds when confronted with adversity. The procedure in its consistency with both the
preferred male image of American society and the general

approach of this society to major life issues, vita activa
[24], embodies a profound symbolic power to heal the
"damaged self." The investigator thus concludes that the
phenomenon of cardiac surgery, is in itself a metaphor for
contemporary American society.

REFERENCES

1. J. Toth, The person with coronary artery disease and
    risk factors, in: "Cardiovascular Nursing," C. E.
    Buzetta and B. M. Dossey, eds., C. V. Mosby, St.
    Louis (1984).
2. _____, Hospital discharge survey, unpublished data
    from the National Center for Health Statistics,
    U.S. Department of Health and Human Services.
    Washington, D. C. (1987).
3. I. K. Crosby, J. Chiang, S. Jordan, R. L. Mentzor Jr.,
    I. L. Kron, D. L. Kaiser and G. B. Craddock Jr., The
    influence of economic and society factors, in:
    "Return to Work After Coronary Bypass Surgery,"
    P. J. Walter, ed., Springer-Verlag, New York
    (1985).
4. K. J. Silverman and W. Grossman, Angina pectoris,
    Natural history and strategies for management,
    NEJM. 319:131-135 (1988).
5. G. R. Cutter, A. Oberman, N. Kouchoukos and W. Rogers.
    Epidemiologic study of candidates for coronary
    bypass surgery, Circulation. 66:III-9 (1982).
6. H. L. Edmunds, L. W. Stephenson, R. N. Edie and M. B.
    Ratcliffe, Open-heart surgery in octogenarians,
    NEJM. 319:131-135 (1988).
7. B. J. Gersh, R. A. Kronmal and H. V. Schaff,
    Comparison of coronary bypass surgery and medical
    therapy in patients 65 years of age or older, NEJM.
    313:217-24 (1985).
8. G. C. Kaiser, Lessons from the Randomized Trials,
    Annals of Thoracic Surgery. 42:3-8 (1986).
9. N. Katz, Expectations of Coronary Artery Surgery,
    American Family Practitioner. 35:181-194 (1987).
10. A. J. Roberts, D. D. Woodhull, C. R. Conti, D. W.
    Ellison, R. Risher, C. Richards, R. G. Marks, D. C.
    Knauf and A. J. Alexander, Mortality, morbidity,
    and cost-accounting related to coronary artery
    bypass grafting in the elderly, Annals of Thoracic
    Surgery. 39:426-431 (1985).
11. D. Callahan, "Setting Limits in an Aging Society."
    Simon and Schuster, New York (1987).

12. J. Paterson and L. Zderad, "Humanistic Nursing," John Wiley and Sons, New York (1976).
13. W. C. Schutz, "Joy," Grove Press, New York (1967).
14. B. Toben, "Space-Time and Beyond," E. P. Dutton, New York (1975).
15. A. Kleinman, Medicine's symbolic reality, Inquiry. 16:206-13 (1979).
16. P. Ricouer, "Hermeneutics and the Human Sciences," (J. B.Thompsom, Trans.), Cambridge Univeristy Press, New York (1981).
17. R. C. Bogdan and S. K. Biklen, "Qualitative Research for Education: an Introduction to Theory and Methods," Allyn and Bacon, Inc., Boston (1982).
18. A. K. Jacox and G. Webster, Competing theories of science, in: L. H. Nicoll, ed., "Perspectives on Nursing Theory," Little, Brown and Company, Boston (1986).
19. R. Dubos, "Man Adapting," Yale University Press, New Haven (1980). (Original publication 1965.)
20. A. Bergman, "Technology and Character in Contemporary Life," University of Chicago Press, Chicago (1984).
21. J. Hartog and E. A. Hartog, Cultural aspects of health and illness behavior in hospitals. Western Journal of Medicine. 139:910-916 (1983).
22. E. Becker, "The denial of death," The Free Press, New York (1973).
23. H. Goldberg, "The hazards of being male," New American Library, New York (1976).
24. R. N. Bellah, To kill and survive or to die and become: the active and the contemplative life as ways of being adult. Daedalus. 105(2):57-76 (1976).

GOOD PSYCHOSOCIAL ADAPTATION TO

IMPLANTABLE CARDIOVERTER DEFIBRILLATORS

Colette Pycha
Joseph R. Calabrese

Cleveland Clinic Foundation
Department of Psychiatry & Psychology
9500 Euclid Avenue
Cleveland, Ohio 44195-5192

INTRODUCTION

Sudden cardiac death accounts for approximately 450,000 of all annual cardiac deaths in the United States alone [1], making it one of the leading causes of death today [2]. Although the pathogenesis of sudden cardiac death remains unclear, it has been accepted that the majority of these out-of-the-hospital deaths are caused by ventricular fibrillation related to a malignant ventricular arrhythmia [1]. One year mortality rates (26%) remain high despite the availability of potent antiarrhythmic agents and arrhythmia surgery [1,3].

Mirowski recognized the problem of sudden arrhythmic death in the late 1960s and conceptualized an implantable defibrillator device [4]. The first human implant was performed in 1980 at Johns Hopkins Hospital [5,6]. The original device could detect and treat only ventricular fibrillation, a limitation since most cardiac deaths arise from ventricular tachyarrhythmias. Later improvements in the device allowed it to be responsive to ventricular tachyarrhythmia, transforming the original defibrillator into a cardioverter-defibrillator system [6], delivering pulses of 25-30 joules of electricity directly to the heart muscle when a malignant rhythm occurs, and restoring normal sinus rhythm to the heart.

Impact of Cardiac Surgery on the Quality of Life
Edited by A. E. Willner and G. Rodewald
Plenum Press, New York, 1990

AICD - PSYCHOLOGICAL IMPACT

Arising from technological advances are concerns
about quality of life and psychosocial adaptation. It was
not until recently that these concerns were closely
scrutinized despite mention of the potential problems that
can arise with the AICD [1]. The early literature delin-
eated potential psychological complications related to
implantation, i.e. device dependency, imagined pulsing,
fear of loss of pulsing capability. Echt and Winkle [5]
address the need for psychological support services as
part of the treatment team, routinely evaluating and being
available to all who receive the AICD. They enumerate the
stressors these patients face, i.e. a life threatening
illness, prolonged and difficult hospitalizations,
unsuccessful drug trials, surgery and fear of an electronic
device. They not only face an unpredictable illness but
are vulnerable to unpredictable and uncontrollable device
discharges that are accompanied by physical discomfort.
Consistent with the previous report, Winkle et al. [6]
also recommended a psychiatrist and/or a clinical psychologist as part of the treatment team to aid in the long-
term management of these patients, as rapport established
early on proves valuable in managing any future problems
that arise.

Fricchione and Vlay [7] provide pertinent and helpful
information in understanding the common responses and
useful psychiatric interventions when dealing with a
patient who has a malignant rhythm disturbance. For those
who require the AICD, potential problems are illustrated
via case example to include panic-like symptoms, even in
the face of a device that engenders security in knowing
that it will restore sinus rhythm should a malignant
rhythm occur. Most of what has been written on the AICD
patient clearly identifies the need of psychological
support services as part of the treatment team. It has
only been recently that the unique issues and concerns
related to psychosocial adaptation of patients and their
spouses have been illuminated.

To further explore psychosocial adaptation to the
implantation of the AICD, we retrospectively administered
a psychometric battery designed to systematically assess
adaptation. Of the 69 patients and spouses who were asked
to complete the questionnaires, 42 patients and 38 spouses
returned them. The battery consisted of self-administered
ratings of mood [8], anxiety [9] and the Cleveland Clinic
AICD Psychosocial Inventory. The Psychosocial Inventory

was designed to elicit information concerning demographics, medical history, patient attitudes toward the device, body image, distortions, lifestyle alterations, impact on family and marriage, general quality of life, and device-specific concerns. The mean period of time the device had been implanted was 17.6 months (range = 1-52 months) and the range of device discharges was 0-45, with the majority of patients experiencing between 0-5 discharges. The Beck Depression Inventory was completed by 40 patients (mean $\pm$ SD, 9.2 $\pm$ 7.4, range 0-27) and 37 spouses (mean $\pm$ SD, 7.4 $\pm$ 6.2, range 0-22). Sixty-five percent (26/40) of patients had total scores on the BDI suggestive of mild, 35% (14/40) moderate, and no patients received a rating compatible with severe depression. Over ninety percent (35/37) of spouses had total scores on the BDI suggestive of mild, 5.4% (2/37) moderate, and no spouses received a rating compatible with severe depression. The Self-Assessment Anxiety Scale was completed by 40 patients (mean $\pm$ SD, 34.8 $\pm$ 9.0, range 17-57). Fifteen percent (6/40) of patients had total scores on the SAS suggestive of mild anxiety, whereas no patients exhibited scores suggestive of moderate or severe anxiety. Over twelve percent (4/33) of spouses had total scores on the SAS suggestive of mild anxiety, whereas no spouses yielded scores suggestive of moderate or severe anxiety.

The Cleveland Clinic Psychosocial Inventory was completed by all patients (n = 42) and spouses (n = 38). Of the 42 patients, worry about resuscitation, shock, and death were either lessened or non-existent (78.5%) since implantation. The AICD was perceived by patients as a life-extender (76.2%), source of security (73.8%), and source of anxiety (4.8%). Spouses viewed it similarly as a life extender and source of security (65.8%). Although a greater number perceived the quality of the shock as lightening-like (45.2%), some responded by saying the pulse was "not-so-bad" (21.4%) while others perceived it as terrifying (14.3%) or painful (16.7%). Fifty-two percent of the patients felt reassured or unchanged after the device fired and 73.8% felt tired or nervous. The majority (83.3%) held the belief that they were able to successfully incorporate the device into their body image but altered body perceptions were frequently reported. Over half of our patients thought the size of the device was too large and a third felt self-conscious because of it. The perception that they could be more active since they had a "back-up" device was reported by 64.2% of our patients, although half of our population reported some decrease in activity level since implantation. The implantation reduced the patient's perception of family worry from 50% pre-implant to 16.7% post-implant. Patients also perceived family overprotectiveness as decreased following implantation, from 31% pre-implant to 16.7% post-implant. Similarly, implantation of the AICD reduced the family's perception of patient worry from pre-implant levels of 55.3% to 21.1%. The major homegoing concern of the patients was the availability of experienced local emergency room care (54.7%). Almost half of the patients had additional concerns relative to where they would be when the device discharged (47.6%), when it discharged (45.2%), and if the device was capable of successfully defibrillating their hearts (42.8%). Additional concerns were cost (42.8%), discharge-related pain (40.4%), frequency of follow-up visits (33.3%), and concerns over the device's energy reserves (26.1%). In addition to having concerns similar to the patients', one-third of the spouses reported a query as to whether they could provoke device-discharge by the candid expression of feelings such as anger. A large number of patients and spouses (>40%) were concerned that sexual activity would trigger the device. For some, this was sufficient to refrain from sexual intercourse.

OTHER STUDIES

     Cooper et al. [2] studied the quality of life and psychosocial adaptation of 17 patients with an AICD and concluded that AICD implantation is associated with multiple psychosocial consequences and that fear was the predominant expressed emotion. Of those who received shocks, 85% reported persistent fear and 47% fear of premature battery depletion. Decreased over-all activity as well as sexual activity particularly in the younger population was also reported. Their patients also identified problems with the device being cumbersome and those related to body image changes. Similar to our findings, 88% were pleased to have the AICD and viewed it as vital to their well-being.

     Vlay [3] discusses the personal and social benefits of the device in terms of returning to work and to an active lifestyle. Their patients perceive the device as a source of comfort and as a "safety-net" to protect them. They conclude that the restoration of the ability to lead an active life has a beneficial social impact and is a reasonable economic investment.

     Brodsky et al [10] conducted a survey of 115 patients

and their caretakers and received completed questionnaires from 53 patients and 52 caretakers. They found that lingering fears persist regarding the trustworthiness of the device. The majority of patient's (59%) and spouses (53%) worried about shocks from the device. Patients were concerned about social embarrassment should the device discharge (64%). Negative alterations in lifestyle included loss of physical activity (83%), less sexual activity (51%), depression (47%), and thoughts of death (54%). Among spouses, 37% reported feeling depressed. This study, as was our own, was compromised by the inability to sort out responses to illness versus responses to AICD implantation alone.

Vlay et al [11] studied anxiety and anger in 8 patients with an AICD using the Symptom Checklist-90, the State-Trait Personality Inventory, and a questionnaire specific to the AICD population. The group as a whole manifested higher degrees of anxiety and anger compared to controls. Trait scores of anxiety remained unchanged pre-vs-post implantation but the state of anxiety was markedly reduced following implantation and patient acceptance of the device was high.

In summary, our findings are consistent with the literature and suggest there are a myriad of psychosocial concerns associated with having an AICD. These include: (1) concerns about the reliability of the device, (2) where the person will be when it discharges, (3) the cumbersomeness of the device, (4) its cost, and (5) the availability of experienced local emergency care should the device malfunction or discharge inappropriately. Patients need to feel secure in the face of a life-threatening illness and with an interventional device that is unpredictable and uncontrollable. These views suggest that benefit can be derived from psychological support services and that an interdisciplinary team approach very much enhances patient care.

REFERENCES

1. B. Flores and M. Hildebrandt, The automatic implantable defibrillator, Heart & Lung. 13:608-613 (1984).
2. D. K. Cooper, R. Luceri, R. Thurer, and R. J. Meyerburg, The impact of the automatic implantable cardioverter on quality of life, Clinical Progress in Electrophysiology and Pacing. 4:306-309 (1986).

3. S. C. Vlay, The automatic internal cardioverter-
    defibrillator: Comprehensive clinical follow-up,
    economic and social impact - The Stony Brook
    Experience, <u>Am Heart J.</u> 112:189-194 (1986).
4. M. Mirowski, M. M. Mower, and A. Langer, A chronically-
    implanted system for automatic defibrillation in
    active conscious dogs: Experimental model for
    treatment of sudden death from ventricular
    fibrillation, <u>Circulation</u>. 58:90-94 (1978).
5. D. S. Echt and R. A. Wing, Management of patients with
    the automatic implantable cardioverter defibrillator,
    <u>Clin Progress</u>. 3:4-16 (1985).
6. R. A. Winkle, E. B. Stinson, and D. S. Echt, Practical
    aspects of automatic cardioverter/defibrillator
    implantation, <u>Am Heart J.</u> 108:1335-1346 (1984)..
7. G. L. Fricchione and S. C. Vlay, Psychiatric aspects
    of patients with malignant ventricular
    arrhythmias, <u>Am J Psychiatry</u>. 143:1518-1526 (1986).
8. A. T. Beck. C. H. Ward, and M. Mendelson, An inventory
    for measuring depression, <u>Arch Gen Psychiatry</u>.
    4:561-571 (1961).
9. W. W. K. Zung, A rating instrument for anxiety
    disorders, <u>Psychosomatics</u>. 12:371-379 (1971).
10. A. Brodsky, M. H. Miller, and D. S. Cannon,
    Psychosocial Adaptation to the AICD. Presented at
    the Annual Meeting of The American Heart
    Association, Washington, DC (November, 1988).
11. S. C. Vlay, L. Olson, and G. Fricchione, Anxiety and
    anger in patients with ventricular tachyarrhythmias:
    Responses after automatic internal cardioverter
    defribillator implantation, <u>Pace</u>. 12:366-373
    (1989).

DENIAL AMONG CARDIAC PATIENTS WITH THE AUTOMATIC

IMPLANTABLE CARDIOVERTER DEFIBRILLATOR

Efrain A. Gonzalez
Deborah K. Cooper

Department of Psychology and Behavioral
Medicine, University of Miami/Jackson
Memorial Hospital
1611 N. W. 12th Avenue
Miami, FL 33136

Despite numerous approaches for managing patients with ventricular arrhythmias, sudden cardiac death remains one of the leading causes of death in the United States today [1]. The psychological reactions to such episodes, namely, fear, anxiety and depression, as well as personality variables which may have contributed to the etiology or exacerbation of coronary heart disease, have been well documented [1-9]. However, the psychological aspects among cardiac patients whose lives have been prolonged by artificial devices, e.g., the automatic implantable cardioverter defibrillator (AICD) is an area that remains relatively unexplored [10].

It is important to understand the adaptive psychological mechanisms that cardiac patients utilize in order to promote them in the treatment setting. For example, Mai [11] found high levels of denial among heart transplant recipients towards the graft and the donor. Mai also suggested that denial appears to serve as a "protective and adaptive function in heart transplant recipients." Therefore, it seems that denial may also serve to avoid the prolongation of post-shock fear and depression. Consequently, this study was conducted to assess levels of denial among AICD patients in relation to experienced levels of fear.

Impact of Cardiac Surgery on the Quality of Life
Edited by A. E. Willner and G. Rodewald
Plenum Press, New York, 1990

In an article published by Vlay, et al. [12], the
authors reported a significant decrease in the level of
anxiety among eight AICD patients over time. Although
they included in their discussion several variables that
may have contributed to the decrease of the state of
anxiety, no mention is made of adaptive psychological
defenses as a possible factor.

METHODS

Thirty-five patients who had successfully received
the AICD were interviewed. All patients had a history of
ventricular tachycardia or ventricular fibrillation with
at least three or more drug therapy failures or intoler-
ances. There were twenty-six males and nine females with
a mean age of 61 years. Patients' age ranged between
24-84 years. Twenty-four patients were retired and
eleven were employed. Twenty-eight of the thirty-five
patients were married, five widowed, and two were
divorced. Throughout the interview, patients were asked
about their experience with the AICD, including their
emotional responses, awareness of the device and manner
of coping with the unpleasantness of shocks.

FINDINGS

Of the thirty-five patients interviewed, 29/35
patients (83%) reported high initial awareness regarding
the AICD, and infrequent awareness after a few months
post-implant. As one patient stated, "I thought about it
all the time." "Now I feel I was born with it." Patients
also reported being aware of the AICD after a shock, at
which time they primarily experienced fear (73%). However, they usually resumed their normal activities within
a few hours.

Several patients reported frequent awareness of the
AICD, even up to one year post-implant. For example, one
patient commented, "I think people are looking at me. My
friends' eyes go right to the box." Interestingly,
patients who were frequently aware of the AICD also reported more anxiety and depression, admitted to premorbid
psychiatric symptoms, and were less adjusted post-implant.

Finally, it should be noted that the only patient
who failed to report any post-shock fear or apprehension

has expired. This patient stated, "I'm not really
frightened by it. Nothing really worries me anymore."

DISCUSSION

     With respect to denial, there appears to be a close
similarity between AICD patients and heart transplant
recipients. That is, both patient populations seem to
employ this defense mechanism to ward off feelings of
anxiety, fear and guilt, in order to resume their
activities of daily living.

     Traditionally, psychodynamic theory has emphasized
the importance of transferring unconsciously repressed
and/or denied material into consciousness as a means of
gaining greater awareness and insight into conflictual
areas that may be expressed as pathological symptoms.
Furthermore, it has been our observation at this medical
center that denial among medical patients is very often
perceived as pathological by physicians, nurses, physical
and occupational therapists, psychology interns and other
staff at the Medical Center.

     In fact, psychologists are frequently called to
"break" a patient's denial as it is often believed to
interfere with rehabilitation goals. As clinicians in a
medical setting we must understand that denial, as with
AICD patients, may be adaptive and should not necessarily
be dismantled, particularly in the initial phases post-
implant.

     It has also been our observation that patients who
seek or are referred to our outpatient psychotherapy
service after hospital discharge are experiencing
recurrent thoughts and fear of being shocked, which is
interfering with their interpersonal and social life.
After exploration of these thoughts and emotions,
patients may benefit from further education regarding the
device and assistance in developing more adaptive
mechanisms for adequate adjustment.

     According to Vlay, et al. [12], the level of state
anxiety among AICD patients post-operatively is significantly high and tends to decrease within several months.
Other studies [13, 14], however, have reported a reduced
level of anxiety immediately after cardiac surgery, not
associated with AICD implantation. Therefore, it seems
that the actual implant tends to dramatically raise the

level of anxiety among AICD patients due to their fear of shocks. Possibly, the reduced level of anxiety is related more to psychological defenses than to the implant itself. Perhaps a greater decrease in the level of state anxiety would be obtained if clinicians attempted to promote healthy denial during post-implant counseling.

Results of this study also revealed a relationship between premorbid history of anxiety and depression, and difficulty in post-operative adjustment. Further research should attempt to shed light on this subject as this may have important implications in the screening, follow-up, and treatment of these patients. Although possibly coincidental, additional research should also focus on examining the possible correlation between total lack of fear and concern after ventricular arrhythmia and mor- bidity among AICD patients. An appropriate level of anxiety and fear may also be warranted for optimal functioning and survival.

REFERENCES

1. G. L. Fricchione and S. C. Vlay, Psychiatric aspects of patients with malignant ventricular arrhythmias, Am J Psych. 143:1518 (1986).
2. C. Bass, Psychosocial outcome after coronary artery by-pass surgery, Br J Psych. 145:526 (1984).
3. L. J. Bloom, Psychology and cardiology: collaboration in coronary treatment and prevention, Prof Psychol. 485:490 (1979).
4. J. G. Bruhn, A. Paredes, C. A. Adsett, and S. Wolf, Psychological predictors of sudden death in myocardial infarction, J Psychosom Res. 18:187 (1974).
5. R. B. Case, S. S. Heller, N. B. Case, and A. J. Moss, Type A behavior and survival after acute myocardial infarction, N Engl J Med. 312:737 (1985).
6. D. L. Dunner, Anxiety and panic: Relationship to depression and cardiac disorders, Psychosomatics. 26:18 (1985).
7. R. W. Guynn, Psychiatric presentations of cardio- vascular disease, in: "Psychiatric Presentations of Medical Illness," Spectrum Publications, New York (1980).

8. T. P. Hackett, Depression following myocardial infarction, _Psychosomatics_. 26:23 (1985).
9. R. H. Rosenman, The impact of anxiety on the cardiovascular system, _Psychosomatics_. 26:6 (1985).
10. D. K. Cooper, R. M. Luceri, R. J. Thurer, and R. J. Myerburg, The impact of the automatic implantable cardioverter defibrillator on quality of life, _Clin Prog Electrophysiol Pacing_. 4:306 (1986).
11. F. M. Mai, Graft and donor denial in heart transplant recipients, _Am J Psych_. 143:1159 (1986).
12. S. C. Vlay, L. C. Olson, G. L. Fricchione, and R. Friedman, Anxiety and anger in patients with ventricular tachyarrhythmias. Responses after automatic internal cardioverter defibrillator implantation, _Pace_. 12:366 (1989).
13. P. J. Walter, Quality of life after open heart surgery, _in_: "Impact of Cardiac Surgery on Quality of Life: Neurological and Psychological Aspects," A. Willner and G. Rodewald, eds., Plenum, NY (1990).
14. H. Speidel, Changes in psychopathology after cardiac surgery, _in_: "Impact of Cardiac Surgery on Quality of Life: Neurological and Psychological Aspects," A. Willner and G. Rodewald, eds., Plenum, NY (1990).

NEUROLOGICAL ISSUES

THE SUSCEPTIBILITY OF THE CENTRAL NERVOUS SYSTEM

TO OPEN HEART SURGERY

Thomas Emskoetter, Lutz Lachenmayer

Neurological Department
University of Hamburg
Hamburg, Fed. Rep. Germany

The occurrence of transient or persistent neurological deficits in the perioperative course of open-
heart surgery is one of the potentially most serious
complications limiting a favorable outcome for cardiac
patients. While permanent brain damage is only rarely
encountered in this setting, several studies indicate
that intermittent neurological abnormalities in the
postoperative period are a much more common feature
unique to cardio-surgical procedures [1, 2, 3]. Such
syndromes of impaired cerebral function until now could
not be correlated with a particular type of cardiac
surgery, the obvious presence of metabolic disturbances,
or the type of anesthesia used [4]. The absence of such
an ostensible relationship is further evidenced by the
fact that we do not observe similar neurological
abnormalities after other surgical procedures [5].

The analysis of the neurological symptomatology
observed in these cases provides some evidence for a
somehow hypoxia-mediated pathogenesis, which is further
substantiated by post mortem pathology in fatal cases
[6]. Systemic hypotension can induce a significant
reduction of the intracerebral blood flow (ICBF), and
ischemic thresholds have been defined for reversible and
irreversible changes in the brain tissue as a time-
related consequence of hypoxia [7]. Hematocrit changes,
as another factor, are inversely correlated with changes
in the regional cerebral blood flow [8]. On the cellular
level, complex metabolic interactions are involved

Impact of Cardiac Surgery on the Quality of Life
Edited by A. E. Willner and G. Rodewald
Plenum Press, New York, 1990

postischemically, each of them contributing to a
destabilization of the microenvironment that leads to
functional impairment, and, when corrective mechanisms
fail, finally to structural neuronal damage [9]. In the
ischemic brain, there is a rapid decrease of high-energy
metabolites, increased lactate, and a shift toward a
reduction of mitochondrial respiratory chain metabolites.
In the center of an ischemic zone, the blood flow is
usually reduced below 10 ml/100 g of brain tissue per
minute, with a marked influx of water and sodium into
the cell, lactic acidosis and a greatly diminished
oxygen availability. Deficient autoregulation can be
compensated for some time by an increased oxygen extrac-
tion, but once corrective mechanisms fail, irreversible
neuronal damage occurs. It is well recognized that
cytotoxic edema plays an important role for reducing the
rate of recoveries from transient ischemia. Crucial
factors that influence postischemic neuronal damage
include the duration and completeness of ischemia, the
collateral circulation, the preischemic glucose content
and intracellular calcium, tissue, prostaglandins, and
the generation of free radicals [9].

The human brain requires a constant supply of oxygen
to maintain ionic gradients across axonal and cellular
membranes [10]. Brief episodes of anoxia usually are
well tolerated and patients awaken promptly. Slightly
prolonged periods of anoxia lead to a reversible
metabolic posthypoxic encephalopathy, with coma, if
occurring, only lasting for a few hours and symptoms
resolving within hours to days. Neurons that are
particularly susceptible to even milder degrees of
anoxia are the pyramidal cells in the uncal region of
the hippocampus [11], known to be crucial for memory
functions, and the pyramidal cells of the third and
fifth layers of the cerebral cortex, which presumably
accounts for the states of diffuse encephalopathy
encountered in these patients. In the setting of more
severe anoxia, the basal ganglia, substantia nigra, and
nuclei amygdalae also become involved, which results in
a midbrain syndrome with preserved brainstem reflexes,
sometimes stabilizing and leaving the patient in a
persistent decorticate state. Finally, with profound
anoxia, substantial damage to the brainstem nuclei may
result in irreversible dissociated brain death.

Since obvious incidents leading to hypoxia, like
circulatory arrest or depression, are only seen in a
minority of patients with neurological abnormalities,

either localized or disseminated embolism of air or particles must be taken into account as a possible etiologic factor. Multiple microemboli can in fact be demonstrated in retinal vessels after open-heart surgery has been performed. It is tempting to assume that similar events might take place in the brain parenchyma as well. CBF measurements during extracorporeal circulation (ECC) procedures indeed reveal brain hyperperfusion during steady-state hypothermic ECC and signs of impaired autoregulation following subsequent rewarming to steady-state normothermic ECC, compatible with multiple brain micro-embolization [12].

Stroke-like focal lesions can occur in the same way by direct embolic damage to particular brain areas or by disproportionate ischemia in susceptible areas after prolonged systemic hypotension. Those susceptible areas are either boundary zones between major cerebral arteries or preexistent, until then asymptomatic, vascular stenoses. Brierley [6] reported predominant ischemic damage to the boundary zones of the cerebral cortex at autopsy in all of nine cases dying within hours after cardiac surgery with extracorporeal circulation. Price reported cholesterol emboli with an identical distribution pattern in a further case [13]. In a controlled study of primates subjected to cardiac arrest, Miller observed that the brainstem was regularly affected but cerebral infarcts did not occur as long as prolonged hypotension before and after circulatory arrest was prevented [14]. Brainstem involvement was also pathologically confirmed in humans by other authors [15].

Typical boundary zone syndromes include vision disorders due to dysfunction of both occipital poles, tetrapareses, or the man-in-the-barrel syndrome with bi-brachial paresis due to motor cortex dysfunction in the boundary between the anterior and middle cerebral arteries. If the medulla is primarily involved, a spinal cord syndrome may ensue after posthypoxic damage to watershed zones of the medulla [16]. A progressive neurological deterioration resulting in final coma or death days to weeks after the operation can also occur due to a delayed posthypoxic leukoencephalopathy primarily involving the subcortical white matter of the posterior parts of the brain [17].

Although it is not clear whether the pathogenetic mechanisms presented here are in fact responsible for the bulk of neurological abnormalities observed in the

setting of extracorporeal bypass surgery, the symptomatology associated with it clearly argues in favor of
such an underlying relationship on pathophysiological
grounds. Nevertheless, prospective MRI follow-up studies
indicate that other factors like e.g. intracranial
hemorrhage may also play a role, at least in children
[18].

The diagnosis of cerebral dysfunction is mainly
based upon the clinical neurological examination.
Computed tomography and cross-sectional EEG are of
little help to identify brain lesions or dysfunctions
in most of these cases. Nevertheless, in a study on
long-term follow-up, a persistently abnormal EEG has
been related to prolonged perfusion times [19]. The
potential role of computerized EEG monitoring and MRI is
subject to current investigations. Since most of the
symptoms relating to a pre-damaged or only marginally
compensated brain area are only transient in the first
instance before irreversible damage occurs, the neurologist has to screen the patient's history thoroughly,
especially focusing on potential risks for vascular
lesions. On examination, particular attention is directed to fine symptoms of abnormal CNS functioning. The
findings in previous studies and preliminary data of the
multicenter study presented at this symposium suggest
minor disturbances in exactly those brain areas that are
also affected when more serious complications occur, i.e.
most of these neurologically abnormal patients exhibit
minor signs of brainstem effects, mnestic disturbances
or abnormalities relating to focal cortical irritation.

One aim of this multicenter study is to identify
factors that still expose some of our patients to
potentially serious complications. Considering the participation of centers from many different parts of the
world in this study, a number of biases regarding the
comparability of results is anticipated: The percentage
of neurological abnormalities, especially in terms of
fine symptoms found, depends heavily upon the accuracy of
clinical examination, even if it is done by neurologists
in every single case. A considerable disparity in the
percentage of abnormal neurological findings between
centers thus could emerge that would give a false impression of non-existent differences in the respective groups
of patients. But even given a comparable quality of the
clinical neurological examination between centers, some
other unanticipated methodological problems can arise:
Does the dependence of the regional cerebral blood flow

on the hematocrit values influence the outcome of a patient on ECC exposed to a standardized reduced hemato- crit, but used to much higher values than for example Europeans, like the patients in Bogota, living at 12,000 feet altitude? How does the apparently much higher incidence of delirium due to alcohol withdrawal in Finland influence our statistics? Many of these ques- tions will be subject to further discussions as the evaluation of the data proceeds.

Over the years, severely disabling focal or global brain lesions on the whole have become rare since the introduction of extracorporeal circulation procedures, and the overall incidence of marked transient deficits has declined steadily from 30-50 percent in the sixties [20, 21] to under 10 percent after 1975 [22]. The improved results presumably reflect more sophisticated techniques, including extracorporeal perfusion, filtra- tion, hypothermic protection, and an optimized pre- vention of air embolism.

Beyond the diagnosis of neurological complications, the ultimate goal of sophisticated analysis of possible etiologic factors should serve the definition of predict- ing such complications. A number of predictive factors for neurological complications after open-heart surgery are already known and emerge from previous studies [11, 23, 24]. An increased risk for patients over the age of 60 is likely to reflect an impaired auto-regulation due to atherosclerotic cerebrovascular disease [25]. The same applies for patients with preoperative evidence of neurological dysfunction. Heikkinen saw substantial neurological complications in 4 percent of 50 patients undergoing coronary bypass surgery and concluded from his data that preoperative neurological events increase the frequency of neurological complications [26]. Zisbrod [29] on the other hand did not observe a worse postoperative outcome of patients with a cardiogenic embolic stroke within a mean of 12 days prior to the operation as compared to more remote neurological events. The duration of extracorporeal circulation can be a factor with the risks of microembolization, intra- vascular coagulation and suboptimal perfusion pressure. Fat emboli may not be influenced by the filters used [28, 29], and like intraoperative hypotension [23], can turn out to be a significant feature.

In conclusion, there are a considerable number of variables rendering the central nervous system susceptible

to noxious influences imposed by extracorporeal bypass
surgery. Even nowadays, with greatly improved techniques,
the risk of neurological complications is not eliminated.
Minor, although usually transient, still potentially
hazardous neurological symptoms in many patients indicate
that we need studies like these in our attempt to further
elucidate the pathogenetic mechanisms underlying those
risks in order to optimize the already favorable outcome
of our patients undergoing open-heart surgery.

References

1.   F. A. Freyhan, S. Gianelli, R. A. O'Connell, and J.
      Mayo, Psychiatric complications following open-
      heart surgery, Compr Psychiatr, 12:181 (1971).

2.   R. Meyendorf, Psychische und neurologische Storungen
      bei herzoperationen. Pra- und postoperative
      Untersuchungen, Fortschr Med, 94:315 (1976).

3.   J. P. Mohr, Neurological complications of cardiac
      valvular disease and cardiac surgery including
      systemic hypotension, in: "Handbook of Clinical
      Neurology Vol 38," P. J. Vinken and G. W. Bruyn,
      eds., North-Holland Publ., Amsterdam (1979).

4.   R. Gattiker and R. Pescia, Kardiopulmonale
      Komplikationen, Beatmungsdauer und arterielle
      Sauerstoffspannung nach Operationen am offenen
      Herzen, Herz, 3:191 (1978).

5.   G. Huse-Klienstoll, B. Dahme, B. Flemming, A. Haag,
      J. Meffert, M. J. Polonius, G. Rodewald, and H.
      Speidel, Einige somatische und psychologische
      Pradiktoren fur psychopathologische
      Aufalligkeiten nach Herzoperationen, Thoraxchir,
      24:386 (1976).

6.   J. B. Brierley, Brain damage complicating open-
      heart surgery: a neuropathological study of 46
      patients, Proc R Soc Med, 60:858 (1967).

7.   T. H. Jones, R. B. Morawetz, and R. M. Crowell,
      Thresholds of focal cerebral ischemia in awake
      monkeys, J Neurosurg., 54:773 (1981).

8.   J. H. Wood, and D. B. Kee, Clinical rheology of
      stroke and hemodilution, in: "Stroke", H. J. M.
      Barnett, H. P. Mohr, B. M. Stein, and F. M.
      Yatsu, eds., Churchill Livingstone, New York
      (1986).

9.   K. M. Welch , and G. L. Barkley, Biochemistry and
      pharmacology of cerebral ischemia, in:
      "Stroke", H. J. M. Barnett, J. P. Mohr, B. M.
      Stein, and F. M. Yatsu, eds., Churchill
      Livingstone, New York (1986).

10. J. J. Caronna, Neurologic syndromes following cardiac arrest and cardiac bypass surgery, in: "Stroke", H. J. M. Barnett, J. P. Mohr, B. M. Stein and F. M. Yatsu, eds., Churchill Livingstone, New York (1986).

11. E. Vasquez, and W. R. Chitwood, Postcardiotomy delirium: An overview, Int J Psychiat Med, 6:373 (1975).

12. L. Henriksen, E. Hjelms, and T. Lindeburgh, Brain hyperperfusion during cardiac operations. Cerebral blood flow measured in man by intra-arterial injection of xenon 133: evidence suggestive of intra-operative microembolism, J Thorac Cardiovasc Surg, 86:202 (1983).

13. D. L. Price and J. Harris, Cholesterol emboli in cerebral arteries as a complication of retrograde aortic perfusion during cardiac surgery, Neurology, 20:1209 (1970).

14. J. R. Miller and R. E. Myers, Neuropathology of systemic circulatory arrest in adult monkeys, Neurology, 22:888 (1972).

15. C. Boisen and E. Siemkowicz, Six cases of cerebromedullospinal disconnection after cardiac arrest, Lancet, 1:1381 (1976).

16. J. R. Silver and P. H. Buxton, Spinal stroke, Brain, 97:539 (1974).

17. M. D. Ginsberg, Delayed neurological deterioration following hypoxia, in: "Advances in Neurology 26", S. Fahn, J. N. Davis, and L. P. Rowland, eds., Raven Press, New York (1979).

18. D. McConnell, Brain magnetic resonance imaging in children before and after cardiac surgery: a prospective study, Third International Symposium on the impact of cardiac surgery on the quality of life, New York (paper) (1989).

19. K. Sotaniemi, Five-year neurological and EEG outcome after open-heart surgery, J Neurol Neuro-surg Psychiat, 48:569 (1985).

20. H. Javid, Neurological abnormalities following open heart surgery, J Thorac Cardiovasc Surg., 58:509 (1969).

21. H. M. Tufo, Central nervous system dysfunction following open-heart surgery, JAMA, 212:1333 (1970).

22. M. A. Branthwaite, Prevention of neurological damage during open-heart surgery, Thorax, 30:258 (1975).

23. H. R. M. Johnson, Complications of cardiac surgery, Forensic Sci., 9:99 (1976).

24. R. Meyendorf, Zur Frage psychischer und neurologischer Storungen bei Herzoperationen, Thorax-chirurgie, 25:339 (1977).

25. M. A. Branthwaite, Neurological damage related to open-heart surgery, Thorax, 27:748 (1972).

26. L. Heikkinen, A. Harjula, and S. Mattila, Neurological events in cardiac surgery, Ann Chir Gynaecol, 74:118 (1985).

27. Z. Zisbrod, D. M. Rose, I. J. Jacobowitz, M. Kramer, A. Acinapura, and J. N. Cunningham, Results of open-heart surgery in patients with recent cardiogenic embolic stroke and central nervous system dysfunction, Circulation, 76:109 (1987).

28. R. Frick, H. Schmidt and R. Leutschaft, Die cerebrale Fettembolie bei Operationen mit der Herz-Lungen-Maschine, Verh Dt Ges Pathol, 56:544 (1972).

29. N. R. Ghatak, R. J. Sinnenberg, and G. G. deBlois, Cerebral fat embolism following cardiac surgery, Stroke, 14:619 (1983).

NEUROLOGICAL ASSESSMENT OF EARLY CEREBRAL OUTCOME AFTER CORONARY BYPASS SURGERY

Hans Strenge

Department of Neurology
University of Kiel
Federal Republic of Germany

Neurological complications after open heart surgery have been the subject of many recent studies [1]. However, there are only a limited number of prospective studies [2-6] which have been devoted to the occurrence of neurological abnormalities including all degrees of severity following coronary artery bypass surgery (CABS). Even in these studies, detailed information about the clinical course of minor signs in the early postoperative phase is not available. Therefore, it seemed worthwhile to define the incidence and severity as well as the dynamics of new clinical abnormalities in the early stage after CABS and to look at possible connections with pre- and intraoperative parameters.

We studied the cases of 78 consecutive patients admitted to the Department of Cardiovascular Surgery of the University of Kiel from May 1987 to October 1988. The group included 61 males and 17 females, the ages ranged from 39 to 74 years (mean 59.5, S. D. 8.2). Anaesthesia and surgery were standardized. Nonpulsatile extracorporeal perfusion was performed with a bubble oxygenator in 45 patients, with a membrane oxygenator in 33 cases. The flow was maintained at 2.5 litres/m^2/min. Moderate hypothermia (27 - 32°C) was used. The median values of bypass time and aortic cross-clamping time were 80 min (39 - 140) and 39 min (20 - 112) respectively.

After informed consent each patient underwent a detailed neurologic history and examination to a standard-

Impact of Cardiac Surgery on the Quality of Life
Edited by A. E. Willner and G. Rodewald
Plenum Press, New York, 1990

ized protocol 2-3 days prior to surgery. Repeat neurologic
assessments were done by the same investigator 2-3 days
(t_1) and 6-8 days (t_2) after CABS. All observable
disturbances were registered. Thirty of the 78 patients
(38%) had previous histories of vertigo, nausea, dizzy
and/or fainting spells. Hearing disorders and chronic
headaches were reported by 18 patients each. In 14 cases
there had been prior fleeting signs or strokes.

Preoperative assessment revealed clinically detectable
abnormalities in 35 out of 78 cases. In 28% of the whole
study group (22 patients) these findings were attributable
to the central nervous system (CNS). Many patients had
isolated signs, in 10 patients the abnormalities were
compatible with brain lesions affecting circumscribed
parts of the brain stem, the hemispheres, or the spinal
cord.

New neurological signs could be found in 40 patients
(51%) at any time after CABS (at t_1 and/or at t_2). Among
these patients 26 (33%) had new developmental reflexes
(palmomental, snout, extensor-plantar); 24 (31%) had
motor hemisyndromes, cranial nerve disturbances and/or
unilateral hyperreflexia. Three patients died of cardiac
disease but did not display any CNS sign in the examinations
during the first postoperative week. A summary of the
frequencies and dynamics of different new signs of CNS
dysfunction is given in Fig. 1. Considering the time
course of the new findings the highest rate of reversibility during the first week (percentage of cases with
negative findings at t_2) was found for the Babinski's
sign. In 56% of all cases involved, this reflex had
disappeared after one week. Both a unilateral hyperreflexia and an abducens nerve dysfunction were totally
reversible in 40%. On the other hand, a unilateral
weakness of the lower facial muscles seemed to be the
symptom with the least fluctuation during the early stage
(detectable at t_1 and t_2 in 75%). In general, there was
no clear-cut difference between the early clinical course
of the newly developed focal signs and the developmental
reflexes.

The clinical course during the first postoperative
week on an individual basis are demonstrated in Table 1.
There are many subpopulations with different development
processes of neurological signs which, however, do not
correlate with a special type of CNS manifestation.

To study possible relationships between history, pre-
and intraoperative data and immediate outcome, a con-

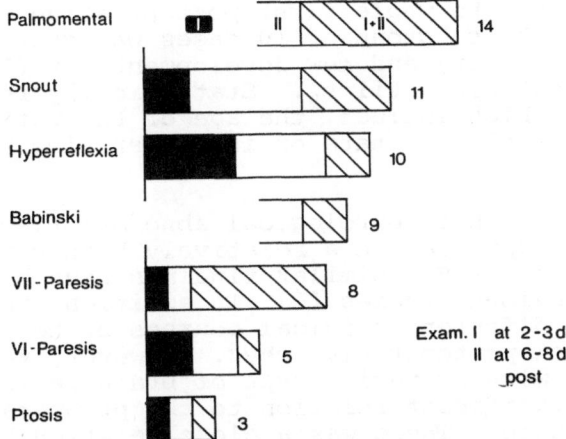

Fig. 1.   Frequencies and dynamics of new neurological
          signs after surgery.

figural frequency analysis [7] was performed. Statistical
associations between triples of variables were examined by
comparing the observed number of patients exhibiting
specific combinations of features with the number predicted from the overall incidence rates. A significant
relation (P<0.05) was found between a previous history of
cardiovascular symptoms and new focal signs after CABS,

Table 1.   Clinical course of neurological abnormalities
           after CABS.

Clinical Course During 1st Post- operative week	Number of Patients	Area of CNS dysfunction		
		Hemisphere	Brainstem	Uncertain
1. Complete Recovery	8 (20%)	1	4	3
2. Incomplete Recovery	5 (13%)	1	2	2
3. No Change	12 (30%)	0	3	9
4. Progression and/or addi- tional new signs.	9 (22%)	2	5	2
5. Late signs	6 (15%)	1	2	3
Total Number	40 (100%)	5	16	19

persisting during the whole first postoperative week in 10
patients. Another subgroup of 10 cases was characterized
by an abnormal history and new developmental reflexes
constantly detectable until t_2. Statistically reliable
configurations which include the age of the patient,
preoperative neurologic state or intraoperative variables
were not found.

In summary, minor neurological abnormalities due to
CNS dysfunction appeared in a relatively high percentage
of patients after CABS. Similar findings have been
reported in previous studies [2]. In addition, we were
able to define different clinical courses of new CNS signs
during the first postoperative week. However, they were
not associated with a special type of brain lesion and did
not show any significant relation to the preoperative
neurological state. There was a close relation between a
history of cardiovascular symptoms or signs and the
occurrence of lasting post-operative focal signs or
development reflexes in the very early stage. The significance of these findings to the search for predictive
factors of neurological complications after CABS has to be
determined in future studies with multivariate data
analysis.

ACKNOWLEDGMENTS

The author gratefully acknowledges the help of V.
Lindner, M.D., G. Paulsen, M.D., S. Tiemann and all
colleagues of the Dep. Cardiovas. Surg., Kiel, who have
organized the neurological examinations.

REFERENCES

1. T. Åberg, Cerebral injury during open heart surgery:
    Studies using functional, biochemical, and
    morphological methods, in: "Brain Injury and
    Protection During Heart Surgery," M. Hilberman,
    ed., Martinus Nighoff, Boston (1988).
2. A. C. Breuer, A. J. Furlan, M. R. Hansen, R. J.
    Lederman, F. O. Loop, D.M. Cosgrove, R. L.
    Greenstreet, F. G. Estafanous, Central nervous
    system complications of coronary artery bypass
    graft surgery: Prospective analysis of 421
    patients, Stroke, 14: 682-687 (1983).

3. F. Carella, G. Travaini, P. Contri, S. Guzzelli, M. Botta, E. Pieri, A. Mangoni, Cerebral complications of coronary bypass surgery. A prospective study. Acta, Neurol. Scand., 77: 158-163 (1980).
4. P. Gotze, B. Dahme, Psychopathological syndromes and neurological disturbances before and after open heart surgery, in: "Psychic and Neurological Dysfunctions After Open Heart Surgery," H. Speidel and G. Rodewald, eds., Thieme, Stuttgart, New York (1980).
5. P. J. Shaw, D. Bates, N. Cartlidge, D. Heaviside, D. Julian, D. Shaw, Early neurological complications of coronary artery bypass surgery, Brit. Med. J., 291: 1384-1387 (1985).
6. P. L. Smith, T. Treasure, S. P. Newman, P. Joseph, P. J. Ell, A. Schneidau, M. J. Harrison, Cerebral consequences of cardiopulmonary bypass, Lancet, 1: 823-825 (1986).
7. A. Von Eye, Some multivariate developments in nonparametric statistics, in "Handbook of Multivariate Experimental Psychology," J. R. Wesselroade and R. B. Cattel, eds., Plenum Press, New York, London (1988).

AUTOMATIC EEG MONITORING IN CARDIAC SURGERY

E. H. J. F. Boezeman, A. J. R. Simons
Department of Clinical Neurophysiology

J. A. Leusink
Department of Anesthesiology

St. Antonius Hospital
Nieuwegein
The Netherlands

INTRODUCTION

EEG monitoring during cardiac surgery has achieved clinical significance because the brain is very sensitive to alterations in metabolism, and possibly the organ most sensitive to hypoxia. A circulatory arrest of more than 3 minutes may lead to irreversible damage to neurons [1]. The brain generates continuous electrical signals which are in direct relation to metabolism [2, 3]. Thus measuring the EEG is a potent method to monitor the level of metabolism of the brain during such procedures and to determine whether its condition becomes marginal. In fact the only source of real and continuous information on brain function is the EEG [4, 5, 6]. This observation paved the way for EEG monitoring from very early in the history of cardiac surgery [6-19]. Besides the amount of anaesthetics, a number of patient parameters such as blood pressure are of importance in stabilizing brain function. So are temperature, PO2 and to lesser extent PCO2 and electrolytes [20, 21]. Deterioration of any one of these parameters does not necessarily imply clinical importance as far as brain function is concerned, unless the EEG is also deteriorating. The EEG reflects whether or not the combined effect of all those factors remains adequate for good brain function and whether the worsening of a certain parameter may be tolerated for some time, assuming a constant level of anaesthesia [17A].

Impact of Cardiac Surgery on the Quality of Life
Edited by A. E. Willner and G. Rodewald
Plenum Press, New York, 1990

Observing EEGs during surgery remains a daunting task because of the enormous amount of EEG information generated during 3 to 4 hours from several cases simultaneously. Automatic analysis is essential to interpret the information within the limited period of the surgical procedure. Automatic analysis of the EEG during cardiac surgery is focussed on three hallmarks. First, to detect brain dysfunction in relation to anesthesiological and surgical parameters with the shortest possible delay so that its cause can be discovered and the efficacy of the course of action can be checked. Second, it is essential to have a built-in warning system to indicate when the margins of safety have been reached. Automatic analysis without such a system is useless and brings one no further than that given by conventional strip chart recording. Such a warning system is based on the experience of the clinical neurophysiologist and can be considered as an artificial intelligence system. Third, documentation of brain function in relationship to all other parameters being monitored has the capacity to evaluate the impact of new anesthesiological and surgical procedures on brain function in this fast developing field. Over the years, a number of discussions have been published concerning the importance of using EEG monitoring during surgery [22-26, 18, 19]. These papers present data about the outcome of the surgical procedure in terms of cerebral morbidity and possible prevention of morbidity by using the EEG, but nearly no one asks how much more information about the state of the patient may be gained by using this technique. The brain may be seen as a sensitive transducer, which reacts to many alterations in homeostasis via changes in metabolism and EEG. In relation to this question, an editorial paper by Block [24] is very clear. His proposed minimum standards for monitoring equipment to be used during anaesthesia including the EEG which gives so much value for the money that it is worth the necessary expenditure. We completely agree with this opinion. If EEG monitoring is based on procedures such as A.I. (Expert System) as we have advocated already, and as others [27] now envisage, we are convinced that this may optimize treatment during the course of surgery. This article demonstrates such an approach and pays attention to crucial moments during surgery, and preliminary results of outcome at the intensive care unit. The system has been running now for 9 years. This paper reflects our experience in 10,749 cases.

THE MONITORING SYSTEM

One of the main features of the system is the

capacity to produce warnings and alarms on which actions can be taken [17A]. This setup can be considered as an on-line automatic EEG interpreter during anaesthesia and surgery (Expert System). It is based on clinical experience obtained from the ongoing EEG. The zero-crossing rates and amplitudes of the two recorded EEG signals are checked every 15 seconds for 3 types of abnormal EEG activity:

1) Slow waves (slow EEG); i.e. if the average number of zero-crossings falls below 52 (about 1.0 Hz).

2) Slow waves of low amplitude (low EEG); i.e. a slow EEG but with an average amplitude that falls below 15 uV.

3) Unilateral slow wave and/or low amplitude activity, i.e. an asymmetry exceeding 8% which is called slight, or an asymmetry exceeding 14%, which is called severe.

The warning and alarm signal are presented in this order of priority. The computer program has a logical decision tree structure. After checking the zero-crossing rates as well as the amplitude values, the software tests whether the patient is on cardiopulmonary bypass, i.e., cooled or rewarmed or has been given anesthetics that affect the EEG. If no explanation is found, a visual warning, i.e., SLOW EEG, is generated on the VDU. This is followed by an auditory alarm if the user does not respond by pressing an attention key on the special function keyboard. If simultaneously the blood pressure falls below 50 torr, an additional LOW PRESS signal appears. The warnings are presented only after a steady state of 2 minutes. This software makes the immediate supervision of an expert in this field, i.e., a clinical neurophysiologist, unnecessary. If artifacts occur that are difficult to distinguish from biological activity, the neurophysiologist can attend to slave monitors situated in the EEG department outside the operating complex, showing the histograms and the ongoing EEG.

Figure 1 shows the presentation of the data on the VDU monitor in the operating room. The EEG wavelength histograms of successive 1-minute time intervals are presented from the bottom to the top showing a trend analysis. For signalling relatively fast changes in the patient, instantaneous numerical values of the parameters are determined and displayed every 15 seconds at the top

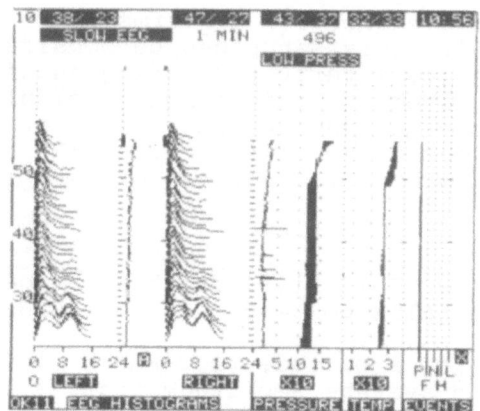

Fig. 1   Warning for SLOW EEG and LOW BLOODPRESS at
            10.54. Read the time scale from the bottom to
            the top. The quantitative EEG profiles from
            the two hemispheres are shown. Print-out
            every minute, the numerical values (top line)
            every 15 seconds. The channel in between shows
            the mean rectified EEG amplitudes. The next
            channels represent, from left to right,
            pressure, pump flow, temperature (naso-
            pharyngeal and perfusion), and events like
            bypass or administration of drugs.

line of the VDU. There is a visually displayed warning
for SLOW EEG (< 52 zero-crossings) and LOW PRESS (< 50
torr) during one minute at the end of the bypass around
10.54. At this point interventions causing increased
perfusion of the brain should follow to restore brain
function.

RESULTS AND DISCUSSION

     We investigated the mortality and morbidity rate in
a population of 4,500 cases from the last 3 years undergoing coronary artery bypass grafting (CABG) and/or
replacement of heart valves. We looked only for gross
abnormalities like stroke, encephalopathy, cardiac and
renal failure. Because we monitor nearly all our
patients, many EEG data are available. Table 1 shows the

outcome in relationship to such factors as operation, age, cause, and the peroperative EEG findings. The combined rate was 47/4500 (1%). If one looks to milder abnormalities, the combined rate is of course very much higher [28]. CABG procedures do not produce significantly higher morbidity and mortality rates compared to other procedures because the total number performed is 4 times as high. Increasing age (> 60) is a striking factor because the combined rate is 2 times as high as compared to the younger group (< 60), while the total number of patients in each group are more or less the same. Cardiac failures, i.e., low output syndrome, infarction, cardiac arrest, or arrhythmia, were the main causes for the mortality rate followed by neurological and renal failures. As for morbidity, neurological injury like stroke and encephalopathy prevailed. The peroperative EEG findings were normal in 16 cases. These cases, however, sustained organ failures following the intervention from hours to days later at the intensive care unit. From a neurophysiological point of view they came through the operation very well. For 8 cases, EEG recordings were not available because those were emergency operations.

For 23 cases the peroperative EEG findings were abnormal during the procedure. These peroperative EEG findings can be divided into two types, those with diffuse abnormalities (13 cases) and those with focal abnormalities (10 cases). Table 2 shows the relationship with the specific events that caused these abnormalities.

Diffuse EEG abnormalities in our material generally lead to a diffuse encephalopathy caused by a hemodynamic instability. This instability has been found by others as well [29]. A sudden decrease in perfusion during cardiopulmonary bypass is the main cause of diffuse abnormalities in the EEG. Automatic analysis has the capability to detect this on line and gives insight into the efficacy of the protective measures that have to be taken. There are diffuse abnormalities during bypass (6 cases) whose causes are uncertain. In the literature [30] suggestions have been made that defective cerebral autoregulation in hypertensive patients with arteriolar disease may be responsible. A partial explanation can be found in the preoperative EEG [31, 32] with diffuse abnormalities such as we observed in 2 cases, the abnormalities increased throughout the whole operation without recovery. Both had encephalopathy.

Table 1

Outcome*

		Morbidity	Mortality	All
	cabg	13	16	29
	cabg/valve	2	2	4
Operation	valve	3	6	9
	vsd	2	3	5
	all	20	27	47
age	<60	5	9	14
	>60	15	18	33
	all	20	27	47
cause	cardiac	1	17	18
	neurological	18	8	26
	renal	1	2	3
	all	20	27	47
per EEG	diffuse	5	8	13
	focal	4	6	10
	normal	10	6	16
	not done	1	7	8
	all	20	27	47

*The numerical data represent the number of cases

      Focal abnormalities in our material are related
mostly to stroke caused by embolization, i.e., air in the
heart or bypass lines, brittle aorta at the site of the
clamping, or cardiac arrhythmia. A few focal abnormalities are not explained by the peroperative EEG findings.
They are mainly based on preoperative EEG abnormalities
like dysfunction of the temporal lobe caused by cerebrovascular disease. A special remark has to be made about
the rewarming procedure. Fast rewarming, i.e., more than
8 degrees, gives rise to more diffuse EEG abnormalities

than slow rewarming. Its significance concerning
clinical outcome is not yet clear. In our material, it
is not taken as a sign for gross clinical abnormalities.

Table 2

Peroperative EEG findings*

	Diffuse	Focal	All
low perfusion	6	2	8
embolism	1	7	8
uncertain	6	1	7
all	13	10	23

* The numerical data represent the number of cases

CONCLUSIONS

1. Automatic EEG monitoring provides an ongoing
   assessment of brain function in relationship to
   hemodynamic and anesthetic variables.

2. The Expert System automatically generates warnings
   based on logical decision making procedures concerning
   the type and the degree of the cerebral change.

3. The Expert System provides guidelines for surgical and
   anesthetic procedures so that one can work within safe
   margins. If these are exceeded, however, it shows the
   nature of the corrective action that must be taken.

4. The anesthesiologist does not need extensive knowledge
   of clinical neurophysiology and experience with EEG
   monitoring.

REFERENCES

1. C. A. F. Tulleken, Circulation of the brain, in:
    "Oxygen supply of heart and brain," Dutch Heart
    Foundation, The Hague (1979).
2. D. H. Ingvar, B. Sjolund, A. Ardo, Correlation
    between dominant EEG frequency, cerebral oxygen

uptake and blood flow, EEG Clin. Neurophysiol., 41:268-276 (1976).

3. D. H. Ingvar, Cerebral blood flow and metabolism related to EEG and cerebral functions, Acta. Anaesth. Scand. (suppl), 45:110-114 (1971).

4. R. A. F. Pronk, "EEG processing in cardiac surgery," Thesis, Vrije Universiteit Amsterdam (1982).

5. R. A. F. Pronk, Peri-operative monitoring, in: "Clinical applications of computer analysis of EEG and other neurophysiological signals, revised series, H. F. Lopes da Silva, W. Storm van Leeuwen, A. Remond, eds., Elsevier Science Publishers, Amsterdam (1986).

6. R. A. F. Pronk, Data processing for monitoring brain function during anesthesia and surgery, in: "The London Symposia," R. J. Ellinson, N. M. F. Murray, A. M. Halliday, Elsevier Science Publishers, Amsterdam (1987).

7. G. Arfel, J. Weis, N. Duboucet, EEG findings during open heart surgery with extracorporeal circulation, in: "Cerebral anoxia and the electroencephalogram," J. S. Meyer, H. Gastaut, eds., Thomas, Springfield, Ill. (1961).

8. W. Storm van Leeuwen, K. Mechelse, L. Kok, B. Zierfuss, EEG during open-heart operations with artificial circulation, in: "Cerebral anoxia and the electroencephalogram," J. S. Meyer, H. Gastaut, eds., Thomas, Springfield, Ill. (1961).

9. M. Fischer-Williams, R. A. Cooper, Some aspects of the electroencephalogram changes during open heart surgery. Neurologie, 14:472-482 (1964).

10. P. E. Prior, D. E. Maynard, P. C. Sheaff, B. R. Simpson, L. Strunin, E. J. M. Weaver, D. F. Scott, Monitoring cerebral function: clinical experience with a new device for continuous recording of electrical activity of the brain, Brit. Med. J., 2:736-738 (1971).

11. J. S. Wright, A. K. Lethlean, R. G. Hicks, T. A. Torda, R. Stacey, Electroencephalographic studies during open heart surgery, J. Thorac. Cardiovasc. Surg., 63:631-638 (1972).

12. A. J. R. Simons, Aspects of EEG control during open heart surgery, Electroenceph. Clin. Neurophysiol., 35:105-106 (1973).

13. M. Weiss, J. Weis, J. Cotton, F. Nicolas, J. P. Binet, A study of the electroencephalogram during surgery with deep hypothermia and circulation arrest in infants, J. Thorac. Cardiac. Surg., 70:316-329 (1975).

14. P. E. Prior, "Monitoring cerebral function," Elsevier/North-Holland Biomedical Press, Amsterdam (1979).

15. T. A. Salerno, D. P. Lince, D. N. White, L. R. Beverly, E. J.F. Charette, Monitoring of electroencephalogram during open heart surgery. A prospective analysis of 118 cases, J. Thorac. Cardiovasc. Surg., 76:97-100 (1988).

16. A. J. R. Simons, R. A. F. Pronk, Les données électroencéphalographiques pendant la chirurgie à coeur ouvert leur analyse automatique et son utilisation pour la surveillance peropératoire de la fonction cérébrale, Rev. EEG Neurophysiol., 243-252 (1982).

17. A. J. R. Simons, R. A. F. Pronk, EEG analysis in monitoring anesthesia. Objective medical decision-making. System approach in acute disease, in: "Lecture Notes in Medical Informatics," J. E. W. Beneken, S. M. Lavelle, Springer-Verlag, Berlin, Heidelberg, New York, Tokyo (1983).

17A. A. J. R. Simons, R. A. F. Pronk, Automatic EEG monitoring during anesthesia, in: "Computing in anesthesia and intensive care," O. Prakash, S. H. Mey, R. W. Patterson, eds., Martinus Nyhoff Publishers, Boston, The Hague, Dordrecht, Lancaster (1983).

18. S. N. C. Bolsin, Is the EEG a useful monitor during cardiac surgery?, Anesthesiology, 68:956 (1988).

19. M. El-Fiki, K. J. Fish, Is the EEG a useful monitor during cardiac surgery? A case report, Anesthesiology 67:575-578 (1987).

20. I. Juneja, R. Flynn, R. Berger, The arterial venous pressure and the EEG during open heart surgery, Acta. Neurol. Scandinav., 48:163-168 (1971).

21. I. Juneja, R. Flynn, R. Berger, The arterial Ph, pCO2 and the electroencephalogram during open heart surgery, Acta. Neurol. Scandinav., 48:169-176 (1972).

22. W. K. Hamilton, Do we monitor enough? - We monitor too much, J. Clin. Monit., 2:264-266 (1986).

23. F. E. Block, Do we monitor? - We don't monitor enough, J. Clin. Monit., 2:267-269 (1986).

24. F. E. Block, A proposed standard for monitoring equipment: What equipment should be included?, (editorial), J. Clin. Monit., 4:1-4 (1988).

25. A. D. Zablocki, M. S. Albin, The EEG should be monitored during cardiopulmonary bypass, J. of Cardiothoracic Anaesthesia, 3:119-123 (1989).

26. Chung-Yuang Lin, Con: The EEG should not be
    monitored during cardiopulmonary bypass, J.
    Cardiovas. Anaesth., 3:124-126 (1989).
27. G. D. Rennels, P. L. Miller, Artificial intelligence
    research in anesthesia and intensive care, J.
    Clin. Monit., 4:274-289 (1988).
28. P. C. Shaw, P. Bates, N. E. F. Cartlidge, J. M.
    French, D. Heaviside, D. G. Julian, D. A. Shaw,
    Neurologica and neuropsychological morbidity
    following major surgery: comparison of coronary
    artery bypass and peripheral vascular surgery,
    Stroke, 18:700-707 (1987).
29. E. R. John, L. S. Prichep, R. J. Chabot and W. O.
    Som, Monitoring brain function during cardio-
    vascular surgery: Hypoperfusion vs. microembolism
    as the major cause of neurological damage during
    cardiopulmonary bypass, in: "Heart Brain & Brain
    Heart," H. Refsum, I. Sulg, K. Rasmussen, eds.,
    Springer-Verlag (1989).
30. A. J. Furlan, A. C. Breuer, Central nervous system
    complications of open heart surgery, Stroke,
    15:912-914 (1984).
31. K. Sotaniemi, Clinical and prognostic correlates of
    EEG in open heart surgery patients, J. Neurol.
    Neurosurg. psychiatry, 43:941-947 (1980).
32. K. Sotaniemi, Five-year neurological and EEG outcome
    after open heart surgery, J. Neurol. Neurosurg.
    Psychiatry, 48:569-575 (1985).

MAGNETIC RESONANCE IMAGING OF THE BRAIN IN INFANTS AND CHILDREN BEFORE AND AFTER CARDIAC SURGERY; A PROSPECTIVE STUDY

James R. McConnell *, **, William H. Fleming **, Lynne B. Sarafian **

*Departments of Radiology & Pediatrics,
**Department of Surgery,
University of Nebraska Medical Center
Omaha, NE

INTRODUCTION

The treatment of children with congenital heart disease (CHD) constitutes one of the common reasons for admission to pediatric hospital units. There are approximately 30,000 infants born with CHD in the United States each year. An estimated 10,000 of these infants will require surgical correction of cardiac defects early in life [1,2].

Advances in the technology of open heart surgery (OHS) and cardiopulmonary bypass (CPB) have helped thousands of children with fatal or debilitating and congenital heart disease (CHD) to lead active and productive lives. Neurologic dysfunction developing in the operative or perioperative period still limits favorable outcome in the treatment of CHD [1]. The incidence of neurologic deficit in children is unknown. Subclinical changes of the brain have been demonstrated with computed tomography following cardiac operations in children and clinically unsuspected brain infarction and gliosis have been found in autopsy studies of children with CHD [3,4]. Considering the evidence that subclinical changes occur, we studied the morphology of the brain prospectively before and after cardiac surgery using magnetic resonance imaging (MRI).

Impact of Cardiac Surgery on the Quality of Life
Edited by A. E. Willner and G. Rodewald
Plenum Press, New York, 1990

PATIENTS AND METHODS

Eighteen infants and children with the diagnosis of
CHD were enrolled in a prospective imaging study of the
brain. Patients with previous CPB surgery were excluded
from the study. There were 12 patients with acyanotic
and six patients with cyanotic heart disease. The ages
ranged from 17 days to nine years. Fifteen patients in
the study group were under two years of age. There were
two intercurrent deaths and one patient was lost to
follow-up. The two deaths were in a 17-day old infant
with truncus arteriosus and an 18-month old with severe
Tetralogy of Fallot. They were not included in the study
group. Fifteen patients completed the study.

Brain MRIs were done the day prior to OHS and
repeated in the same manner after the course of clinical
recovery. All postoperative MRIs were done before
discharge from the hospital. The average time interval
from the preoperative to the postoperative MRI was ten
days. The time ranged from five days to four weeks.

All patients in the study group underwent CPB using
a non-pulsatile membrane oxygenator and heparin anti-
coagulation. The surgery was performed under moderate
core cooling hypothermia with body temperatures ranging
from 26-28°C. A 37 micron filter was placed in the
arterial line in all cases. CPB times were recorded from
the anesthesia record. The average CPB time was 100
minutes with a standard deviation of 55 minutes.

MRIs of the brain were done with a 1.5 Tesla
magnetic resonance imaging system (GE-Signa). All
patients had routine spin-echo MRIs in the sagittal and
axial planes of the head. The scanning pulse sequences
included T1 weighting (T1WD), proton density and T2
weighted images (T2WD). The T1WD images used a repeti-
tion time (TR) of 600 milliseconds (ms) and a time to
echo (TE) of 20 ms. The T2WD and proton density images
were obtained at a TR of 2000 ms and a TE of 20 and 80
ms, respectively. Field of views for the scans ranged
from 20 to 24 cm.

Measurements in the study were obtained with the
GE-Signa computer (distance measurement mode) on the
preoperative and postoperative axial T1WD scans.
Multiple measurements were done to insure reproduci-
bility. Measurements of the bicaudate diameter of the
frontal horns of the lateral ventricles and the diameter
of the third ventricle were done in all cases in the

study group. The level of the anterior columns of the
fornix and the anterior commissure and massa intermedia
served as precise anatomic landmarks for the bicaudate
and third ventricular measurements, respectively. The
subcutaneous fat of the skull was used as an endpoint to
measure the largest anterioposterior and biparietal
dimensions. The comparison measurements were done on
preoperative and postoperative scans at the same anatomic
level of the head and with the same radiopulse sequence.

Statistical analysis of the preoperative and postoperative measurements of the ventricles used the paired
T test. The linear regression was used to compare CPB
time with ventricular change. The MRIs were evaluated
independently by two neuroradiologists. One neuro-
radiologist evaluated the studies blindly. There was
100% agreement in the interpretation of the MRIs by the
neuroradiologists.

RESULTS

The ages, cardiac diagnoses, CPB times and results
of the radiologic interpretations are summarized in
Table I. Ten of the preoperative MRIs were normal, but
only two of the postoperative studies were interpreted as
normal. One-third of the preoperative MRIs showed changes
of ventriculomegaly and dilatation of the cerebrospinal
fluids (CSF) spaces. One patient (Case 8) showed preoperative ventriculomegaly and a small focal area of
hyperintense T2 signal in the deep white matter of the
left occipital lobe that was interpreted as a border zone
infarction. The ventriculomegaly and the CSF spaces
increased in volume postoperatively, but the white matter
infarction showed no change and no new infarctions were
found. The infarction was considered subclinical since
no symptomatology referable to the infarction was known.
No border zone (watershed) infarctions were found on any
other postoperative MRI in the study group.

Four patients (Cases 2, 3, 5, 7) developed postoperative subdural hemorrhages (SDHs). The SDHs were
small and caused no demonstrable mass effect on MRI. The
MRI signal characteristics of the SDHS were consistent
with subacute (greater than one week old) hemorrhage. In
addition, Case 12 developed increased ventriculomegaly
and bilateral frontoparietal subdural hygromas on postoperative MRI. The hygromas showed MR signal characteristics consistent with CSF. The SDHs were also considered
subclinical since no symptomatology referable to the
hemorrhage or hygromas was known.

TABLE 1

CASES	AGE	CONGENITAL HEART DISEASE	CARDIOPULMONARY BYPASS TIME (MINUTES)	PREOP MRI	POSTOP MRI
1	1Y	Ventricular Septal Defect	95	Normal	Ventriculomegaly
2	9M	Total Anomalous Pulmonary Venous Return	41	Normal	Left Occipital Subdural Hematoma
3	5M	Ventricular Septal Defect	72	Ventriculomegaly	Increased Ventriculomegaly Right Frontal Subdural Hematoma
4	5Y	Pulmonary Atresia	71	Normal	Left Temporal Parietal Infarction
5	9M	Ventricular Septal Defect	78	Normal	Ventriculomegaly Left Occipital Subdural Hematoma
6	2M	Hemitruncus	73	Normal	Ventriculomegaly
7	1Y	Tetralogy of Fallot	96	Ventriculomegaly	Increased Ventriculomegaly Left Temporal, Sagittal Sinus Subdural Hematoma
8	18M	Tetralogy of Fallot	153	Ventriculomegaly Left Occipital Infarction	Increased Ventriculomegaly, Infarction No Change
9	10M	Ventricular Septal Defect	144	Normal	Ventriculomegaly
10	9M	Ventricular Septal Defect	83	Normal	Ventriculomegaly
11	8Y	Aortic Stenosis	145	Normal	Normal
12	1Y	Tetralogy of Fallot	109	Ventriculomegaly	Increased Ventriculomegaly Subdural Hygromas
13	9Y	Atrial Septal Defect	25	Normal	Normal
14	1Y	Transposition of Great Vessels	250	Ventriculomegaly	Increased Ventriculomegaly
15	1Y	Ventricular Septal Defect	65	Normal	Ventriculomegaly

Case 4 had a normal preoperative MRI, but showed a left temporoparietal hyperintense T2 signal on postoperative MRI. The abnormal area was interpreted as an infarction most likely due to a left middle cerebral artery embolus. The patient developed a right hemiparesis post-OHS and was the only patient in the study group with a clinically diagnosed neurologic deficit.

The comparison measurements of the preoperative and postoperative ventricular diameters are summarized in Tables II and III. The measurements showed an increase in the bicaudate and third ventricular diameters in virtually all cases (p < 0.005). The anterioposterior dimensions of the heads showed no statistical difference in the preoperative and postoperative measurements (T value = .339). The biparietal dimensions had a mean preoperative measurement of 117.2 mm and a mean postoperative measurement of 118.5 mm with an average increase of 1.3 mm. This slight increase in the biparietal diameter is not enough to account for the observed increase in the bicaudate (mean 3.1 mm) and the third ventricular (mean 1.6 mm) diameters.

Comparison of CPB time and the ventricular changes in diameter showed no linear correlation between the amount of ventricular enlargement postoperatively and the time on CPB (r correlation coefficient = 0.51). Excluding Case 14 (CPB time = 250 min.), recalculation still showed no definite linear correlation (r = 0.59) (Table IV).

COMMENTS

The study shows that morphologic changes of the brain occur in children after recovery from CPB operations. Fourteen of 15 patients in the study group showed measurable increase in ventricular volumes and subarachnoid CSF spaces. Five of 15 patients showed subclinical SDHs on postop MRI. The ages of the subdural hemorrhages were consistent with occurrence during CPB heparinization. The study also indicates that morphologic changes of the brain occur before CPB operations. One-third of cases in the study group had subclinical changes on MRI before surgery. These cases had severe heart disease with failure to thrive, congestive heart failure or cyanosis.

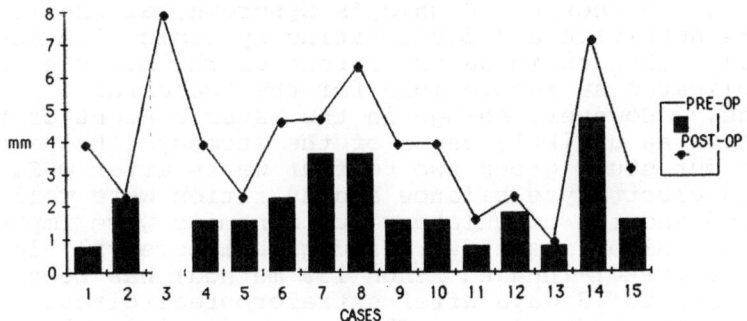

Fig. 1.   Comparison of Third Ventricular Diameter.

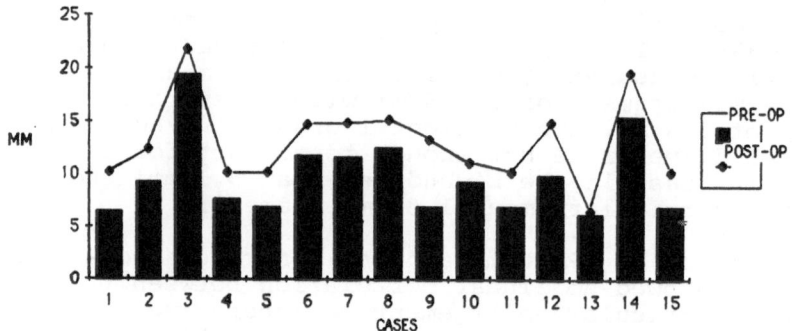

Fig. 2.   Comparison of Bicaudate Ventricular Diameter.

        All infants under two years of age showed marked
ventricular enlargement and larger cisternal and sulcal
subarachnoid CSF spaces two to four weeks after CPB
surgery.   The ventricular changes were not associated
with an increase in the anterioposterior or biparietal
diameters of the cranium.   The measurable ventricular
enlargement and dilatation of the CSF spaces suggest that
brain parenchymal volumes actually diminished since there
was no concomitant change in the cranial dimensions.   If
there is an increase in the volume of one of the intracranial compartments, such as the CSF spaces and ventricles, then in order for the total volume to remain
constant, there must be shrinkage of one of the other
compartments.   Communicating hydrocephalus seems an
unlikely explanation for the dilatation of the ventricles
and CSF spaces since there was no head enlargement or
symptomatic fullness of the fontanelles in the younger
patients.   Reversible "cerebral shrinkage" or atrophy-
like pattern has been reported in association with
corticosteroid therapy, Cushing's Syndrome, alcoholism,
severe malnutrition and debilitating systemic diseases
[5,6,7,8].   Changes in water content of the brain have
been implicated as responsible for the "cerebral
shrinkage."   However, change in the water content of the
brain seems an unlikely cause of the atrophy-like pattern
found in our study group two to four weeks after OHS.
Fluid and electrolyte balance and nutrition were well
controlled and the circulatory hemodynamics were improved
after OHS.   Significant decreased global cerebral blood
flow (CBF) (SPECT-inhaled xenon 133 method) has been
observed six to 13 days after extracorporeal circulation [9].   The reduction of CBF occurred evenly throughout the brain including the border zones.   Microischemia

secondary to decreased CBF during CPB cannot be excluded as a cause for the atrophy-like pattern observed in our study group. Border zone infarctions between brain areas supplied by different major arteries were not found in our postoperative group. The absence of border zone infarctions suggests that the macrocirculation of the brain is adequate during CPB. The pathogenesis of the "cerebral shrinkage" found in our series is unknown and reversibility of the phenomenon has not been established.

Cases 11 and 13 were the oldest children in the study group. These cases showed little or no change on the MRIs as interpreted subjectively (Table I), but measurements showed slight increase in the ventricular dimensions. Case 11 had an increase of 3.1 mm in the bicaudate diameter and 0.8 mm in the third ventricle on MRI eight days post OHS. Case 11 was an 8-year old female with aortic stenosis and underwent 145 minutes CPB for valve replacement. Case 13 showed the least change in the ventricular diameters. Case 13 was a 9-year old male with uncomplicated atrial septal defect and 25 minutes CPB. The patient was the oldest in the study group and had the least CPB time. It is interesting that the best MRI outcome was in the patient with the least CPB time. Although no significant linear correlation of the ventricular change and CPB time was found in our cases, the study group was small and further investigation of the relationship of CPB time and ventricular change is warranted.

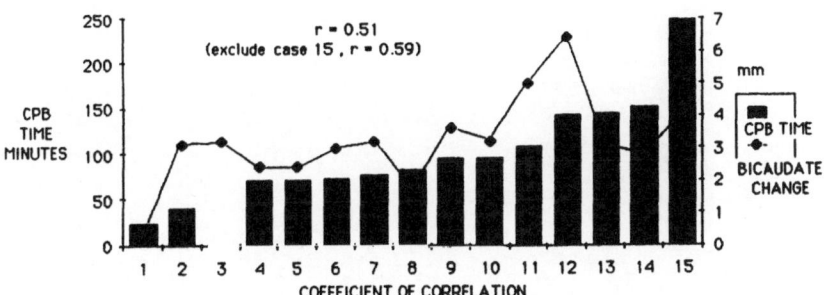

Fig. 3.   CPB Time Comparison With Change in Bicaudate Diameter (Post-op to Pre-op).

REFERENCES

1. J. H. Meuller, Incidence of cardiac malformation, in:
   "Heart disease in infancy," J.H. Meuller, W. A.
   Neal, eds., East Norwalk, Conn., Appleton-Century-
   Crofts (1982).
2. P. C. Ferry. Neurologic sequelae of cardiac surgery
   in children, Am J Dis Child. 141:309 (1987).
3. K. L. Terplan, Brain changes in newborns, infants and
   children with congenital heart disease in association with cardiac surgery, additional observations,
   J Neurol. 212:225 (1976).
4. B. Muraoka, Subclinical changes in brain morphology
   following cardiac operations as reflected by
   computed tomographic scans of the brain, J Thorac
   Cardiovasc Surg. 81:364 (1981).
5. E. R. Heinz, J. Martinez, A. Haenggeli, Reversibility
   of cerebral atrophy in anorexia nervosa and
   Cushing's syndrome, J Comp Assist Tomo., 1:415
   (1977).
6. I. Lagenstein, R. P. Willing, D. Kuhne, Reversible
   cerebral atrophy caused by corticotrophin (letter),
   Lancet, 1: 1246 (1979).
7. K. R. Lyen, I. M. Holland, Y. C. Lyen. Reversible
   cerebral atrophy in infantile spasms caused by
   corticotrophin (letter), Lancet, 2:37 (1979).
8. P. L. Carlen, G. Wortzman, R. C. Holgate et al,
   Reversible cerebral atrophy in recently abstinent
   chronic alcholics measured by computed tomography
   scans, Science, 200:1076 (1978).
9. L. Henriksen, Evidence suggestive of diffuse brain
   damage following cardiac operations, Lancet,
   816-820 (1984).

CEREBRAL DYSFUNCTION IN ELECTIVE CORONARY SURGERY

W. A. Stertmann
Department of Cardiovascular Surgery

C. Lammers
Department of Neurology

R. Moosdorf
Department of Cardiovascular Surgery

C. R. Hornig
Department of Neurology

H. H. Scheld
Department of Cardiovascular Surgery

University Hospital of Giessen
Federal Republic of Germany
D 6300 Giessen, Klinikstr 29

INTRODUCTION

In the sixties and early seventies several authors reported neurological complications following open-heart surgery. A primary matter of discussion was valid pre-operative investigation aimed at preventing neurological complications among the increasing number of patients undergoing elective coronary artery bypass grafting (CABG). Controversy exists as to whether patients with asymptomatic carotid bruits have an increased risk of perioperative stroke at the time of cardiac surgery, especially when prolonged hypotension occurs. Moreover, perioperative strokes often occur in patients who were not suspected of having carotid disease. Furthermore, significant carotid occlusive disease may be present without signs or symptoms, and thus remain undiagnosed.

Impact of Cardiac Surgery on the Quality of Life
Edited by A. E. Willner and G. Rodewald
Plenum Press, New York, 1990

For this reason we prospectively studied a group of
patients undergoing elective coronary revascularization.
In addition to neurological investigations performed
preoperatively, special attention was given to carotid
occlusive disease.

Patients and Methods

Between September 1986 and June 1987, 303 patients
undergoing elective coronary artery revascularization
were neurologically examined pre- and postoperatively.
This also included the Doppler sonographic examination of
the extra-cranial brain arteries. In a standardized
protocol, the cardiological and neurological history of
patients was registered. Postoperative follow-up was
performed on the 2nd and 6th day after operation.

This group consisted of 256 male and 47 female
patients. The ages ranged from 36 to 74 years, with a
mean of 58 years. Cardiac history revealed myocardial
infarctions (MI) in 69.6% (Fig. 1). Fifteen point two
percent of the patients had even experienced two or more
episodes of MI. Ninety-five percent of all patients
complained of angina pectoris at the time of operation.
Angiographic examination showed a restricted contrac-
tility in 74% and heart wall aneurysms in 12%. Disturbances of cardiac rhythm were found in more than 20%
and heart valve disease in 11.9% of the patients.

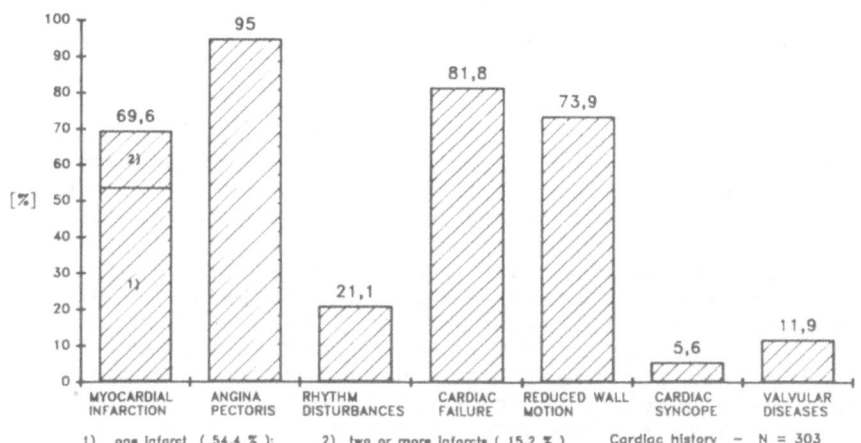

Fig. 1. Cardiac history of 303 patients.

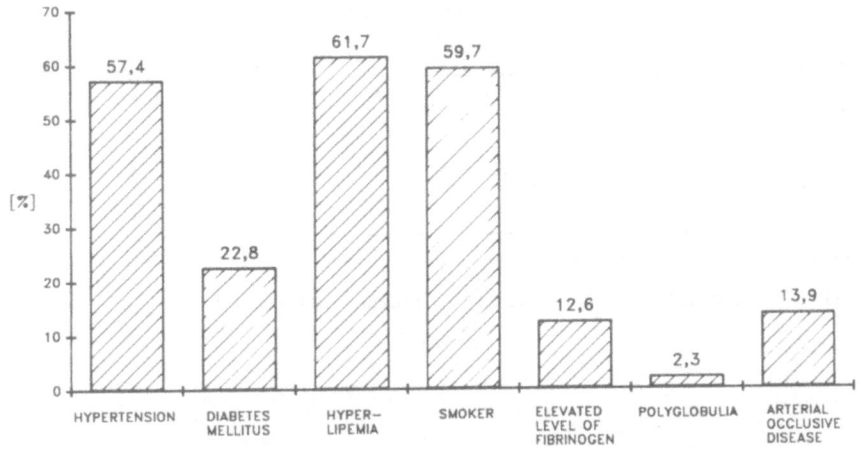

Fig. 2. Cardiovascular risk factors in 303 patients.

The predominant risk factors in our sample were hyperlipidemia in 61.7% (Fig. 2), smoking in 59.7% and arterial hypertension in 57.4% followed by 22.8% of patients with diabetes mellitus.

Neurological investigations, including preoperative Doppler sonographic examination of the extra-cranial brain arteries, revealed pathologic results in 27 (8.9%) of the patients (Table 1). Single lesions were noted in 21 patients and, further, four patients showed bilateral stenoses. In the cardiovascular history, 17 patients had been aware of their illness. Only 5 of the 27 patients had ischemic cerebral insults, due to a stenosed or occluded carotid artery. Cases of suspected carotid stenosis were diagnosed and graded by transvenous or transarterial digital angiography (DSA). The indication for operating upon carotid artery stenosis was a high grade stenosis (>75 grade) and patients having had previous corresponding symptoms. The predominant carotid stenosis was operated in patients with bilateral stenoses.

Surgical Techniques

Coronary revascularization was handled in a standardized manner under extracorporeal circulation and cardioplegic arrest. In 303 electively operated coronary bypass patients, the aorta was cross-clamped for a mean

Table 1.   Pathological results found in 27 patients.

Carotid Artery Disease	Symptomatic	Asymptomatic
Occlusion	1	1
Stenosis		
< 75%	3	13
> 75%	0	5
both sides	1	3
Total	5	22

(Carotid artery disease - preop. examination.)

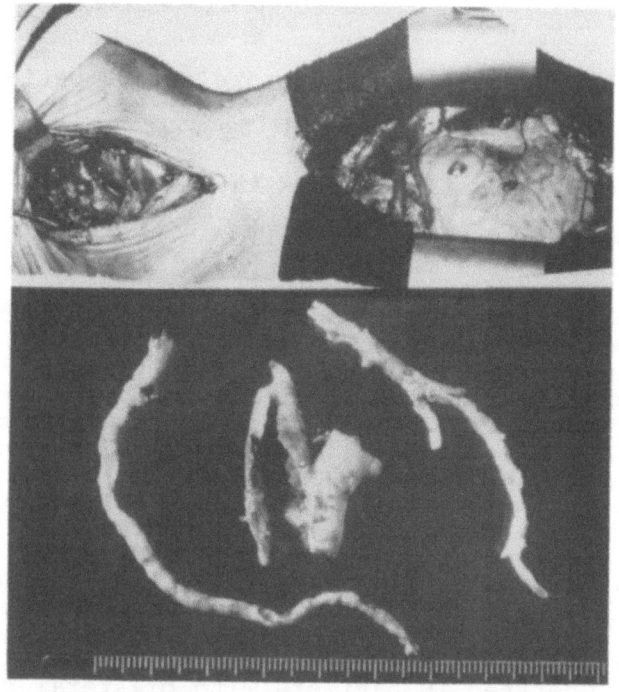

Picture 1.   The upper left side shows the carotid artery endarterectomy and patch plastic.   The upper right shows the perioperative state after endarterectomy of the right and left coronary artery and coronary revascularization with two grafts.   Below is the calcified specimen of the right and left coronary artery and the right carotid bifurcation.

time of 59 minutes. The average number of bypasses per
patient was 3.2. In addition, coronary endarterectomy
was necessary in 18.8% (57/303), heart valve replacement
in 8.9% (27/303) and coronary angioplasty in 5% (15/303).
Nine of 27 (33%) patients with high grade carotid stenoses
underwent simultaneous operation, where after sternotomy,
the endarterectomy of the carotid artery was carried out
first, before institution of cardiopulmonary bypass
(picture 1).

Results

Ischemic cerebral symptoms occurred postoperatively
in 12 of the patients. The neurological deficit was
reversible in 6 patients after CABG (Table 2).   Three
patients had an irreversible neurological deficit: one
of these patients died because of postoperative low
cardiac output. Two of 18 patients with severe asymptomatic carotid artery stenoses prior to surgery who had
only CABG surgery showed a reversible neurological
deficit on the second postoperative day. After CABG and
carotid endarterectomy, one patient developed a reversible neurological deficit on the 6th postoperative day
without any sequelae.

Table 2. Cerebral dysfunction after CABG

Procedure		Neurological Deficit	
		Reversible	Irreversible
CABG	(276/303)	6	3*
CABG + CAEA	(9/303)	1	0
CABG + CAS < 75%	(18/303)	2	0
Total		9	3

Key: *low cardiac output (1); CAEA - carotid artery
endarterectomy; CAS - Carotid artery stenosis

When preoperative risk factors and intraoperative complications were compared for the 12 patients who had a perioperative stroke vs. the remaining patients (58.3% vs. 19.6%), the former showed a greatly increased frequency of cardiac rhythm disturbances. In particular, ventricular extrasystolies occurred more frequently. Six patients had diabetes mellitus (50.0% vs 21.6%).

Patients with cerebral strokes had significantly more episodes of low cardiac output (58.3% vs. 25.4%). The coincidence between insufficient circulation and stroke could be clearly demonstrated in 4 patients. Furthermore, ventilatory insufficiency (33.3% vs. 9.6%) and pericardial effusion (33.3% vs. 2.4%) contributed to circulatory deterioration. Patients with severe carotid artery stenoses or occlusions and patients with pre-operative stroke showed three times as many circulatory complications compared to other patients (25.0% vs. 8.2%). There was no difference between the three patients with severe carotid stenoses having peri-operative stroke, and the other 24 patients with respect to operative data, neurologic, operative and post-operative complications, vascular risk factors, and age.

Summary

After elective CABG, some authors [1-4] have described cerebral dysfunction as the most severe functional complication, with reversible and irreversible sequelae. In retrospective examinations, Coffey and other authors [5-8] found a perioperative risk of stroke in CABG between 0.8% and 1.8%. In prospective studies, Barnes and others [2, 4, 9-11] described values between 1.9% and 4.8%. In our prospective study, 4% of our patients (12/303) suffered from cerebral insults, one patient died because of postoperative low cardiac output and only two patients (0.6%) remained with neurologic symptoms.

The number of patients with coronary heart disease and carotid disease was 8.9% in the present study. In previous studies such as Barnes and other authors [9-11], the incidence ranged from 8.6% to 17.6%. Our results showed that a major portion of cerebral insults probably resulted from cardiac embolism while a smaller number of patients had carotid alterations as well. The cerebral insults suffered by the latter group revealed an association between insufficient circulation and stroke.

While some authors [7, 12, 13] advise that CABG and endarterectomy of asymptomatic high grade carotid stenosis be done simultaneously, Ivey [14] recommends a higher margin of safety. The risk of a cerebral insult by combined CABG and carotid operation runs from 0.0% (Emery [15]) to 7.9% (Bernhard [16]). All authors concluded there is a higher risk in simultaneous operations compared to only coronary surgery.

There were similar findings in the present study; there was no superiority of the simultaneous operation in patients with concomitant severe carotid disease. The Doppler sonographic examination of the extra-cranial brain arteries permitted the identification of a group of patients in danger of carotid disease with a non-invasive technique. We conclude that the decision for a simultaneous operation must be made for each case of coexistent asymptomatic high grade carotid stenosis, individually.

REFERENCES

1. R. M. Bojar, H. Najafi, G. A. Delaria, C. Serry and M. D. Goldin, Neurological complications of coronary revascularisation, Ann. Thorac. Surg. 36: 427-432 (1983).
2. A. C. Breuer, A. J. Furlan, M. R. Hanson, R. J. Lederman, F. D. Loop, D. M. Cosgrove, R. L. Greenstreet and F. G. Estafanous, Central nervous system complication of coronary artery bypass graft surgery: Prospective analysis of 421 patients, Stroke, 14:682-687 (1983).
3. A. J. Furlan and S. C. Jones, Central nervous system complications related to open heart surgery, in: "The Heart and Stroke," A. J. Furlan, ed., Springer, Berlin, Heidelberg (1987).
4. P. J. Shaw, D. Bates, N. E. F. Cartlidge, J. M. French, D. Heaviside, D. G. Julian and D. A. Shaw, Neurologic and neuropsychological morbidity following major surgery: Comparison of coronary artery bypass and peripheral vascular surgery, Stroke, 18:700-707 (1987).
5. C. E. Coffey, W. Massey, K. B. Roberts, S. Curtis, R. H. Jones and D. B. Pryer, Natural history of cerebral complications of coronary artery bypass graft surgery, Neurology, 33: 1416-1421 (1983).

6. F. Gonzales-Scarano and H. I. Hurtig, Neurologic
    complications of coronary artery bypass grafting:
    A casecontrol study, Neurology, 31:1032-1035
    (1981).
7. N. R. Hertzer, F. D. Loop, P. C. Taylor and E. G.
    Beven, Staged and combined surgical approach to
    simultaneous carotid and coronary vascular
    disease, Surgery, 85:803-811 (1978).
8. P. Sergeant, W. Flameng and R. Suy, The cerebral risk
    in coronary surgery, Stroke 19:143 (1988).
9. R. B. Barnes, P. R. Liebman, P. B. Marszalek, C. L.
    Kirk and M. H. Goldman, The natural history of
    asymptomatic carotid disease in patients
    undergoing cardiovascular surgery, Surgery,
    90:1075-1083 (1981).
10. P. J. Breslau, G. Fell, T. D. Ivey, W. W. Bailey,
    D. W. Miller and D. E. Strandness, Carotid
    arterial disease in patients undergoing coronary
    artery bypass operations, J. Thorac. Cardiovasc.
    Surg., 82:765-767 (1983).
11. W. D. Turnipseed, H. A. Berkoff and F. O. Belzer,
    Postoperative stroke in cardiac and peripheral
    vascular disease, Ann. Surg., 192:365-368 (1980).
12. N. R. Hertzer, F. D. Loop and E. G. Beven, Management
    of coexistent carotid and coronary artery disease:
    A surgical viewpoint, in: "The Heart and Stroke,"
    A. J. Furlan, ed., Springer, Berlin, Heidelberg
    (1987).
13. K. Minami, K. S. Sagoo, T. Breymann, D. Fassbender,
    M. Schwerdt and R. Korfer, Operative strategy in
    combined coronary and carotid artery disease,
    J. Thorac. Cardiovasc. Surg. 95:303-309 (1988).
14. T. D. Ivey, D. E. Strandness, D. B. Williams, Y.
    Langlois, G. A. Misbach and A. P. Kurse, Manage-
    ment of patients with carotid bruit undergoing
    cardiopulmonary bypass, J. Thorac. Cardiovasc.
    Surg., 87:183-189 (1984).
15. R. W. Emery, L. H. Cohn, A.D. Whittemore, J. A.
    Mannick, N. P. Couch and J. J. Collins, Coexistent
    carotid and coronary artery disease, Arch. Surg.,
    118: 1033-1038 (1983).
16. V. M. Bernhard, W. D. Johnson and J. J. Peterson,
    Carotid artery stenosis: Association with surgery
    for coronary artery disease, Arch. Surg., 105:
    837-840 (1972).

CEREBRAL BLOOD FLOW REGULATION DURING CARDIOPULMONARY

BYPASS: CORRELATION WITH POSTOPERATIVE NEUROLOGIC

AND NEUROPSYCHOLOGIC DEFICITS

Mark F. Newman, N. Croughwell, William Greeley,
Frank Kern, John Aladj, Gregory Brusino,
Michael Lyth, L. Richard Smith, and J. G. Reves

Department of Anesthesiology
Division of Cardiac Anesthesia
The Heart Center at Duke University Hospital
Durham, North Carolina

INTRODUCTION

Postoperative neuropsychologic deficits after cardiopulmonary bypass for coronary revascularization or open
cardiac procedures remains a disturbing and poorly understood complication. The etiology of postoperative neuropsychologic deficits is being aggressively investigated,
but remains controversial. It has been widely speculated
that these complications are the results of either:
1) embolism of air or particulate matter, or 2) hypoperfusion during cardiopulmonary bypass. Since the
incidence of postoperative neuropsychologic deficits
(PNPD) is significantly higher after cardiac than non-
cardiac surgery, events associated with cardiopulmonary
bypass (CPB) must lead to these complications. The fact
that many of the PNPD are transient and nonfocal lends
credence to the possibility of hypoperfusion or changes in
cerebral autoregulation and cerebral blood flow (CBF) as a
mechanism for these injuries. Therefore, the research on
neurologic and neuropsychologic outcome at The Duke Heart
Center has centered around CBF and changes occurring
during cardiopulmonary bypass.

Impact of Cardiac Surgery on the Quality of Life
Edited by A. E. Willner and G. Rodewald
Plenum Press, New York, 1990

CEREBRAL BLOOD FLOW INVESTIGATIONS

The first cerebral blood flow measurement was made in
1966 by a Fick $AO_2 - VO_2$ method [1]. Using the 133Xenon
washout method for cerebral blood flow determination, our
group was the first to compare CBF with psychometric testing results and report factors which influence CBF in
patients undergoing cardiac surgery [2]. The first study
investigated 67 patients without history of hypertension
or cerebrovascular disease undergoing elective coronary
revascularization and found that cerebral blood flow is
significantly reduced during CPB (See Figure 1). The 55%
decrease in CBF correlated with a similar reduction in
$CMRO_2$. The two factors in this study which were found to
significantly influence CBF were temperature (r=0.54,
p< .0001) and $PaCO_2$ (r=0.36, p<0.05). Perhaps more important was the determination of factors which did not influence CBF, perfusion pressure, hemoglobin, pump flow and
time. A mini-mental status exam examination (MMSE) was
performed preoperatively and postoperatively, and in this
small sample there was no significant change in MMSE after
surgery. There was also no relationship between cerebral
blood flow and MMSE changes. In a similar study of 14
patients we examined the relationship between CBF and
postoperative cognitive function [3]. Although not
significant, a negative trend was noted in the association
of age with changes in MMSE (r=0.36, p<0.20).

The most recent completed investigations at our institution have examined the CBF of patients at the extremes
of age (old and young). Using 133Xe washout CBF in 25
children (age 2 days to 60 months), Greeley found that
factors (nasopharyngeal temperature and $PaCO_2$) that govern
CBF in the adult are the same in children and that autoregulation (defined as no statistical association between
perfusion pressure and CBF) is preserved at moderate hypothermia (>28°C) [4]. We did find however that at deep
hypothermia (18 - 20° C) cerebral autoregulation is lost.
CBF becomes perfusion pressure dependent but responsiveness
to CO_2 is probably maintained. We concluded from these
data that the pediatric and the adult patient have similar
CBF responses to CPB at moderate hypothermia, but that
profound hypothermia alters cerebral blood flow and cerebrovascular responsivity. We also found that circulatory
arrest (n=14) is associated with a significantly (p<0.01)
lower CBF during rewarming and after CPB than in 11
controls (See Figure 2). We are uncertain of the explanation of this finding; however it may be part of the no-
reflow phenomenon. This change in cerebral blood flow was

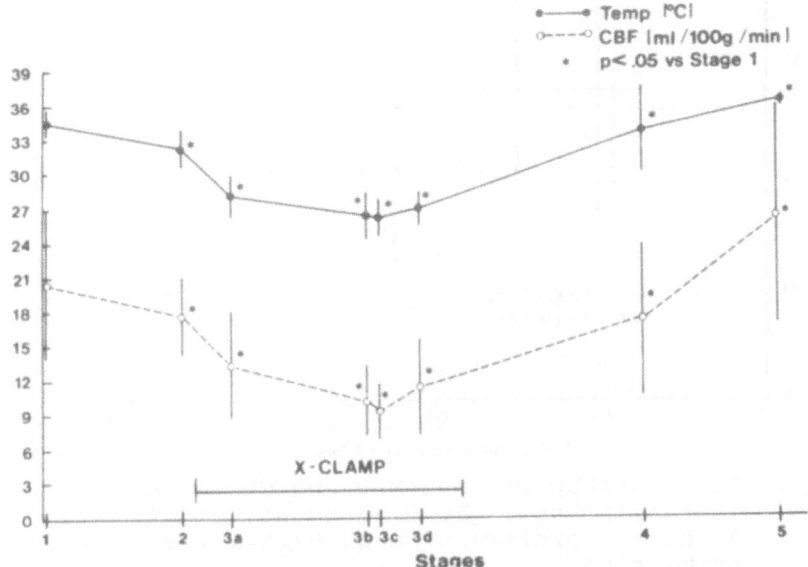

Figure 1. Changes in temperature and cerebral blood flow
during CPB (From A. V. Govier, et al. Ann
Thorac Surg. 38:592 (1984) with permission.)

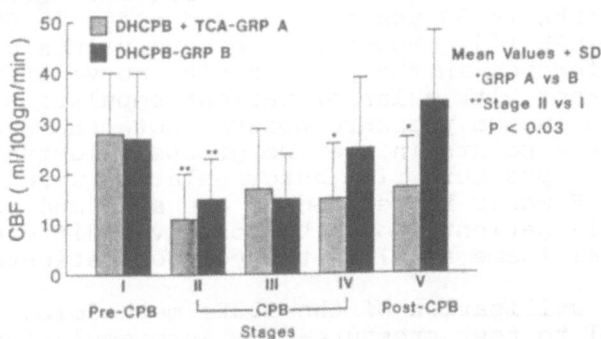

Figure 2. Changes in CBF during deep hypothermic CPB and
deep hypothermia with total circulatory arrest.
(From W. J. Greeley, et al. J Thorac
Cardiovasc Surg. 97:737 (1989) with
permission.)

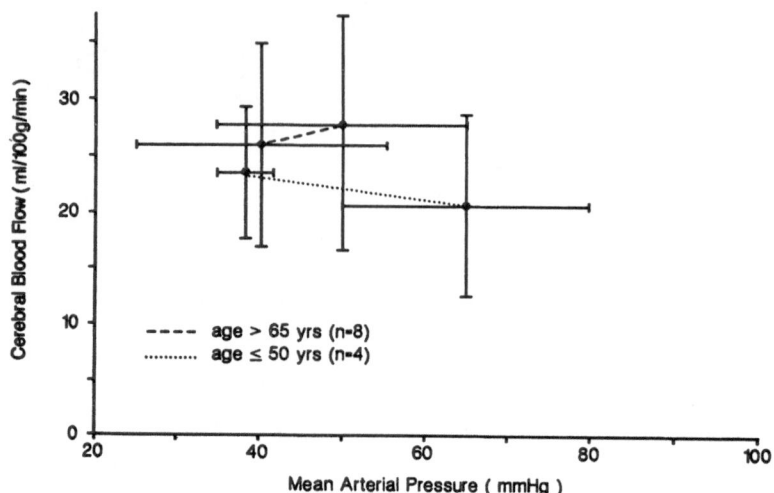

Figure 3.   Relationship between MAP and CBF with
             increasing age. F. G. Brusino, et al.
             J Thorac Cardiovasc Surg. 97:541 (1989) with
             permission.

tested by measurement of CBF with constant temperature,
CO_2, pump flow and perfusion pressure.

     We also have limited data on the other age extreme,
the elderly. These data on 20 elective CABG patients show
that mean CBF is not significantly different between
younger patients (< 50 years, n=9) and older (> 65 years,
n=11) during CPB [5]. However, the mean values suggest a
possible difference in the pressure-CBF curve that might
be more apparent with a larger patient population and with
equivalent perfusion pressure points (note the upper perfusion pressure points in the two groups illustrated in
Figure 3). If pressure flow autoregulation were disrupted
by age the CBF would be related to pressure and the slope
of the elderly patients would be positive (different from
0) and neutral (same as 0) in the younger patients.

     Further utilization of the 133Xe methodology has lead
us to a model to test pressure-flow autoregulation. Under
identical conditions of nasopharyngeal temperature, pH,
and pump flow, cerebral blood flow determinations are made
prior to and after phenylephrine (shown not to increase
CBF during bypass by Rogers et al [6]) is used to increase
the mean pressure 20%. This allows two points for determination of the lower end of the pressure-CBF relationship
in normotensive patients without cerebrovascular disease.

Using this method in 21 patients, Aladj tested the
hypothesis that isoflurane abolished cerebral autoregulation [7]. He found that the addition of isoflurane to a
background anesthetic of automated continuously infused
fentanyl and midazolam during CPB, significantly (p<0.02)
reduces the CBF, but autoregulation remains intact (See
Figure 4).

DISCUSSION

       The ability to quantitate cerebral blood flow by the
133Xe method has led to as many questions as answers in
relation to changes with cardiopulmonary bypass and their
signficance. Many postulates, including those of our own
mentioned in the previous pages, require investigation.
Larger patient populations are needed to produce correlates
between CBF and neuropsychologic or neurologic outcome, if
any exist. The possible risk groups including the elderly,
hypertensives and diabetics require larger randomized
trials to evaluate their cerebral autoregulation during
CPB and the signficance of these factors on outcome.

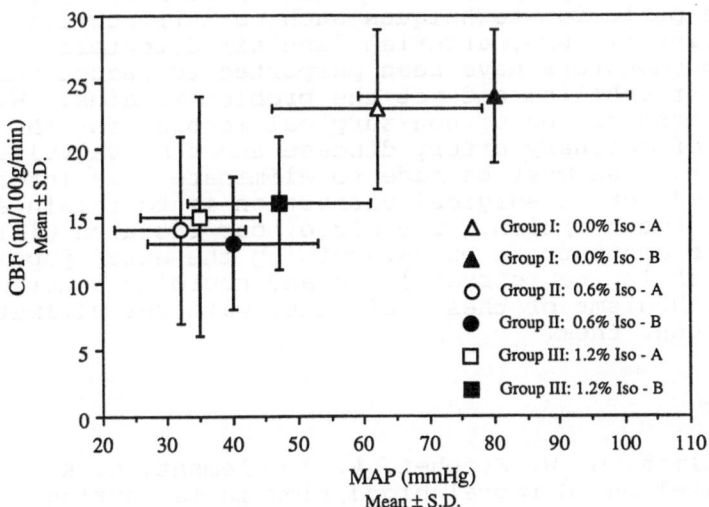

Figure 4.   CBF compared to MAP with varying concentrations
            of isoflurane. J. Aladj, et al. Anesth Analg.
            68:S7 (1989) with permission.

The other area of increasing interest is that of cerebral protection agents such as thiopental, isoflurane and the burgeoning group of calcium channel blockers including nimodipine and flunarizine. Large trials with these medications are also necessary to determine the significance of the CBF changes and neurologic and neuropsychologic function improvement that can be realized.

Lastly, since much research is now spent in the evaluation of postoperative neuropsychologic deficits after cardiac surgery, it seems important that further long-term follow-up be undertaken to determine any signficant impact on the quality of life and cerebral function. Sotaniemi showed that in a small group of patients followed for five years after cardiac surgery, those patients who developed transient neuropsychologic deficits perioperatively had significantly poorer global cerebral function after five years [8]. Larger patient populations are obviously required to see if this long term association holds.

As continued improvements have been made in myocardial preservation during cardiopulmonary bypass (CPB), neuropsychologic and neurologic deficits have projected even larger as complications of cardiopulmonary bypass. Changes in perfusion techniques such as introduction of arterial line filters, arterial line air detectors, and membrane oxygenators have been purported to reduce the incidence of embolism and yet the problem remains. With the rapid progression of non-surgical methods for the treatment of coronary artery disease and some valvular lesions, progress must be made to eliminate this intolerable side effect if surgical correction is to remain a viable treatment option. Therefore, our research will continue to concentrate on determining the exact population at risk for neuropsychologic and neurologic deficits and the mechanisms of these deficits, with the ultimate aim to prevent them.

REFERENCES

1. H. Wollman, G. W. Stephen, A. J. Clement, C. K. Danielson, Cerebral blood flow in man during extracorporeal circulation, J Thorac Cardiovasc Surg. 52:558 (1966).
2. A. V. Govier, J. G. Reves, R. D. McKay, R. B. Karp, G. L. Zorn, R. B. Morawetz, L. R. Smith, M. Adams, A. M. Freeman, Factors and their influence of

regional cerebral blood flow during cardiopulmonary bypass, Ann Thorac Surg. 38:592 (1984).

3. A. M. Freeman, D. G. Folks, R. S. Sokol, A. V. Govier, J. G. Reves, E. L. Fleece, K. R. Hall, G. L. Zorn, R. B. Karp, Cognitive function after coronary bypass surgery: Effects of decreased cerebral blood flow, Am J Psychiatry. 142:110 (1985).

4. W. J. Greeley, R. M. Ungerleider, L. R. Smith, J. G. Reves, The effects of deep hypothermic cardio-pulmonary bypass and total circulatory arrest on cerebral blood flow in infants and children, J Thorac Cardiovasc Surg. 97:737 (1989).

5. F. G. Brusino, J. G. Reves, L. R. Smith, D. S. Prough, D. A. Stump, R. W. McIntyre, The effect of age on cerebral blood flow during hypothermic cardiopulmonary bypass, J Thorac Cardiovasc Surg. 97:541 (1989).

6. A. T. Rogers, D. A. Stump, G. P. Gravlee, D. S. Prough, K. C. Angert, J. Phipps, J. Hinshelwood, Preservation of cerebral autoregulation during cardiopulmonary bypass, Anesth Analg. 66:S149 (1987).

7. L. J. Aladj, J. G. Reves, J. R. Jacobs, L. R. Smith, The effects of isoflurane on cerebral blood flow during hypothermic cardiopulmonary bypass, Anesth Analg. 68:S7 (1989).

8. K. A. Sotaniemi, H. Mononer, T. E. Hokkanen, Long-term cerebral outcome after open-heart surgery, Stroke. 17:410-16 (1986).

ELECTROENCEPHALOGRAM-BASED PROGNOSIS OF CARDIAC SURGERY -

A LONG-TERM FOLLOW-UP STUDY

Phiroze L. Hansotia, Percy N. Karanjia,
Richard D. Sautter, William O. Myers,
Jefferson F. Ray, III, Betty Ann Becker,
and Willard E. Pierce

Marshfield Clinic and
Marshfield Medical Research Foundation
Marshfield, WI

INTRODUCTION

Hansotia et al. [1] reported on the use of electroencephalogram (EEG) in determining the immediate outcome
of cardiac surgery. During a two year period between
1970 and 1972, 117 patients undergoing cardiac operations
were studied. EEGs were recorded pre-operatively, in the
recovery room (up to 12 hr. post-operatively), 24 hr., 2
days, 7 days, and at regular weekly intervals if abnormal.
Operative and anesthesia data were correlated with EEG
findings. All patients had normal EEGs pre-operatively.
On the basis of EEG criteria, four groups were identified:
Group I - The EEG remained normal throughout the postoperative period (41 patients); Group II - Diffuse,
nonspecific EEG abnormalities in the recovery room,
followed by a normal EEG thereafter (25 patients); Group
III - Abnormal EEG in the recovery room with essentially
no change throughout the remainder of the hospital stay
(40 patients); and Group IV - Abnormal EEG in the
recovery room with a progressively worsening pattern
until the patient died (11 patients).

Bypass time appeared directly related to outcome by
group but not individually. Hypotension prior to pumping
occurred most often and mean blood loss was greatest in
the patients who had abnormal EEGs in the recovery room

Impact of Cardiac Surgery on the Quality of Life
Edited by A. E. Willner and G. Rodewald
Plenum Press, New York, 1990

with progressively worsening patterns until death. The
level of consciousness was not as prognostic as was the
EEG. The pattern of EEGs in the first few post-operative
days was more important in prognosis than any other
single record. All those who showed progressive deterioration in the first two or three days (all Group IV
patients) died shortly thereafter [1].

      The patients in Groups I, II, and III who survived
the immediate post-operative state constitute the basis
for this study. These patients have been followed for 10
years at the Marshfield Clinic. The present cross-
sectional retrospective analysis is aimed at reviewing
the mortality and morbidity of these patients. Unfortunately, detailed mental status examinations or neuropsychological evaluations had not been performed earlier
and therefore were not necessarily performed for the
present study. The central question being addressed is
whether the prognostic criteria developed for the immediate post-operative state following cardiac surgery, using
EEG criteria, were also valid for the long term morbidity
and mortality of these patients.

METHODS

      Adequate follow-up examinations and records were
available for 105 of the 106 subjects. The EEGs were
reviewed 'blind' and earlier interpretations confirmed.
Of these, 42 subjects belonged to Group I, 25 to Group
II, and 38 to Group III. Mortality data was obtained for
each patient for the 10 consecutive years following their
cardiac surgery (Table 1). The cause of death was identified as cardiac, cerebral, renal, or other, whenever
identified, preferably by autopsy data. The present
health of the survivors residing in the area was determined from the medical records, if the patients had been
evaluated with appropriate physical examination with
laboratory tests within six months by one of us (authors).
Those patients who had not been examined between July and
December of 1984 were contacted and scheduled for a
complete medical and neurological examination with appropriate laboratory tests. There were 2 patients in Group
I, 4 in Group II, and 6 in Group III who were examined.
If the patients had moved away from the area, information
was obtained by telephone interview either with the
patient or a close relative (17 patients). The patients
are defined as being alive and well, ill with either
cerebrovascular, cardiac, renal, or other diseases, or

living but with an undetermined health status. Most of
these 17 patients were residing remote from our area and
were difficult to examine or obtain accurate medical
information on.

Table 1.   Status of Cardiac Surgery Patients Ten Years
           Post-Surgery, Grouped According to EEG
           Responses Following Surgery

EEG Group	No. of Pts.	Died in Hosp.	Died Within 10 Yr.	Alive With Cardiac Disease	Alive and Well	Alive, Status Unknown	Unknown
I	41	0	17	7	12	6	
II	25	0	10	3	9	3	
III	40	0	15	4	11	8	
IV	11	11	-	-	-	-	
TOTAL	117	11	42	14	32	17	1

RESULTS

     The status of these patients 10 years post-surgery
is shown in Table 1. The mortality at 10 years in Groups
I, II, and III is similar (40%). Cardiac causes of death
accounted for 40% in Group 1, 25% in Group II, and 54.5%
in Group III subjects. No significant differences in the
mortality figures between Groups I, II, and III are
detected (Fig. 1). Table 2 depicts the number of deaths
in each group with no significant differences seen.
Interestingly, there were no deaths reported from cerebrovascular disease. The morbidity table in Groups I,
II, and III shows a similar profile (Fig. 2) to the
mortality.

Table 2.   Mortality table

| | Time of Death | |
	1st Five Years	2nd Five Years
Group I	5	12
Group II	5	5
Group III	9	6

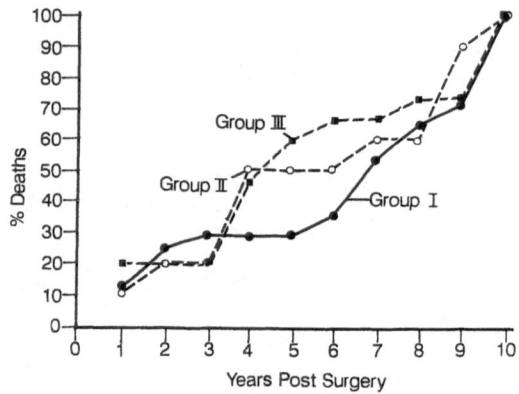

Fig. 1   Accumulative percentage of patients dying by
           year post surgery.

DISCUSSION

        There are several reports of EEG monitoring during
cardiac surgery [2-13], but only one, to date, of
long-term follow-up of these patients to indicate if the
prognostic value of the EEG criteria extend beyond the
immediate post-operative state.   Sotaniemi [14] carried
out a five year neurological and EEG follow-up on 55
patients who had undergone open heart surgery for valve
replacement.   The five year survival rate was 89%.   The
prevalence of permanent neurological abnormality after
surgery was 9%.   Also, the five year EEG outcome was
encouraging;   the prevalence of abnormal EEGs had fallen
from the value before operation of 45% to 25%.   The
correspondence between the clinical and EEG course
established immediately after surgery remained also in
the later course.   Our data indicates that it does not do
so.   The outcome of patients who had normal EEGs and
neurological findings pre-operatively, during surgery,
and post-operatively was virtually identical to that of
patients who developed complications during surgery and
left the hospital with an abnormal EEG and some neurological deficit.   Despite their varying immediate
outcomes following cardiac surgery, the mortality or the
morbidity of Groups I, II, and III was the same past the
first years of survival.

        Sotaniemi et al. [10] suggested that multi-parameter
investigation using neuropsychological testing together
with clinical and EEG follow-up is useful in the assessment of cerebral disorders attributable to open heart
surgery.   They confirmed our earlier observations of the

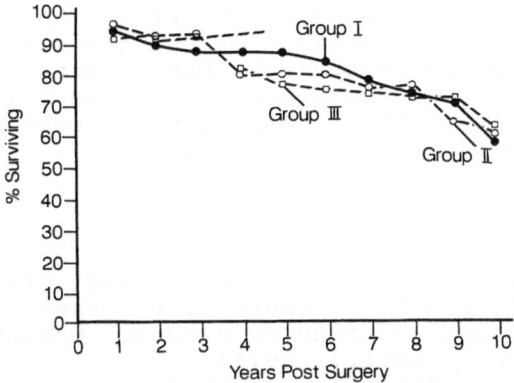

Fig. 2   Percent patients surviving by year post surgery
          by diagnostic group.

operative variables, perfusion time, and unexpected intraoperative events were the most important factors leading
to post-operative, neuropsychological, and clinical
impairment. In a later study, Sotaniemi [15] showed that
approximately 35% of the survivors of cardiac surgery
patients studied showed EEG, neuropsychological, and
subtle clinical evidence of cerebral dysfunction following
cardiac surgery. This observation again was similar to
that made by Hansotia et al. [1]. Since our initial
study in 1972, other studies [12, 15] have shown the high
frequency of subtle mental changes and neuropsychological
findings following cardiac surgery. Our study was unable
to explore this dimension and relates to the issues of
cardiovascular, renal and system health, and mortality
only.

     Coronary bypass surgery can be performed with a low
morbidity and operative mortality dependent on patient
mix and surgical experience. Operative mortality is
generally higher in elderly patients, in patients with
impaired left ventricular function, symptoms of heart
failure, severe left main coronary artery stenosis, or
unstable (versus stable) angina, in women, and in urgent
or emergency surgery [16, 17]. It is important to
remember that coronary artery disease is a dynamic
process and the progression of old lesions, the appearance of new ones, and graft patency can be expected to
influence outcome. Graft patency rates of 75 to 90% from
one to two years after surgery [18-20] have been reported
with an average annual graft attrition rate of 2.2%
between one and six years after surgery [21]. All of
these factors seem to apply equally to our patients, both

in terms of survival as well as in terms of health and disease later on. On the basis of our observations, we conclude that the EEG criteria we use to determine prognosis of cardiac surgery are applicable only for the immediate operative period. They are not helpful in determining prognosis in the long term.

REFERENCES

1. P. L. Hansotia, W. O. Myers, J. F. Ray, III, C. Greehling, and R. D. Sautter, Prognostic value of electroencephalography in cardiac surgery, Ann. Thorac. Surg. 19:127 (1975).
2. T. Aberg and M. Kihlgren, Cerebral protection during open-heart surgery, Thorax. 32:525 (1977).
3. M. A. Branthwaite, Prevention of neurological damage during open-heart surgery, Thorax. 30:258 (1975).
4. I. Juneja, R. E. Flynn, and R. L. Berger, The arterial, venous pressures and the electro-encephalogram during open heart surgery, Acta Neurol. Scand. 48:163 (1972).
5. P. E. Kritikou and M. A. Branthwaite, Significance of changes in cerebral electrical activity at onset of cardiopulmonary bypass, Thorax. 32:534 (1977).
6. R. R. Myers, J. J. Stockard, and L. J. Saidman, Monitoring of cerebral perfusion during anesthesia by time-compressed Fourier analysis of the electro-encephalogram, Stroke. 8:331 (1977).
7. T. A. Salerno, D. P. Lince, D. N. White, R. B. Lynn, and E. J. P. Charrett, Monitoring of electro-encephalogram during open-heart surgery. A prospective analysis of 118 cases, J. Thorac. Cardiovasc. Surg. 76:97 (1978).
8. K. A. Sotaniemi, Clinical and prognostic correlates of EEG in open-heart surgery patients, J. Neurol. Neurosurg. Psychiatry. 43:941 (1980).
9. K. A. Sotaniemi, The benefits of open-heart surgery as reflected in the EEG, Scand. J. Thorac. Cardio-vasc. Surg. 15:205 (1981).
10. K. A. Sotaniemi, A. Juolasmaa, and T. E. Hokkanen, Neuropsychologic outcome after open-heart surgery, Arch. Neurol. 38:2 (1981).
11. K. A. Sotaniemi, I. A. Sulg, and T. E. Hokkanen, Quantitative EEG as a measure of cerebral dysfunction before and after open-heart surgery, Electroencephalog. Clin. Neurophysiol. 50:81 (1980).

12. M. M. Witoszka, H. Tamura, R. Indeglia, R. W. Hopkins and F. A. Simeone, Electroencephalographic changes and cerebral complications in open-heart surgery, J. Thorac. Cardiovasc. Surg. 66:855 (1973).

13. J. S. Wright, A. K. Lethlean, R. G. Hicks, T. A. Torda, and R. Stacey, Electroencephalographic studies during open-heart surgery, J. Thorac. Cardiovasc. Surg. 63:631 (1972).

14. K. A. Sotaniemi, Five-year neurological and EEG outcome after open-heart surgery, J. Neurol. Neurosurg. Psychiatry. 48:569 (1985).

15. K. A. Sotaniemi, Cerebral outcome after extra-corporeal circulation: Comparison between prospective and retrospective evaluations, Arch. Neurol. 40:75 (1983).

16. B. J. Gersh, R. A. Kronmal, R. L. Frye, H. V. Schaff, T. J. Ryan, A. J. Gosselin, G. C. Kaiser, T. Killip, III, and Participants in the Coronary Artery Surgery Study, Coronary arteriography and coronary artery bypass surgery: Morbidity and mortality in patients ages 65 years or older: A report from the coronary artery surgery study, Circulation, 67:483 (1983).

17. J. W. Kennedy, G. C. Kaiser, L. D. Fisher, J. K. Fritz, W. Myers, J. G. Mudd, and T. J. Ryan, Clinical and angiographic predictors of operative mortality from the collaborative study in coronary artery surgery (CASS), Circulation. 63:793 (1981).

18. M. G. Bourassa, L. Campeau, J. Lesperance, and C. M. Grondin, Changes in grafts and coronary arteries after saphenous vein aortocoronary bypass surgery: Results at repeat angiography, Circulation 65 (Suppl II):II90 (1982).

19. J. R. Kramer, Y. Matsuda, J. C. Mulligan, M. Aronow, and W. L. Proudfit, Progression of coronary atherosclerosis, Circulation. 63:519 (1981).

20. A. V. G. Bruschke, T. S. Wijers, W. Kolsters, and J. Landmann, The anatomic evolution of coronary artery disease demonstrated by coronary arteriography in 256 non-operated patients, Circulation. 63:527 (1981).

21. D. M. Cosgrove, F. D. Loop, and W. C. Sheldon, Results of myocardial revascularization: A 12-year experience, Circulation 65 (Suppl II): II37 (1982).

PSYCHOMETRIC ISSUES

THE USE OF COGNITIVE TESTS TO ASSESS COGNITIVE IMPAIRMENT

IN CARDIAC SURGERY PATIENTS: WITH EMPHASIS ON THE CLAT

ANALOGY TEST

Allen Willner

Hillside Hospital
Glen Oaks, NY

Cognitive impairment has frequently been reported in cardiac surgery patients, both preoperatively and post-operatively [1-38]. In preoperative impairment, the severe cardiac illness for which the surgery is required can impair cerebral circulation in some patients, with consequent tissue damage and impaired cerebral functioning. In postoperative cognitive impairment, cerebral damage can be related to perioperative conditions such as problems with the extracorporeal perfusion equipment, e.g. arterial line filters and/or oxygenators [35, 36].

Both neurological examination and psychometric tests are used to assess possible cerebral damage. Neurological examination is sensitive to abnormal reflex patterns, motor weakness, sensory impairment, but less sensitive in assessing complex higher mental functions. Psychometric tests make a contribution in assessing higher mental functions such as: abstract reasoning, memory, language, visual spatial ability, visual motor abliity, etc.

There are many psychometric tests. The specific cognitive test battery employed in this study was selected by the neuropsychology committee of the International Consortium, chaired by Dr. Ralph Reitan. The test battery was selected as likely to be sensitive to cognitive dys-function in cardiac surgery patients. Three tests (WAIS Block Design, WAIS Digit Symbol, Trailmaking test) are frequently used in cognitive assessments. The other three

Impact of Cardiac Surgery on the Quality of Life
Edited by A. E. Willner and G. Rodewald
Plenum Press, New York, 1990

have been used effectively in studies of the cognitive
effects of cardiac surgery: the Åberg Figure Rotation
Test, Willner's CLAT Analogy Test, and the Bethune-
Williams Visual Memory Test.

Because of the central role of the CLAT test in the
cognitive assessment used here, we will emphasize the
discussion of the CLAT in this chapter. Nancy Feys-Dunne
describes the other 5 tests in the next chapter.

DEVELOPMENT OF THE CONCEPTUAL LEVEL ANALOGY TEST (CLAT)

Willner constructed the CLAT to remedy two major
weaknesses in tests of the ability for analogical reasoning: insufficient psychometric purity and assessment of
irrelevant variables [36, 37].   Tests in which variables
extraneous to the abstraction process are confounded with
abstraction are deficient in psychometric purity. Tests
in which the basic variables assessed have little relevance to abstraction suffer from assessment of irrelevant
variables. Willner demonstrated in 1964 that 50% of items
drawn from American analogy tests were solvable by word
association. For example, in the analogy "Vinegar-Sour:
Sugar - ?, the correct answer "sweet" was a frequent
association to "sugar" independent of the analogy. Since
such items are solvable either by word association or by
analogical reasoning, they have insufficient psychometric
purity. A second type of confounding variable has the
opposite effect, the subject fails the analogy item
although he is quite capable of the reasoning processes
required. This usually happens when the vocabulary level
is too high. Difficult items on analogy tests are very
often difficult because of the vocabulary or information
required, rather than analogical reasoning. Subjects with
excellent analogical reasoning ability but weak vocabulary
or information background are penalized on such tests.

Relevant Variables

These considerations raised the question of what are
the relevant variables in analogical reasoning. Willner
[36, 37] proposed that the major relevant variables are
logical complexity level (LCL) and relationship availability level (RAL). Logical complexity level is based
only upon the use of categories in the analogy test item
(see Table 1). Relationship availability level is based
upon the empirical availability of the relationships
required to solve the analogy item, independent of logical
complexity levels (see Table 2).

Table 1. LOGICAL COMPLEXITY LEVELS (LCL)

LCL 1 -- Opposites	Black-White: Old-New
LCL 2 -- Functional	Hay-Horse: Bread-Man
LCL 3 -- Member-Class	Dog-Animal: Bible-Book
LCL 4 -- Coordinate Relations	January-March: Submarine-Sailboat
LCL 5 -- Opposite Categories	Diamond-Steel: Pillow-Jello
LCL 6 -- Two-Category Contrast	Wolf-Dog: Hurricane-Breeze

Table 2. RELATIONSHIP AVAILABILITY LEVEL (RAL)

Higher Availability	Diamond-Steel: Pillow-Jello
Lower Availability	Cat-Oak: House-Book

Highly significant correlations were found between the difficulty of analogy test items and both logical complexity level and relationship availability level, supporting the hypothesis that both were related to the difficulty of analogy test items. Moreover, each of these two variables remained significantly related to item difficulty when the effect of the other was partialled out.

The CLAT Test

The CLAT [25] consists of 42 multiple choice analogy items, thoroughly screened for solvability by word association and requiring vocabulary and information at or below the capability of the average 4th grade student. However, the conceptual functioning required ranges from simple to complex, as may be noted in the following two items:

Bird - Sings: Dog - (Cat, Song, Florida, Barks, Dances)

Cat - Oak: House - (Poison Ivy, Family, Dog, Book, Pony)

The test was standardized on a sample of 150 subjects (75 male, basic airmen and 75 female WAFS) at Lackland Air Force Base, Texas. Standard Scores were constructed on the model of Wechsler Adult Intelligence Scale scaled scores, with the mean set equal to 10, and standard deviation (SD) to 3. The corrected split-half reliability (odd vs. even items) is 0.83.

Several studies demonstrate a significant relationship between analogy test scores and other criteria for brain damage: 1) EEG abnormality [40] in a psychiatric hospital population, 2) neuro-psychological test battery scores for both a psychiatric and a neurologic sample, 3) neurological soft signs and 4) Bender-Gestalt test findings in a psychiatric hospital sample.

Kelleher et al. [41] studied the internal consistency and factorial composition of the CLAT. They found it to be an "unidimensional scale" with 41 of 42 items contributing significantly to the measurement of a "global ability."

Several studies have used a "devastated" CLAT score to predict poor outcome. The "devastated" score is obtained by the lowest one percent of the standardizing population, and can easily be obtained by random response on this multiple choice test. Patients whose abstraction ability was so gravely impaired were predicted to have unfortunate outcomes.

STUDIES WITH PATIENT SAMPLES

Prospective Cardiac Surgery Studies

A signficant relationship was found between pre-operative CLAT test score and in-hospital psychiatric complications and mortality in a prospective study of 100 cardiac surgery patients [42]. Subsequent studies extended these findings to 18 months [43] and 5 years [44] postoperatively.

The test-retest reliability of preoperative CLAT scores with one week, 18 months, and 5 years postoperative scores is substantial: r=0.81, 0.85 and 0.70, respectively. These correlations suggest a minimal effect of preoperative anxiety upon CLAT scores. This was directly investigated by correlating scores on the Spielberger State-Trait anxiety test with CLAT scores. The correlations were essentially zero, both preoperatively and postoperatively.

Prospective Studies of Vulnerability of Other Patient Samples

Other prospective studies have shown a relationship between devastated CLAT test scores and:

(1) Vulnerability to subsequent development of tardive dyskinesia and other movement disorders in psychiatric patients treated with psychotropic medications [45-47].

(2) Vulnerability to mortality over the next 9 years in a sample of community living elderly members of senior citizens clubs [48].

Impaired Verbal Abstraction in Alcoholics

Yohman and Parsons, in a series of three experiments, showed that alcoholics had significantly lower CLAT scores than carefully matched controls, which they took to represent an impairment of verbal abstraction ability by the effects of excessive alcohol [49].

Relationship between Preoperative CLAT Scores and Variables Relevant to Cardiac Illness. International Study Data

We examined the relationship between preoperative CLAT scores and several variables presumably related to severity of cardiac illness.

Age. The mean preoperative CLAT score showed a highly significant decline with increasing age (p < .001) for a group of 450 patients in this study.

Diagnosis. The mean preoperative CLAT score also declined signficiantly according to medical diagnosis for Ss diagnosed as having the following conditions: coronary artery disease, cardiac valvular disease, and both conditions (p = .03) for a group of 450 Ss. The number of Ss having cardiac valvular disease (37) and both conditions, (15) was small however.

Diabetes. There was a trend (p = .06, n = 371) for patients having diabetes to have lower preoperative CLAT scores than non-diabetic patients.

Sex. Female patients had significantly lower preoperative CLAT scores (p < .005, n = 459) than males.
There was no evidence that this difference was attributable to differences in age of the patients. However,
there was evidence that the difference was attributable to
an interaction between sex and medical diagnosis. Specifically, there was no significant difference between the
preoperative CLAT Scores of male and female coronary
artery disease patients, whereas female cardiac valvular
disease patients had significantly lower CLAT scores than
their male counterparts, p = .03. This finding was
observed despite the much larger number of coronary artery
disease patients (306 males, 50 females) than cardiac
valvular disease patients (27 males, 22 females).

Hypertension. There was no significant difference in
preoperative CLAT scores for patients with hypertension or
normal blood pressure (p = .15, n = 371).

History of myocardial infarction. There was no
relationship between a history of myocardial infarction
and preoperative CLAT scores (p = .52, n = 361).

The CLAT as a Measure of Postoperative Change.

The studies cited above, however, did not use the
CLAT prospectively to assess postoperative changes in the
patient's cognitive functioning. One purpose of the
International Study is to identify aspects of cardiac
surgery related to postoperative impaired cognitive
functioning. It is essential to define cognitive impairment to accomplish this purpose. In this study, impairment
is defined as a drop of one standard deviation or more in
CLAT score. Since, ordinarily one might expect that
scores would rise by practice effect when patients are
retested after a short interval, a drop of one standard
deviation seems substantial enough to use as a definition
of impairment. Many authors have in fact used a drop of
one standard deviation as their definition of impairment.
They, however, usually use the standard deviation of the
subjects in their study as their criterion. Another
possibility is to use the standard deviation of the
standardizing sample as the criterion. The writer [36]
chose the latter as a criterion for several reasons:

(1) Uniformity of measures. Different studies will
obtain different values for the standard deviation. A

standard deviation which changes from study to study is
inconsistent with the principle of using a common yardstick when one compares results across studies.

(2) Normal parameters as a reference point. When
tests are well-standardized, it seems useful to employ
parameters of the standardizing sample as a reference
point rather than the scores of clinically abnormal populations. Thus, in studying the cognitive functioning of
retarded patients, one uses normal population parameters
as reference points rather than in effect renorming the
test for each sample of patients. In essence, one derives
"norms" from normal, not pathological, samples. In
practice, moreover, patient samples usually have larger
standard deviations than normal samples, so that using
patient-derived standard deviations results in fewer
people being classified as abnormal.

None of this is intended to discourage the use of new
tests, since they represent the potential for improvement
in the field. Since no established norms may be available
for a new test, one may simply administer it to a normal
population, establish norms for that sample, and then use
it provisionally in clinical research. Should it prove
promising, more rigorous norming of the test would follow.

Prospective Study of Postoperative Drop in CLAT Score With Two Different Arterial Line Filters

Willner et al [36] studied the relationship between
the use of two different arterial line filters and postoperative brain dysfunction as assessed by a postoperative
drop of one standard deviation or more in CLAT test scores.
They found a significant difference in the incidence of
patients whose CLAT scores dropped postoperatively, 5% for
one filter and 24% for the other. The postoperative
change in CLAT scores correlated significantly with pump
time for one filter, but there was no correlation for the
second filter. Moreover, there is evidence that impaired
CLAT scores are stable over a period of several years and
related to poor outcome during that period.

One problem with the use of the CLAT in such studies
is its very sensitivity, that it is sensitive to impaired
cerebral functioning that can occur before the surgery.
Many cardiac surgery patients have extremely low scores
before the surgery, scores so low that they can no longer
drop by one standard deviation postoperatively. For this
reason, we used a battery of three tests to assess possi-

ble brain dysfunction after the surgery. This test
battery consisted of two subtests from the Wechsler Adult
Intelligence Scale (WAIS), the WAIS Block Design and WAIS
Digit Symbol tests as well as the CLAT. Since these tests
are not as difficult as the CLAT, they provided coverage
for patients whose CLAT scores were so low preoperatively
that there was no room for them to drop further. The
CLAT provided coverage for those patients with better
retained preoperative cognitive functioning.

Relationship Between Several Parameters of the Cardio-Pulmonary Bypass Pump and Postoperative Drop in CLAT Score International Study Data

Bypass time. Time on the bypass pump was signficantly related (p < .01, n = 277) to the postoperative
drop in CLAT score.

Predominant hematocrit level. Predominant hematocrit
level was signficantly related (p < .05, n = 276) to the
postoperative drop in CLAT score.

Venous Oxygen Saturation. There was a significant
effect (p=.05, n = 239) for venous oxygen saturation to be
related to postoperative drop in CLAT score.

Other perfusion variables. No significant relationship was found between drop in CLAT score and three other
perfusion variables: hypothermia, lowest systemic
temperature and mean perfusion pressure.

REFERENCES

1. F. A. Freyhan, S. Gianelli Jr., R. A. O'Connel and
      J. A. Mayo, Psychiatric complications following
      open heart surgery, Comprehen Psychiatry
      12:181-195 (1971).
2. C. P. Kimball, The experience of open heart surgery
      III, Toward a definition and understanding of
      postcardiotomy delirium, Arch Gen Psychiatry.
      27:57-63 (1972).
3. D. M. Quinlan, C. P. Kimball and F. Osborne, The
      experience of open heart surgery IV: Assessment of

disorientation and dysphoria following cardiac surgery, Arch Gen Psychiatry. 31:241-244 (1974).

4. S. S. Heller, K.A. Frank, J. R. Malm, F. O. Bowman, P. D. Harris, M. H. Charlton, and D. S. Kornfeld, Psychiatric complications of open heart surgery: A re-examination, New Eng J Med. 283:1015-1020 (1970).

5. D. S. Kornfeld, S. S. Heller, K. A. Frank and R. Moskowitz, Personality and psychological factors in postcardiotomy delirium, Arch Gen Psychiatry. 31:249-253 (1974).

6. H. M. Tufo, A. M. Ostfeld and R. Shekelle, Central nervous system dysfunction following open heart surgery, JAMA. 212:1333-1340 (1970).

7. P. H. Blachly and A. Starr, Post-cardiotomy delirium. Am J Psychiatry. 121:371-375 (1964).

8. N. Egerton and J. H. Kay, Psychological disturbances associated with open heart surgery, Brit J Psychiatry. 110:433-439 (1964).

9. S. Gilman, Cerebral disorders after open heart operations, New Eng J Med. 272:489-498 (1965).

10. P. Gotze and B. Dahme, Psychopathological syndromes and neurological disturbances before and after open heart surgery, in: "Psychic and Neurological Dysfunctions after Open Heart Surgery," H. Speidel and G. Rodewald, eds., Georg Thieme Verlag, Stuttgart (1980) pp 48-67.

11. W. Spehr and P. Gotze, Computerized encephalogram before and after open heart surgery (preliminary results) in: "Psychic and Neurological Dysfunctions After Open Heart Surgery," H. Speidel and G. Rodewald, eds., Georg Thieme Verlag, Stuttgart (1980), pp. 67-73.

12. H. Pokar and G. Huse-Kleinstoll, Possible intra-operative influences by anesthesia and ECC on postoperative psychic dysfunctions, in "Psychic and Neurological Dysfunctions After Open Heart Surgery," H. Speidel and G. Rodewald, eds., Georg Thieme Verlag, Stuttgart (1980) pp. 130-134.

13. D. B. Longmore, The value of protacyclins in cardio-pulmonary bypass, in: "Towards Safer Cardiac Surgery," D. B. Longmore, ed., G. K. Hall Medical Publishers, Boston (1981), pp 355-377.

14. R. Meyendorf, Psychopathology in heart disease aside from cardiac surgery: A historical perspective of cardiac psychosis, in: "Psychic and Neurological Dysfunctions After Open Heart Surgery," H. Speidel and G. Rodewald, eds., Georg Thieme Verlag, Stuttgart (1980), pp 14-19.

15. R. Meyendorf, Psychopathology in heart disease aside from cardiac surgery: A historical perspective of cardiac psychosis, Comprehen Psychiatry 20: 326-331 (1979).
16. K. A. Sotaniemi, A. Juolasmaa and E. T. Hokkanen, Neuropsychologic outcome after open heart surgery, Arch Neurol. 38:208 (1981)
17. T. Åberg and J. Kihlgren, Effect of open heart surgery on intellectual function, Scand J Thor Cardiovasc Surg (Suppl. 15), 1974.
18. T. Åberg and M. Kihlgren, Effect of open heart surgery on intellectual function, Comments, Scand J Thor Cardiovasc Surg. 10:221 (1976).
19. T. Åberg and M. Kihlgren, Cerebral protection during open heart surgery: A comparison between a disk oxygenator and two bubble oxygenators. Thoraxchirug. 25:146 (1977a).
20. T. Åberg and M. Kihlgren, Cerebral production during open heart surgery, Thorax. 32:525 (1977b).
21. T. Åberg and M. Kihlgren, The use of psychometric testing as a quality criterion in open heart surgery, in: "Psychic and Neurological Dysfunctions After Open Heart Surgery," H. Speidel and G. Rodewald, eds., Georg Thieme Verlag, Stuttgart, (1980), pp. 107-111.
22. H. Gilberstadt and Y. Sako, Intellectual and personality changes following open heart surgery, Arch Gen Psychiatry. 16:210-214 (1967).
23. W. S. Priest, M. S. Zaks, G. K. Yacorzynski and B. Boshes, The neurological psychiatric and psychologic aspects of cardiac surgery, Med Clin American. 41:155-169 (1957).
24. M. S. Zaks, Longitudinal research studies of effects of heart disease and cardiac surgery on psychologic and neurologic functioning, in: "Research Approaches to Psychiatric Problems," T. T. Toulentes, S. I. Pollack, and H. E. Himwich, eds., Grune and Stratton, New York (1962) pp 164-178.
25. A. E. Willner, C. J. Rabiner, B. G. Wisoff, M. Hartstein, F. A. Struve and D. F. Klein, Analogical reasoning and postoperative outcome, Arch Gen Psychiatry. 33:255-259 (1976).
26. A. E. Willner, C. J. Rabiner, B. G. Wisoff, J. Fishman, B. Rosen, M. Hartstein and D. F. Klein, Analogy tests and psychopathology at follow-up after open heart surgery, Biological Psychiatry. 11:687-696 (1976).
27. A. E. Willner and C. J. Rabiner, Psychopathology and cognitive dysfunction five years after open heart surgery, Comprehen Psychiatry. 20:409-418 (1979).

28. D. W. Bethune, The Assessment of organic brain damage following open heart surgery, in: "Psychic and Neurological Dysfunctions After Open Heart Surgery," H. Speidel and G. Rodewald, eds., George Thieme Verlag, Stuttgart (1980). pp 100-106.

29. D. W. Bethune, Psychometric testing in the evaluation of the postoperative cardiac patient, in: "Towards Safer Cardiac Surgery," D. B. Longmore, ed., G. K. Hall Medical Publishers, Boston (1981), pp. 613-617.

30. W. H. Lee, W. Miller Jr., J. Rowe, P. Hairston and M. P. Brady, Effects of extracorporeal circulation on personality and cerebration, Ann Thor Surg. 7: 562-570 (1969).

31. K. A. Frank, S. S. Heller, D. S. Kornfeld and J. R. Malm, Long-term effects of open heart surgery on intellectual functioning, J Thor Cardiovasc Surg 64:811 (1972).

32. A. Joulasmaa, J. Outakoski, R. Hirvenoja, P. Tienari, K. Sotaniemi and J. Takkunen, Effect of Open Heart Surgery on Intellectual Performance, J Clin Neuropsychol. 3:181-197 (1981).

33. P. Smith, T. Treasure, S. P. Newman, P. Joseph, P. Ell, M. Harrison, Cerebral consequences of cardiopulmonary bypass, Lancet. 1:823-825 (1986).

34. S. P. Newman, P. Smith, T. Treasure, P. Joseph, P. Ell and M. Harrison, Acute neuropsychological consequences of coronary bypass surgery, Curr Psychol. Res. Rev. 6:115-124 (1987).

35. J. W. Garvey, A. E. Willner, A. Wolpowitz, L. Caramante, C. J. Rabiner, D. Weiss and B. J. Wisoff, The effect of arterial filtration during open heart surgery on cerebral function. Circulation (Suppl. II). 68:125-128 (1983).

36. A. E. Willner, L. Caramante, J. W. Garvey, A. Wolpowitz, C. J. Rabiner, D. Weiss and B. G. Wisoff, The relationship between arterial filtration during open heart surgery and impaired mental abstraction ability. Proceedings of the American Academy of Cardiovascular Perfusion, Volume 4 (1983).

37. A. E. Willner, Towards development of more sensitive clinical tests of abstraction: The analogy test. Proceedings, 78th Annual Convention, American Psychological Assocation, 553-554 (1970).

38. A. E. Willner, An experimental analysis of analogical reasoning. Psychological Reports Monograph Supplement. 15:479-494 (1964).

39. A. E. Willner, Conceptual Level Analogy Test. Copyright, 1971.

40. A. E. Willner, F. A. Struve, An analogy test that
    predicts EEG abnormality: use with hospitalized
    psychiatric patients. <u>Archives of General
    Psychiatry</u>. 23:428-437 (1970).
41. W. J. Kelleher, B. D. Townes, and D. C. Martin,
    <u>Psychological Reports</u>. 54:971-976 (1984).
42. A. E. Willner, C. J. Rabiner, B. Wisoff, M. Hartstein,
    F. A. Struve and D. F. Klein, Analogical reasoning
    and postoperative outcome: predictions for
    patients scheduled for open heart surgery.
    <u>Archives of General Psychiatry</u>. 33:255-259 (1976).
43. A. E. Willner, C. J. Rabiner, B. G. Wisoff, J.
    Fishman, B. Rosen, M. Hartstein, and D. F. Klein,
    Analogy tests and psychopathology at follow-up
    after open heart surgery, <u>Biological Psychiatry</u>.
    11:698-705 (1976).
44. A. E. Willner and C. J. Rabiner, Psychopathology and
    cognitive dysfunction five years after open heart
    surgery, <u>Comprehensive Psychiatry</u>. 20:409-418
    (1979).
45. F. A. Struve and A. E. Willner, Cognitive dysfunction
    and tardive dyskinesia. <u>British Journal of
    Psychiatry</u>. 143:597-600 (1983).
46. F. A. Struve and A. E. Willner, A long term prospective
    study of electroencephalographic and neuropsycho-
    logical correlates of tardive dyskinesia: Initial
    findings at five year follow-up, <u>Clinical
    Electroencephalography</u>. 14:186-201 (1983).
47. F. A. Struve, P. P. Ramsey, J. Kane and A. E. Willner,
    Neuropsychological and electroencephalographic
    correlates of neuroleptic induced involuntary
    mov ments: Implications for tardive dyskinesia,
    <u>in</u>: "Neurospychology and Cognition," Volume 2,
    R. N. Malatesta and L. C. Hartlage, eds., NATO
    Advanced Study Institute Series, Martins Nijhoff
    Publishers, The Hague, Holland, (1982).
48. B. Burns, The Conceptual Level Analogy Test, the
    Bender-Gestalt Test and the WAIS Vocabulary Test as
    predictors of death and of level of cognitive
    functioning in the community-living elderly.
    Unpublished Doctoral Dissertation, Hofstra
    University (1985).
49. R. J. Yohman, O. A. Parsons, Verbal reasoning deficits
    in alcoholics, <u>The Journal of Nervous and Mental
    Diseases</u>. 175:219 (1987).

CHANGES IN PSYCHOMETRIC TEST SCORES AFTER CARDIAC SURGERY

Nancy Feys-Dunne   and   Allen E. Willner

Project Coordinator   Department of Psychiatry
St. Francis Hospital   Hillside Hospital
Evanston, Illinois   Long Island Jewish
                        Medical Center
                        Glen Oaks, New York

Five hundred patients were entered into the study "Neurological and Psychological Aspects of the Impact of Cardiac Surgery on the Quality of Life." When the study is complete, another five hundred patients will have been entered. At that time the data reported herein will be altered, perhaps significantly. We ask that you reflect upon these data as indicators, providing direction and guidance as to the definition of the distinct subgroup of patients whose established, but undefined, existence provided the impetus for this study.

Each hospital in the study followed the same protocol although the selection for surgery, amount of time between being informed of the need for surgery and the actual surgery, and hospital admission procedures varied greatly. Patients participated in psychometric testing on three occasions - before surgery, before release from the hospital, and one year later. The test results used for this presentation reflect only the pre- and postoperative scores. Although five hundred cases were entered for preliminary results, the number of patients who participated in both pre- and postoperative testing varied both for the testing sessions and for the individual tests administered at each session. Many variables interfered with complete patient participation, and all examiners learned to adapt to each patient and family. Interference arose from every posible innocuous situation (glasses

Impact of Cardiac Surgery on the Quality of Life
Edited by A. E. Willner and G. Rodewald
Plenum Press, New York, 1990

missing, early release, upset family member, ad infinitum)
to emotional, neurological, and physical factors. The
session itself lasted between one and two hours, with some
exceptions.

The psychometric tests were the Bethune-Williams
Visual Memory Test, CLAT analogy test, Figure Rotation,
Trails B, WAIS Block Design, and WAIS Digit Symbol. The
CLAT analogy test has been described by Dr. Willner in
the preceding chapter [1, 2].

The Bethune-Williams Visual Memory Test assesses
delayed memory recall. The patient is shown pictures of
commonplace objects and required to recall them from
memory. Recall occurs at three levels: first, spon-
taneously; second, the recall of still unremembered
items is encouraged with verbal cues; and finally, the
remaining items are sought from among many items on a
card. Performance on this test is affected by organicity,
anxiety, and distractibility. Low scores indicate better
performance.

The Aberg Figure Rotation Test is a test of visual
spatial ability in which the patient is required to
specify which of several figures represent rotations of
the sample figure. Figure rotation is a complex cognitive
function. It requires verbal comprehension in order to
understand the directions. It is responsive to right
brain functioning, and deals with distinguishing essential
from non essential items. Performance is subject to
anxiety and organicity (both or either could affect concentration or comprehension), time pressure, a certain
level of distractibility, and visual scanning. Scoring is
done on a correct-incorrect basis and higher scores
indicate better performance.

The Trailmaking Test Part B is a test of mental
flexibility in which one is required to connect a set
of circles in an alternating number and letter sequence,
e.g., 1, A, 2, B, 3, C, etc. Trails B is a test of visual-
motor coordination, which involves integrated brain
function and tests the ability to do sequencing and
immediate recall. Performance is subject to organicity,
anxiety, distractibility, and psychomotor speed. Errors
affect the score and lower scores indicate better
performance.

The WAIS Block Design subtest requires the patient
to put together colored blocks so that they match the geo-

metric pattern on a display card. The WAIS Block Design
tests visual-motor coordination and visual perception of
abstract stimuli. It is an integrated brain function task
requiring the ability to synthesize. It is affected by
cognitive style (field-dependent versus field-independent),
time constraints, anxiety and organicity. Higher scores
indicate better performance [3].

     The WAIS Digit Symbol subtest requires the patient
to write in symbols next to numbers according to a given
code. WAIS Digit Symbol tests new learning ability, visual
perception of abstract stimuli, visual-motor coordination,
and paper-pencil skills. It requires integrated brain
functioning. It is affected by anxiety, organicity,
distractibility, and time constraints. The higher scores
indicate better performance [3].

     The results of simple mean comparisons pre- and
postoperatively for the psychometric tests are shown in
Table 1. For the CLAT analogy test there was a very small
non-significant decrease in mean score postoperatively.
The mean preoperative test score was quite low, only 57%
of the mean in the normative sample. The WAIS Digit
Symbol test showed a highly significant decrease in mean
score postoperatively, a drop of about one sixth of a
standard deviation. The mean preoperative score was low,
only 70% of the mean normative sample score. No postoperative change was found in WAIS Block Design scores.
The mean preoperative score was almost identical to the
mean normative sample score, at 98% of the normative
value. The Trails B test showed a significant worsening
postoperatively, a change of 0.12 standard deviations.
The Figure Rotation test, however, showed a highly
significant <u>increase</u> in scores postoperatively. Finally
the Bethune-Williams Visual Memory Test showed no change
in scores postoperatively.

DISCUSSION

     The results of these simple mean comparisons were as
follows: two tests showed a modest but highly significant
worsening in score (WAIS Digit Symbol and Trails B), one
showed a modest but highly significant improvement in
scores (Figure Rotation) and the remaining three showed
no significant change. These results indicate no major
changes in cognitive functioning for the sample as a
whole.

However, as was be discussed by Dr. Willner in the preceding chapter, there is a substantial subgroup of patients who show a postoperative drop in test scores of at least one standard deviation. The presence of this subgroup is obscured when one studies only mean differences. This subgroup requires close investigation to see whether their drop in cognitive test scores is related to parameters of the cardiac surgery as well as to neurological symptoms and psychopathology.

Table 1

SIMPLE MEAN COMPARISONS FOR PRE AND
POSTOPERATIVE PSYCHOMETRIC TEST SCORES

Test	X Preop	X Postop	X Diff.	P	N	r
CLAT	5.72	5.55	-0.17	.17	408	.86
WAIS D.Symb.	6.96	6.42	-.054***	.000	373	.74
WAIS B.D.	9.76	9.74	-0.01	.93	368	.72
Trails B	2.14	2.26	0.12*	.013	396	.68
Figure Rot.	14.53	15.70	1.17***	.000	241	.68
B-W	25.53	25.91	0.38	.58	355	.52

CLAT = 57% of preoperative mean score in norm. sample.
D.Sym. = 70% of preoperative mean score in norm. sample.
B.D. = 98% of preoperative mean score in norm. sample.

REFERENCES

1. A. E. Willner, C. J. Rabiner, B. G. Wisoff, M. Hartstein, R.A. Struve, D. F. Klein, Analogical reasoning and postoperative outcome. Archives of General Psychiatry, 33:255, 1976.
2. A. E. Willner, C. J. Rabiner, Psychopathology and cognitive dysfunction five years after open heart surgery. Comprehensive Psychiatry. 20:409 (1979).
3. A. S. Kaufman, "Intelligence Testing with the WISC-R." John Wiley & Sons, New York (1979).

2. A. E. Willner, C. J. Rabiner, Psychopathology and
        cognitive dysfunction five years after open heart
        surgery. Comprehensive Psychiatry. 20:409 (1979).
3. A. S. Kaufman, "Intelligence Testing with the WISC-R."
        John Wiley & Sons, New York (1979).

THE PERSISTENCE OF NEUROPSYCHOLOGICAL DEFICITS TWELVE

MONTHS AFTER CORONARY ARTERY BYPASS SURGERY

Stanton Newman, Louise Klinger, Graham Venn,
Peter Smith, Michael Harrison and Tom Treasure

University College & Middlesex School of
Medicine
(University of London) & Middlesex Hospital

INTRODUCTION

That some cardiac surgery results in brain damage
has been known for some time and has been demonstrated in
pathological findings [1,2]. Much current attention has
focused specifically on coronary artery bypass surgery
(CABS) which has seen a dramatic increase in recent
years. The techniques and time on extracorporeal circulation have, however, changed considerably over the years
and studies performed some time ago may not provide an
accurate picture of the frequency of deficits with
current surgical practice [3].

Neuropsychological assessment provides a sensitive
technique with which to evaluate brain functioning
following CABS, although care needs to be exercised in
the nature and number of assessments performed. In particular, tests which are sensitive to diffuse cortical
damage and not overly susceptible to practice effects
should be applied. In addition, a sufficient number of
different forms of tests need to be applied in order to
sufficiently sample a range of cognitive behaviors. The
analysis of the data also needs to be performed with
care. This issue will be discussed in more detail below.

We have been studying the neuropsychological consequences of CABS for some time and have demonstrated that
a significant proportion of patients show deficits in the

Impact of Cardiac Surgery on the Quality of Life
Edited by A. E. Willner and G. Rodewald
Plenum Press, New York, 1990

period immediately following surgery. When assessed 8
days following surgery, 73% of CABS patients showed significant neuropsychological deficits [4]. Both age and
the duration of bypass were found to be associated with
neuropsychological deficit at this time. When the patients
were assessed 8 weeks after surgery, the frequency of
neuropsychological deficits was found to have dropped to
37%. These findings suggested that the 8 day assessments,
rather than reflecting long term disturbance, appeared to
be due to the short term effects of surgery.

This present study was performed to consider whether
the neuropsychological deficits observed up to 8 weeks
after surgery persisted up to 12 months after surgery.

Subjects

The sample studied to 12 months consisted of 66
patients undergoing routine CABS with a mean age of 55
years. Sixty-one were male and five female. This
comprises 96% of the sequential routine patients entered
into the study. Two patients died and one patient
declined to attend the 12 month assessment.

PROCEDURES

Surgery

Anesthesia and surgery were standardised as far as
possible for all patients. Volatile agents were avoided.
The CABS technique included a Stockert pump in pulsatile
mode, a bubble oxygenator (Bentley) primed with Hartmans
solution and no arterial line filtration. Flow was maintained at 2.4 litres/square meter/minute, dropping to 75%
of this value after core cooling to 28°C.

Neuropsychological Assessment

Verbal memory was assessed using the Rey Auditory
Verbal Learning Test. This test consists of a free
recall task of a fifteen item word list. The list is
repeated on 5 occasions followed by a new list. The
final section of the test involves an additional recall
of the original list.

Nonverbal memory was assessed by means of a computerised recognition test which consisted of a checker-

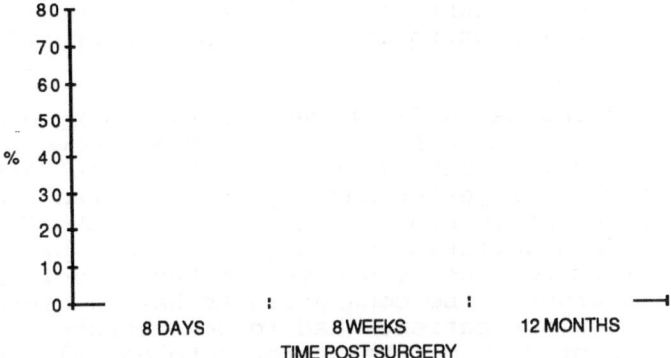

Fig. 1. Neuropsychological Deficits in CABS Patients.

board design presented to the patient for 10 seconds followed by three designs, one of which was identical to the original. Two tests were perfomed at different levels of difficulty, each with fifteen designs. The number of correct responses and the speed of response were recorded.

The Trail Making Tests A and B were administered to assess attention and concentration. These tests require the individual to draw lines to connect consecutively numbered circles (Part A) and consecutively numbered and lettered circles (Part B) as rapidly as possible.

A Letter Cancellation Task required the subject to work as quickly as possible through an array of 90 letters crossing out every occurrence of the letter 'p.'

The Purdue Pegboard where the subject places, one at a time, as many pegs as possible into a ine of holes in thirty seconds. The first trial using preferred hand, the second trial with the non-preferred and both hands simultaneously on the last trial.

A computerised two choice reaction time task.

A Symbol Digit Replacement Test automated on an Apple 2e microcomputer in which the subject has 'to type' the appropriate number which corresponds to a particular symbol. After 20 practice trials, 50 test items were presented.

The Block design subtest of the Wechsler Adult
Intelligence Test was performed to assess visuospatial
functioning.

Neuropsychological deficit was calculated by considering the change in performance from the preoperative
assessment to the 12 month assessment. For each test a
standard deviation of performance was constructed from
all of the preoperative scores. Any patients showing a
drop of 1 standard deviation or more from their preoperative performance was considered to have a deficit in
that test. In order to be considered to have a neuropsychological deficit patients had to demonstrate
deficits in two or more of the neuropsychological tests.

Statistical analysis was non-parametric with the
Mann Whitney U test.

RESULTS

Twenty-nine percent of patients showed deficits at
the 12 month assessment. In order to compare this
percentage to the numbers of patients with deficits at
earlier assessments they are displayed together in Figure
1. These findings suggest the deficits observed at 8
weeks represents relatively stable neuropsychological
deficits which tend to persist up to 12 months after
surgery.

The major explanations for the neuropsychological
deficits observed in CABS are embolic in nature and/or
perfusion related. Whichever cause is considered the
most likely, it should be expected that the tendency for
deficits should increase as the duration of bypass
increases simply because the cumulative effects of emboli
and/or extracorporeal circulation should, over time,
increase the probability of detectable neuropsychological
deficits. An analysis of bypass time between those
patients showing deficits at 12 months and those without
deficit indicated a significantly longer bypass in the
group with neuropsychological deficits (p<0.05). In
addition, the duration of the operation was found to be
longer in those with deficits (p<.02). These results are
displayed in Table 1.

Our previous research has demonstrated that older
patients appear to be more susceptible to neuropsychological deficits in CABS. This was confirmed in this

Table 1. Preoperative and Surgical Differences Between
          Those Patients With and Without Neuro-
          psychological Deficits Twelve Months After CABS

	DEFICIT	NO DEFICIT	
AGE (median)	58.0 years	53.0 years	p < .01
10-90th %ile	47 - 68	42 - 64	
OPERATION TIME			
(median)	270 mins	240 mins	p < .02
10-90th %ile	180-348	174-348	
BYPASS TIME			
(median)	95 MINS	80 MINS	p < .05
10-90th %ile	65-119	51-130	

study where the patients with deficit were significantly
older than those without deficit (p<0.01).

DISCUSSION

     This study has confirmed that neuropsychological
deficits persist to twelve months after CABS. These
findings also emphasize the value of a sensitive battery
of neuropsychological tests to detect the deficits
observed in these patients. The validity of the data is
supported by the associations found with the duration of
bypass and surgery. These are associations that have
been reported in other studies with different assessment
procedures and definition of deficit [2, 4-7]. In
addition, the increased vulnerability with age has been
reported in other studies [2, 6].

     The technique of analysis used in this study is to
be contrasted with some recent reports where it has been
claimed that no neuropsychological deficits are discern-
ible following CABS [8]. When analysing neuropsychological data some other authors have chosen to compare
group data rather than analysing individual data. The
difficulty with group data analysis is that it assumes
deficits in all patients and denies the possibility of
some learning which is common in neuropsychological

tests. To take a hypothetical example, if approximately
20% of patients show some deterioration and approximately
60% show some learning effects, with the remaining
showing no change, then the overall trend will be towards
some improvement. Group data analysis consequently fails
to detect those patients with deficits and it is only by
considering individual performance that the deficits may
be detected.

The findings in this paper support the belief that
there are imperfections in the current practice of CABS
and that deficits persist despite the reduction in time
on extracorporeal circulation.

Acknowledgments

We would like to acknolwedge the generous support of
the Jules Thorn Charitable trust.

REFERENCES

1. J. D. Brierly, Brain damage complicating open heart
    surgery: A neuropathological study of 46
    patients, Proc R Soc Med. 60:858-859 (1967).
2. T. Aberg, and M. Kihlgren, Effect of open heart
    surgery on intellectual function, Scand J Thorac
    Cardiovasc Surg. Suppl 15 (1974).
3. S. P. Newman, The incidence and nature of neuro-
    psychological mobidity following cardiac surgery,
    Perfusion, 4:93-100 (1989).
4. W. H. Lee, M. P. Brady, J. M. Rowe, and W. C. Miller,
    Effects of extracorporeal circulation upon
    behaviour, personality, and brain function:
    Part 2, Haemodynamic, metabolic, and psychometric
    correlations, Ann Surg. 173:1013-1023 (1971).
5. T. Aberg, and M. Kihlgren, Cerebral protection during
    open heart surgery, Thorax. 27:748-753 (1977).
6. J. A. Savageau, B. Stanton, C. D. Jenkins, M. D.
    Klein, Neuropsychological dysfunction following
    elective cardiac operation. 1. Early assessment,
    J Thorac Cardiovasc Surg. 84:585-594 (1982).
7. J. W. Garvey, A. Willner, A. Wolpowitz, L. Caramante,
    C. J. Rabiner, D. Weisz, and B.G. Wisoff, The
    effects of arterial line filtration during open
    heart surgery on cerebral function, Circulation.
    68:125-128 (1983).

8. H. Klonoff, C. Clark, D. Kavanagh-Grey, H. Mizgala, and I. Munro, Two-year follow-up study of coronary bypass surgery, <u>J Thorac Cardiovasc Surg.</u> 97:78-85 (1989).

NEUROPSYCHOLOGICAL FUNCTIONING FOLLOWING

CARDIOPULMONARY BYPASS

Maud van Foreest

Medical Centre "De Klokkenberg"
Breda
The Netherlands

INTRODUCTION

Since the beginning of heart surgery (about 30 years ago) neurological and psychiatric complications have been mentioned. During the past decade serious complications have decreased considerably, thanks to great improvements in surgical equipment and techniques. Mortality rates have steadily fallen: in recent years fatal cerebral damage of 0.3 - 2% has been found [1]. In many subsequent studies neurological morbidity has been recognized using different methods of assessment. Despite the many improvements there is still little reason for complacency. Extracorporeal circulation (ECC) still implies a risk for cerebral functioning. Incidence of cerebral damage has been estimated at many different percentages depending on its classification and the criteria that are used. The classification may vary from fatal cerebral damage to mild cognitive changes.

This study focuses on the less dramatic but more common syndromes of cerebral dysfunction seen after cardiopulmonary bypass (CPB), which tends to result in cognitive changes. These disturbances may be mostly reversible but in a number of cases they may be permanent; so there is clearly a major cause for concern. Neuro-psychologic testing is very well suited for measuring the effects of heart surgery on postoperative functioning.

Impact of Cardiac Surgery on the Quality of Life
Edited by A. E. Willner and G. Rodewald
Plenum Press, New York, 1990

CAUSES FOR CEREBRAL DYSFUNCTIONING

The understanding of cerebral events related to CPB is far from complete, despite extensive literature on the subject during the past 2 decades. Clinical and neuro-pathological data implicate the following possible causes for cerebral dysfunctioning.

Macroembolization

In the case of macroembolization, the cellular damage in the brain is associated with a massive cerebral embolism of air, calcium and other small particles. Recovery from the focal lesions is often incomplete and residual neurological deficits may appear. Nowadays macroembolism is fortunately rare in heart surgery [1, 2].

Microembolization

The occurrence of microembolism is still regarded as an important cause for postoperative cerebral dysfunction. Microembolism may be due to air embolization, particle embolization, embolization from blood products and fat embolization.

Gaseous microemboli may result from oxygenation, from air injected with cardioplegic solutions, from air injected with pressure in measuring needles and cannulae, from air suspended in cold blood causing bubbles when the blood is rewarmed, from areas of low pressure in the perfusion circuit or from air left behind or introduced into the heart by the surgeon [1, 2, 3].

Particle microemboli that enter the patient during bypass may consist of: silicone and polivinyl chloride tubing fragments, precipitates and particles in the prime and added fluids, etc. Whatever the source of these microemboli may be, all are equally dangerous and can be the center of thrombus formation [1, 2,].

Embolization from blood products may consist of platelet, leukocyte and fibrine aggregates, which may develop during ECC despite adequate heparinization. These aggregates are also present in donated, stored blood. When blood passes over a foreign surface (such as extracorporeal tubing), the clotting systems are stimulated. Platelet adhesion and activation occurs and thus results in formation of platelet and cellular aggregates. These aggregates are always present in blood from the extracorporeal circuit and can be responsible for thrombotic occlusion of the microvasculature.

The use of micropore filters has gained considerable attention in attempting to remove potentially harmful debris in the blood passing back to the patient. Although filtration still remains a controversial subject with regard to clinical need, there is little controversy regarding the efficacy of modern filters to remove microemboli [4].

Duration of Perfusion

The duration of perfusion seems to be a clearly defined determinant of postoperative cerebral outcome. A number of investigators agree on the fact that the duration of perfusion, longer than 2 hours, should be considered as a significant cause for cerebral damage after CPB.

Inadequate Cerebral Perfusion

There seems to be an obvious role for hypoperfusion in the pathogenesis of CPB related cerebral injury. Hypoperfusion may result from low flow, non-pulsatile bloodflow, incorrect placement of the aortic cannula and cerebrovascular occlusive disease.

Age

Most authors agree that advanced age is a serious risk factor in the development of cerebral complications following cardiac operations. One may assume that these patients have a higher degree of arteriosclerosis in their cerebral vessels. Diminished neuronal reserve may also be a factor. The age of 60 years and above is often mentioned as risky. Sotaniemi (1980) concludes that age itself is not a matter of importance but rather the state of the regulatory mechanisms of circulation [5].

Intraoperative Hypotension

The onset of ECC causes an abrupt and sometimes profound reduction in cerebral perfusion. In the literature there is conflicting evidence regarding the importance of low mean arterial pressure (MAP) levels in the pathogenesis of cerebral injury. When the perfusion of certain brain areas falls below critical ischaemic thresholds, irreversible hypoxic brain damage may occur.

Several studies have suggested cerebral cellular damage
when MAP levels fall below 50 mmHg. Taylor (1982) argues
that the brain is probably much more resistant to reduced
perfusion pressures and that hypothermia offers considerable protection under low-flow, low-pressure perfusion
conditions [2]. It appears that pharmacological support
is not necessary to maintain a constant CBP between a MAP
of 30 and 110 mmHg during CPB. This is probably due to
autoregulation of cerebral blood flow (CBF) during
hypothermic CPB [6].

Type of Oxygenator

     The oxygenator is known to be an important source for
emboli. It has been proven that membrane oxygenators
produce less emboli than bubble oxygenators. Several
studies report less cerebral impairment in patients
perfused with a membrane oxygenator compared to those
perfused with a bubble oxygenator [7].

Existence of Previous Cerebral Disturbances

     Pre-existing even slight cerebral dysfunction makes
the brains of the patients especially vulnerable to the
strains of surgery. A history of neurological disease
and its type, severity and duration are preoperative
factors that may influence postoperative outcome [8].

Intraoperative Anticoagulation

     Heparin is used routinely as an anticoagulant. It
interrupts clotting at various levels, but stimulates
platelet aggregation. During bypass a 60% fall in platelet count is usual. Prostacyclin (PGI_2) is probably the
most platelet stabilizing substance yet discovered. In
several studies it has been shown to preserve platelet
number during CPB. Despite these promising results, there
seems to be no role for PGI_2 in CPB because of its powerful
vasodilatory effect, possibly causing a dangerous drop in
blood pressure. Future developments in prostaglandin
synthesis may result in better compounds [9].

     Until better anticoagulants are available, it might
be useful to administer drugs to protect the brain during
CPB. Barbiturates have been postulated to improve the
outcome of focal ischaemia by protecting cells that are
damaged but still capable of recovery. In 1986,
Nussmeyer, et al. published the first demonstration of
cerebral protection by a barbiturate in humans. They

found that patients pretreated with thiopental had a significantly lower incidence of neuropsychiatric complications than those who did not receive the drug. However,
they recommend searching for equally effective drugs
without the hemodynamic consequences and persistence of
thiopental [10].

Postoperative Factors

Cerebral complications have been closely attributed
to intraoperative factors. However, some postoperative
factors should not be overlooked. There have been reports
of postoperative cardiac arrhythmia as potential causes
for stroke.

A number of authors have stressed the importance of
postoperative factors, such as sensory and sleep depriva-
tion during the stay in the intensive care unit. These
factors may influence psychiatric derangement.

MATERIAL AND METHODS

The study in the Medical Centre De Klokkenberg,
Breda, the Netherlands, was set up to get further insight
in neuropsychologic functioning following CPB. Aspects of
memory (short term and long term), psychomotor functions,
visuo-spatial organization, orientation, concentration,
attention and response speed were investigated. The
patients were tested at: 14 days preoperatively and 8
days postoperatively. The characteristics of the treatment group are listed in Table 1.

Table 1. Characteristics of the treatment group

Sex: male	33	
female	10	
Age: mean $\pm$ sd	62.42 ± 5.42	
Symptom duration		
< 3 months	4	
3 - 6 months	14	
6 - 12 months	6	
> 12 months	19	
NYHA classification		
class I	2	
class II	5	
class III	36	

The selection criteria were the following:

- age 55 years and above.
- NYHA classification I, II, or III.
- no pre-operative evidence of neurospsychological lesions.
- no renal and/or hepatic dysfunction.
- no carotid problems.
- B-blockers : preoperatively   metoprolol
                postoperatively sotalol

A neurological check-up was done by a neurologist at both test periods.

The chosen protocol used the following tests in order of presentation to the patients:

- The Utrecht 15 word test, for short term memory, left hemisphere (LH).
- Luria's pictures I, for short term memory, right hemisphere (RH).
- Verbal fluency, regarding frontal functions which concern motor organization and higher integration (LH).
- WAIS block design, for visuospatial organization (RH). (This test is also sensitive to any kind of brain damage).
- Trail Making Test (TMT), version A and B, for orientation and concentration (LH and RH).
- Number Letter Substitution, a test which is comparable to the digit-symbol subtest of the WAIS. It measures psychomotor performance, attention and response speed (LH and RH), and is at the same time sensitive to any kind of brain damage.
- Luria's pictures II, for long term memory (RH).
- Delayed recall of the 15 word test, for long term memory (LH).
- Spielberger State-Trait Anxiety Inventory (STAI-DY), an anxiety scale.

At the end of the test battery some questions were asked about depression, tiredness, aggressiveness and motivation to join the investigation.

RESULTS

Since several investigators found that vigilance went down and reaction time went up with the use of B-blockers, an on-line search was done concerning the influence of

B-blockers on psychomotor performance. There turned out
to be a wide variation in the results of studies on the
subject. In general it appears that the use of B-blockers
produces effects on performance that may be comparable to
ordinary day-to-day variation. Nevertheless it was
decided to give the same B-blockers to all patients in the
trial.

    Four of the neuropsychological response variables had
significant differences between pre- and postoperative
results, as listed in Table 2.

Table 2. Significant test-results.

	F	df	P
Verbal fluency	9.567	1/41	< 0.01
WAIS Block Design	40.386	1/41	< 0.001
Number-Letter Substitution	9.211	1/40	< 0.01
Delayed Recall	17.986	1/42	< 0.001

    Consequently, these results point out a signficant
decline in long term memory, response speed, attention,
concentration and psychomotor performance. Concerning the
emotional function assessment with regard to anxiety,
depression, aggressiveness, tiredness and motivation to
join the investigation, no significant treatment effects
were found. So these factors had little or no overall
effect on cognitive performance.

DISCUSSION AND CONCLUSIONS

    One of the great difficulties in this kind of
investigation is the lack of time for a profound
neuropsychologic investigation. To screen a patient
thoroughly one needs a working day. Therefore it is very
important to have a combination of test materials that
best suit the purpose. Looking at the literature on the
subject, different investigators have used a great variety
of test materials. There is still little agreement, so

that communication about this subject is of utmost
importance. Moreover, studies regarding neuropsychologic
functioning following CPB have their pre-operative
baseline-measurement one or two days preoperatively. The
stress elicited by admission to the hospital and the fear
of the forthcoming operation may have influenced the
neurobehavioral response of the patients.

In order to prevent this baseline-problem as much as
possible, the tests in the study at hand were presented 14
days preoperatively. This may be the reason that there
were no signficant treatment-effects on the emotional
variables, as shown in the results. When the same tests
are presented a few weeks after each other, there is
always the risk of learning effects. In order to avoid
this problem as much as possible, parallel versions of
some tests were used (15 word test, verbal fluency,
number-letter substitution).

Postoperative brain injury is permanent in some
cases. There are several investigations indicating that
many patients recover two months, six months and even one
year postoperatively. Permanent brain injury should be
prevented as much as possible. Moreover, even transient
disturbances should be considered as potentially harmful.
A multidisciplinary approach is required involving
surgeons, anesthesiologists, perfusionists, cardiologists,
psychologists and manufacturers to study, identify and
eliminate the causes.

Acknowledgements

The author would like to thank those who contributed to
this study, especially J. Bach Kolling and C.H.M. Brunia;
and Mrs. E. Koornwinder for the preparation of this
typescript.

REFERENCES

1. P. J. Shaw, Neurological complications of cardio-
    vascular surgery: II. Procedures involving the
    heart and thoracic aorta, in: "Neurological and
    Psychological Complications of Surgery and Anes-
    thesia," B. J. Hindman, ed., Little, Brown and
    Company, Boston (1986).
2. K. N. Taylor, Brain damage during open heart surgery,
    Thorax 37 : 873 (1982).

3. A. G. Hill, R. C. Groom, R. P. Vinansky, et al.
    Gaseaous microemboli and extracorporeal
    circulation, Proceed Am Acad Cardiovasc Perfusion.
    7:131 (1986).
4. L. Marshall, Filtration in cardiopulmonary bypass:
    past, present and future, Perfusion, 3:135
    (1988).
5. K. A. Sotaniemi, Brain damage and neurological outcome
    after open heart surgery, J. Neurosurg Psychiatry.
    43:127 (1988).
6. A. V. Govier, J. G. Reves, Cerebral blood flow:
    autoregulation during cardiopulmonary bypass, in:
    "Brain Injury and Protection During Heart Surgery,"
    M. Hilberman, ed., Martinus Nijhoff Publishing,
    Boston, Dordrecht, Lancaster (1988).
7. R. C. Groom, A. G. Hill, R. P. Vinansky, et al.
    Hollow fiber membrane and bubble oxygenation: A
    comparison of psychometric test results, Proceed Am
    Acad Cardiovasc Perfusion. 6:70 (1985).
8. R. Kolkka, M. Hilberman, Neurologic dysfunction
    following cardiac operation with low-flow, low-
    pressure cardiopulmonary bypass, J Thoracic
    Cardiovas Surg. 79:432 (1980).
9. K. J. Fish, Microembolization: etiology and
    prevention, in: "Brain Injury and Protection
    During Heart Surgery," M. Hilberman, ed., Martinus
    Nijhoff Publishing, Boston, Dordrecht, Lancaster
    (1988).
10. N. A. Nussmeyer, C. Arlund, S. Slogoff, Neuro-
    psychiatric complications after cardiopulmonary
    bypass: Cerebral protection by a barbiturate.
    Anesthesiology. 64:165 (1986).

REPORTS OF COGNITIVE CHANGE, MOOD STATE AND ASSESSED

COGNITION FOLLOWING CORONARY ARTERY BYPASS SURGERY

Stanton Newman, Louise Klinger, Graham Venn,
Peter Smith, Michael Harrison and Tom Treasure

University College & Middlesex School of Medicine
(University of London) & Middlesex Hospital

INTRODUCTION

The impact of coronary artery bypass surgery (CABS) on the amelioration of angina and breathlessness has been dramatic with approximately 90% of patients reporting symptomatic improvement. In recent years this success has been clouded by studies which have indicated a deterioration in cognitive performance with formal neuro-psychological testing performed preoperatively and post-operatively [1, 2]. Studies investigating neuropsychological changes have confirmed that approximately 35% of patients show deficits 8 weeks post surgery [3], still detectable in 33% at one year [4].

Besides the formal studies showing cognitive change, some clinicians, whose patients are encouraged to discuss their own experiences at follow up visits, claim that some patients complain of a reduction in their ability to perform complex cognitive tasks. The question tackled in this study is whether the patients who complain of cognitive changes are the same as those who on testing are found to have deteriorated in their cognitive functions. In this way it considers the status of the reports of cognitive change that are presented in the clinic.

The likelihood of reporting symptoms is influenced by a range of psychological and social factors including mood

Impact of Cardiac Surgery on the Quality of Life
Edited by A. E. Willner and G. Rodewald
Plenum Press, New York, 1990

state. Although systematic prospective studies have
reported little change in psychiatric morbidity when
assessed 12 months after surgery, some have noted a transient depression to occur in a proportion of patients
[5-7]. One of the issues addressed in this paper is the
extent to which mood state influences the reports of
cognitive change.

Subjects

The sample consisted of 62 coronary artery bypass
surgery (CABS) patients (57 male and 5 female). The mean
age for the male group was 55.2 (s.d. 7.8) with a range of
between 37 and 71 and the mean age for the female group
was 54.5 (s.d. 8.8) with a range of between 44 and 65.

Procedures

The patients were seen and assessed before surgery
and at approximately one year for follow-up (mean 13.13
months, sd=1.54 months, range=11-16 months). On each
occasion a series of neuropsychological tests were
performed. The tests and the functions they examined are
described below:

1. The Rey Auditory Verbal Learning Test (verbal memory)
2. Two computerized non-verbal memory tests
3. The Trail Making Tests A and B (attention and
   concentration)
4. A Letter Cancellation Test (attention and
   concentration)
5. The Purdue Pegboard (perceptuomotor skills)
6. Two choice reaction time tests (attention and
   concentration)
7. A Symbol Digit Replacement Test (attention and
   concentration)

Two mood state measures were administered. State
anxiety was assessed by the Spielberger State 40-item
Inventory (STAI) and depression was assessed by the Beck
Depression Inventory (BDI). In addition to these measures
patients were also given a semi-structured interview which
included questions on perceived cognitive changes. These
questions looked at 9 areas of cognitive function;
patients indicated whether the particular aspect of
cognitive functioning had improved, deteriorated or showed
no change from before surgery.

RESULTS

Subjective Reports

The patients' responses to the nine item questionnaire on perceived cognitive function are shown in
Table 1. In order to see if perceived cognitive deficit
coincides with actual deficit in this group of patients,
the data from the self reported changes have been
collapsed into "improved" and "no change" versus "worse."

The most frequently reported area of difficulty is
memory, with 28% reporting that they were worse after
surgery (see Table 1). Problem solving (18%) is the next
most common cognitive complaint, followed by clarity of
thinking (16%) and concentration (16%).

Subjective Reports and Neuropsychological Assessment

Five particular questions related to the neuropsychological assessment; these are reported separately
below. The questions on problem solving ability, decision
making, clarity of thinking and making more mistakes are
either too broad or were not specifically addressed in the
neuropsychological tests. Complaints about specific cognitive functions were considered in relation to the appropriate neuropsychological test both in the form of absolute
performance at 12 months post surgery and as change scores
from the preoperative measures. In each case the patients
who reported a deterioration were compared to those who
reported an improvement or no change.

TABLE 1. Number of patients reporting reduced cognitive
abilities following CABS

		%	(No.)
1.	MEMORY	27.4	(17)
2.	PROBLEM SOLVING	17.7	(11)
3.	CLARITY OF THINKING	16.1	(10)
4.	CONCENTRATION	16.1	(10)
5.	MAKING MISTAKES	14.5	(9)
6.	ATTENTION	12.9	(8)+
7.	CLUMSINESS	9.7	(6)
8.	DECISION MAKING	8.1	(5)+
9.	SPEED OF RESPONSE	6.5	(4)*

*=2 patients failed to respond
+=1 patient failed to respond

The 17 (27%) patients who complained at 12 months of a deterioration in memory were found to be no different in their performance on the Rey Auditory Verbal Learning Test from the remaining subjects on either absolute scores at 12 months or change scores from their pre-operative performance. The performance between those with and without complaints of poor memory was not sig-nificantly different on either of the two non-verbal memory tests for either absolute or change scores.

Ten patients (16%) complained that their ability to concentrate had deteriorated since surgery. Their per-formance was compared to the remaining 52 patients on the five tests considered to reflect concentration. These are the Letter Cancellation Test, Trail Making A and B tests, The Symbol Digit Replacement Test and the Two Choice Reaction time task. On the absolute scores at 12 months only the findings on the Letter Cancellation Test approached significance where those reporting a deterioration in the ability to concentrate produced a longer mean time to complete the test (mean = 178. msec., s.d. 36.3) in contrast to the remaining subjects (mean 149, s.d. 42.4; t=1.99, p = 0.051). The two groups showed similar change scores from their preoperative performance in all five tests concerned with concentration at 12 months.

Thirteen percent of patients (n = 8) reported that their attentional abilities had deteriorated. On comparison of these subjects with the remaining 53 patients no significant differences were found in either absolute scores at 12 months post surgery or in change scores on the Letter Cancellation Test, Trail Making A and B tests, The Symbol Digit Replacement Test and the Two Choice Reaction Time task.

The subjective complaints of clumsiness were compared to performance on the Purdue Pegboard. The 6 subjects (10%) who complained of being more clumsy were not found to have performed differently to the remaining subjects at 12 months, and the change in their performance from before the operation to twelve months post surgery was also found to be similar to that of the remaining subjects.

Only four subjects (6.5%) complained of slowing since surgery. The low number makes statistical tests of little value but their performance on all the time tasks showed little or no difference to the remaining subjects.

Mood State Measures

1. **Anxiety**: The relationship between subjective complaints of cognition and state anxiety measures performed at 12 months post surgery is shown in Figures 1 & 2. Figure 1 shows the relationship between those reporting a deterioration (-VE) in thinking, memory, clumsiness and speed of response in relation to level of anxiety and those reporting either no change or an improvement (+OR=) 12 months following surgery. Figure 2 indicates the level of anxiety associated with complaints of problem solving, decision making, making mistakes, attention and concentration.

In all cases those patients who felt a deterioration in a particular aspect of cognitive ability had higher levels of anxiety than those who felt their cognition was unaltered or improved. For memory and concentration these differences were significant, while in all the other cases the differences failed to reach significance.

2. **Depression**: The relationship between the subjective complaints of deterioration of cognition and depression as measured on the Beck Depression Inventory is shown in Figures 3 & 4. In all cases the score on the Beck Depression Inventory was higher for those who considered their cognition had deteriorated. In all but three cases the differences were highly significant.

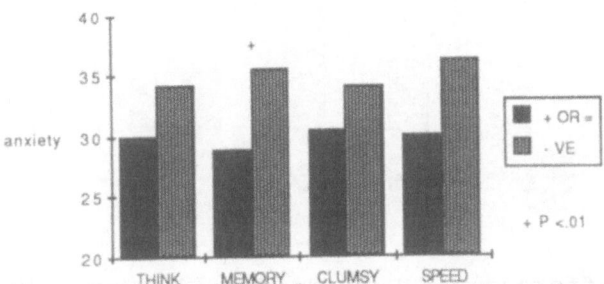

Fig. 1.   Differences in Anxiety Between Those Reporting Change and No Change in Cognitive Function.

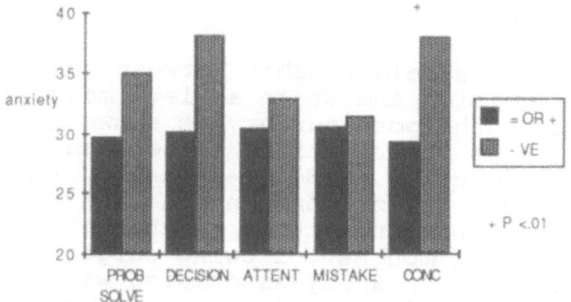

Fig. 2.   Difference in Anxiety Between Those Reporting
           Change and No Change in Cognitive Function.

DISCUSSION

    A number of studies have now shown that in a
proportion of patients CABS does produce deleterious
effects on the brain (See e.g. Newman, et al., this
volume). The question addressed in this paper was whether
those individuals who complain of some cognitive deterioration following surgery are the same as those detected
by formal neuropsychological assessment. Specifically, if
patients are able to identify themselves as showing
cognitive deterioration then the need for elaborate neuropsychological assessment will disappear. It is also
important that the complaints that some patients make at
follow-up clinics constitute the only information regarding cognitive functioning that is available to many
clinicians.

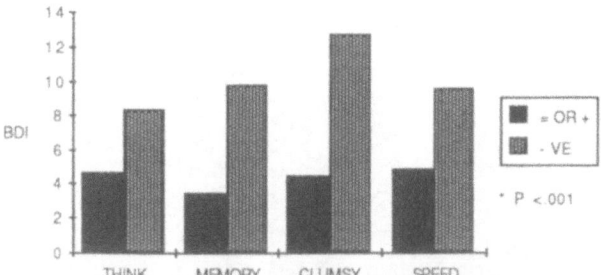

Fig. 3.   Difference in Depressed Mood Between Those
           Reporting Change and No Change in Cognitive
           function

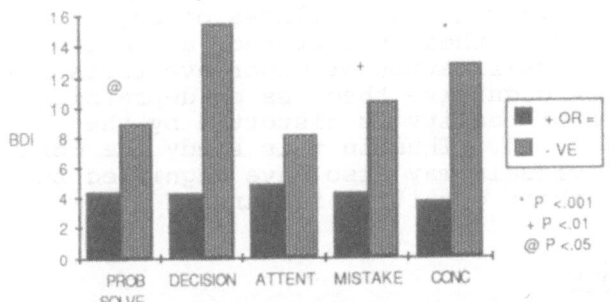

Fig. 4.   Difference in Depressed Mood Between Those
          Reporting Change and No Change in Cognitive
          Function

     The results of this study clearly indicate that
there is little relationship between self-reported changes
in cognitive function and assessed cognitive function.
The patients' complaints of cognitive change were not
reflected in their absolute performance or the change in
their performance from before surgery.

     The mood state of the patients, however, was found to
be associated with reports of deterioration in cognitive
function.   In all cases those patients who reported a
deterioration in a cognitive function were more depressed
and anxious that those who reported no change or an
improvement.   Difficulty in concentration is another
frequent complaint of patients who are depressed.   In this
study the patients who complained of difficulties in
concentration were found to be more depressed and more
anxious than the others in the sample.

     The mechanisms by which patients who are anxious and
of low mood report cognitive deficits after surgery in the
absence of assessed deterioration in cognition, may be
related to other research on the influence of mood on
memory and judgment [8, 9].   These studies have shown that
experimental manipulations of mood state influence
judgments of performance [10].   When judging health status
both memory (saliency of symptoms) and decision making
(appraisal of health status) are involved.   When mood is
manipulated perceptions of health status change in a
concurrent fashion [11].   One may speculate that the
patients in this study with low mood and/or higher levels
of anxiety may have had increased accessibility to their

memories of everyday normal failures of cognition and
consequently judged their performance as having deteriorated. The magnification of minor events is also
consistent with cognitive theories of depression where
the evaluation of reality is distorted by the
individual [12, 13]. Thus in this study the more
depressed individuals may also have magnified the
importance of their cognitive failures.

Acknowledgments

We would like to acknowledge the generous support of
the Jules Thorn Charitable trust.

REFERENCES

1. P. Smith, T. Treasure, S. P. Newman, P. Joseph, P.
   Ell, and M. Harrison, Cerebral consequences of
   cardiopulmonary bypass, Lancet 1: 823-825 (1986).
2. P. Shaw, D. Bates, N. Cartlidge, D. Heaviside, D.
   Julian, and D. Shaw, Early neurological complications of coronary artery bypass surgery, Br. Med
   J, 291:1384-1387 (1985).
3. S. P. Newman, P. Smith, T. Treasure, P. Joseph. P.
   Ell, and M. Harrison, Acute neuropsychological
   consequences of coronary artery bypass surgery,
   Curr Psychol Res Rev., 6:115-124 (1987).
4. G. Venn, L. Klinger, T. Treasure, S. P. Newman, M.
   Harrison, and P. Ell, Neuropsychological sequelae
   of bypass twelve months after coronary artery
   surgery, Br. Heart J., 57:565 (1987).
5. C. Bass, Psychosocial outcome after coronary artery
   bypass surgery, Br J Psychiat. 145:526-532 (1984).
6. R. S. Blacher, and R. J. Cleveland, Paradoxical
   depression after heart surgery, in: "Psychic and
   Neurological Dysfunctions after Open Heart
   Surgery," H. Speidel and G. Rodewald., eds.,
   Thieme Stratton, New York (1980).
7. S. P. Newman, P. Joseph. P. Smith, L. Klinger, G.
   Venn, M. Harrison, and T. Treasure, Psychiatric
   and self rated mood state changes after coronary
   artery bypass surgery, in preparation.
8. B. A. Marcopoulos, Self-reported memory, health and
   cognitive test performance in depressed and
   nondepressed elderly, J Clin Exp Neuropsychol.
   9:260 (1987).

9. A. M. Isen, Toward understanding the role of affect in cognition, in: "Handbook of Social Cognition, (Vol. 3)," R. Wyer and T. Scrull, eds., Lawrence Erlbaum, New Jersey (1984).

10. A. M. Isen, T. E. Shalker, M. S. Clark and L. Karp, Affect, accessibility of material in memory, and behaviour: A cognitive loop? J Pers Soc Psychol. 36:1-12 (1978).

11. R. T. Croyle and M. B. Uretsky, Effects of mood on self-appraisal of health status, Health Psychol., 6:239-253 (1987).

12. A. T. Beck, "Depression: Clinical, Experimental and Theoretical Aspects," Harper, New York (1967).

13. R. E. Ingram, and S. D. Hollon, Cognitive therapy of depression from an information processing perspective, in: "Information Processing Approaches to Clinical Psychology," R. E. Ingram, ed., Academic Press, New York (1986).

MEMORY FUNCTIONING AFTER CARDIAC SURGERY WITH CARDIO-PULMONARY BYPASS: COMPARISONS BETWEEN HEART AND BACK PATIENTS

Gregory W. Harter

Arkansas Rehabilitation
Institute
Little Rock, AR

J. Michael Williams

Hahnemann University
Philadelphia, PA

Wilburn E. George

Methodist Hospital
Memphis, TN

Murry Mutchnick
Ivan Torres

Memphis State
University
Memphis, TN

The risks for complications in CNS functioning following CPB-assisted cardiac surgery are reportedly higher than in other types of thoracic surgery without CPB assistance [1]. Neurological sequellae range from frank symptoms such as coma, seizures, or hemiparesis to less severe manifestations such as abnormal reflexes. In addition, many studies [2 - 6] have reported changes in neuropsychological functions such as visual-perceptual-motor skills, visual-spatial problem solving, and psychomotor speed. Often these changes are subclinical in nature, but nevertheless statistically significant.

Memory functioning has also been assessed in a number of studies, but the effects of CPB-assisted cardiac surgery on memory are less well understood. While a number of studies included memory measures, they frequently only compared subgroups of cardiac patients (e.g., those with frank neurological impairment versus those without

Impact of Cardiac Surgery on the Quality of Life
Edited by A. E. Willner and G. Rodewald
Plenum Press, New York, 1990

201

symptoms), reduced memory functions to a single measure
(e.g., MQ), or were methodologically flawed by poorly controlled practice effects or attrition. As it is now well-
established that memory is not a unidimensional function
[7], the use of single measures and screening devices may
exclude more specific memory effects of CPB surgery.

One particular area of memory functioning that has
been neglected in this literature is delayed recall. Many
patients with amnestic disorders will perform adequately
on immediate recall tasks, but if assessed in a delayed
recall format (e.g., 30 minutes later), these patients
manifest significant memory losses [8]. In looking for
patterns of subtle or early memory loss, such as might
occur after CPB, delayed recall tests might be expected to
be among the most sensitive measures.

In the literature on outcome from CPB surgery, a
comprehensive study of memory functioning, including
delayed recall measures, has been missing. This appears
to be a salient omission in light of data on patients with
transient ischemic attacks which suggest that memory
functions, particularly delayed recall functions, may be
among the first abilities to be compromised after cerebral
ischemic events [9 - 11]. Since one of the suspected
mechanisms of CNS compromise after surgery is inadequate
cerebral perfusion due to low arterial pressures and (or)
blood gas irregularities [12, 13], these patients may be
at risk for ischemic-based memory changes. In particular,
the hippocampus, a structure critical to memory consolidation processes, because of its location in a boundary zone
between the supply areas of the major cerebral arteries,
appears to be selectively vulnerable to partial ischemia
[14].

The purpose of this study was to comprehensively
assess memory functioning following CPB-assisted cardiac
surgery. Anecdotal reports, as well as limited survey
data, suggest that memory deficits after CPB procedures
may be an under-estimated CNS complication. CPB-assisted
cardiac surgery patients were compared with another
hospital patient group for pre-to-post changes in memory
functioning as assessed by a comprehensive memory battery.
A particular focus was delayed recall abilities. It was
expected that CPB patients would manifest significantly
more memory disruption than non-CPB patients, and that
delayed recall measures would prove especially sensitive
in detecting subtle, subclinical memory decrements.

METHOD

Subjects

The cardiac surgery group consisted of 38 patients who completed the study out of 47 patients who were randomly recruited between December 1986 and March 1988 at Methodist Hospital in Memphis. All potential subjects were briefed as to the purpose of the study, and those agreeing to participate signed informed consent forms. All patients in this group underwent elective coronary artery bypass graft (CABG) surgery, and three patients received additional heart surgery procedures as well. All of these procedures required cardiopulmonary bypass (CPB). Pediatric heart surgery cases (CA < 20) and emergency cardiac surgery patients who were too ill to undergo pre-operative psychological testing were excluded from the study.

The back patient comparison group consisted of 17 patients who completed the study out of 24 who were randomly selected and recruited from August, 1987 to March, 1988 at Methodist Hospital. All subjects signed informed consent forms after being briefed about the study. All of these patients had entered the hospital for myelograms to diagnose back pain problems and the possible need for back surgery (e.g., laminectomy). They were assessed using the memory tests prior to receiving myelograms to eliminate any deleterious confounding effects of that procedure (e.g., headache) on memory performance. Subsequently, 11 of the patients who completed the study had laminectomies, typically the day after their myelogram. Back patients with a history of heart surgery were excluded from the study.

The inclusion of back patients as a comparison group was dictated by the need for a relatively homogeneous group of patients who had a similar medical experience to the cardiac patients but without undergoing CPB. The only group at Methodist Hospital that met this general criterion in sufficient numbers were the back patients. Demographic comparisons between the two groups revealed one significant difference (see Table 1). On the average, the back patients were 10 years younger than the cardiac patients. In subsequent comparisons between cardiac and back patients, this difference was controlled statistically by treating age as a covariate.

Table 1. Group Comparisons on Demographic Variables

	Cardiac Group (N = 38)	Back Group (N = 17)	Test of Significance
Sex			
Males	27	10	$x^2 = 1.547$
Females	11	7	(df = 1, n.s.)
Race			
Whites	36	14	$x^2 = 0.027$
Blacks	2	3	(df = 1, n.s.)
Age			
Mean	57.34	47.00	t = 3.370**
S.D.	11.02	9.29	(df = 53)
Education			
Mean	12.37	11.35	t = 0.132
S.D.	3.30	2.64	(df = 53, n.s.)

**p < .01   n.s. = Not significant at .05 level

Procedure

Pretesting. Cardiac patients were tested one to two days prior to surgery. Back patients were tested either the day before or the same day as their scheduled myelograms. All patients were tested in their hospital rooms.

Posttesting. Six to eight weeks after their hospitalization, patients were retested in their own homes. Subjects were given the alternate form of the memory scale they received at pretesting with order effects controlled by counterbalancing.

Measures

Vermont Memory Scale (VMS). This comprehensive memory scale in alternate forms A and B, assesses verbal and visual-spatial consolidation using immediate and delayed recall formats. Subtests measure list learning ability, story recall, digit span, spatial span, recognition of geometric designs, reproduction of geometric

designs from memory, and a names-faces recognition task
[15, 16]. Based on percentage correct scores, composite
scores for immediate verbal memory, immediate spatial
memory, delayed verbal memory, and delayed spatial memory
were computed for each subject. These composite scores
were further aggregated to form a VMS verbal summary score
(immediate + delayed recall) and a VMS spatial summary
score (immediate + delayed recall). A previous investigation [16] of the verbal and spatial subscales found
alternate forms and test-retest reliabilities that ranged
from .62 to .88. In a validity study using discriminant
analysis, the VMS was found to classify 95 per cent of
organically amnestic patients (n = 12) and normal subjects
(n = 62) as compared to an 88 per cent classification rate
for the Wechsler Memory Scale [16].

Statistical Analyses

A multivariate analysis of variance (MANOVA) with one
between group factor and one within subject (repeated
measures) factor was performed using VMS summary scores
(based on percentage correct scores). In this analysis,
the cardiac group was compared with the back group for
change, pre-to-post, in 4 areas of memory functioning:
immediate verbal, delayed verbal, immediate spatial, and
delayed spatial. This required 8 dependent variables
(pre- and posttest scores for each of the 4 memory
measures) to be entered into the analysis. Because there
was a significant mean difference in age between groups,
age was treated as a covariate with the grouping factor.
The effect of attrition within each group was assessed by
chi square and t tests on selected variables.

RESULTS

A total of 38 cardiac patients and 17 back patients
completed pre- and posttesting on the VMS. Overall, both
groups scored in the average range for both assessments
[16, 17] without any signficant clinical findings.
Descriptive data for these groups are summarized in Tables
2 and 3. Except for the Screening Test, higher scores
signified better performances.

The results of the between group repeated measures
comparison by MANOVA, with age as a covariate, on VMS
scores for immediate verbal, delayed verbal, immediate
spatial, and delayed spatial abilities failed to demon-

strate a significant overal difference in pre-to-post
memory functioning (i.e., change scores) between cardiac
and back patients (Wilks' Lambda Approximate F [4, 49] =
1.13, p = .35). Consequently, no follow-up tests on
specific memory measures were conducted. The effect of
the age covariate was signficant in accounting for pre-
post differences in memory functioning between groups
(Wilks' Lambda Approximate F [4, 49] = 3.29, p = .02).
Overall, both groups scored in the average range for these
measures at pre- and posttesting.

     Attrition rates for the cardiac and back groups were
19 and 29 per cent, respectively. One heart patient died
during surgery. The remainder of the patients dropped out
of the study voluntarily. The typical reason given was
that they did not have time to continue in the study. A
few patients indicated that they found test-taking to be
an unpleasant task that they did not care to repeat. Comparisons were made between drop-outs and those completing
the study within each group on demographic variables and
VMS summary scores at pretesting to determine if attrition
signifcantly altered the representativeness of the groups
at posttesting. A major finding was that within the
original cardiac group, those who dropped out achieved
significantly lower VMS verbal (p < .05, df = 43) and
spatial (p < .01, df = 38) summary scores than those who
remained in the study. No significant demographic
differences were found.

Table 2.   Means and Standard Deviations for Cardiac Group

Measures	Pretesting Mean	S.D.	Posttesting Mean	S.D.
VMS Composite Scores[a]				
Immediate Verbal	.63	.12	.63	.13
Delayed Verbal	.69	.16	.68	.16
Verbal Summary	.66	.13	.66	.14
Immediate Spatial	.69	.17	.72	.17
Delayed Spatial	.70	.15	.67	.17
Spatial Summary	.70	.15	.70	.14

Table 2 (continued)

Measures	Pretesting Mean	S.D.	Posttesting Mean	S.D.
VMS Selected Subtests				
Screening (No. wrong)	1.00	1.68	1.11	1.27
List-Direct Recall	8.49	2.46	9.32	2.78
List-Cued Recall	8.97	2.18	9.59	2.68
List-Delayed Recall	9.84	2.20	10.11	2.82
Story-1st Recall	5.34	1.83	5.05	1.75
Story-Delayed Recall	5.00	1.94	4.73	1.61
Digits Forward	6.05	1.01	6.47	1.13
Digits Backward	4.13	.93	4.47	1.16
Star Span	4.62	.82	4.97	.88
Designs-Same/Different	3.84	1.15	4.16	.83
Designs-Multiple Choice	7.94	2.01	8.27	2.13
Drawing 1	2.76	1.14	2.56	1.40
Drawing 2	2.84	1.48	3.07	1.54
Names/Faces-2nd Trial	8.19	1.75	8.24	1.83
Names/Faces-Delayed	7.97	1.87	8.00	2.01

[a] Based on percentage correct scores

DISCUSSION

This study compared cardiac surgery patients with another hospital group of back patients and found no significant differences between the groups in pre-to-post memory functioning on the VMS. Although the groups were not perfectly matched, and it was necessary to statistically control for age differences, it is notable how little the two groups differed from each other across two assessments on a wide array of verbal and spatial memory tasks. This study failed to demonstrate any signficant clinical or subclinical decrements in memory functioning after CPB, despite the inclusion of delayed recall measures which have been found to be highly sensitive to many forms of subtle memory loss. While these findings appear to attest to the general cerebral protectiveness of currént CPB and cardiac surgical procedures, and in that sense are quite significant, there are, nevertheless, some important qualifications to this overall finding.

Table 3.   Means and Standard Deviations for Back Group

Measures	Pretesting Mean	S.D.	Posttesting Mean	S.D.
VMS Composite Scores[a]				
Immediate Verbal	.58	.19	.63	.19
Delayed Verbal	.69	.21	.71	.20
Verbal Summary	.63	.20	.67	.19
Immediate Spatial	.73	.15	.72	.13
Delayed Spatial	.73	.18	.71	.16
Spatial Summary	.74	.14	.72	.13
VMS Selected Subtests				
Screening (No. wrong)	1.18	1.42	1.06	1.68
List-Direct Recall	9.47	2.37	9.53	2.48
List-Cued Recall	9.36	2.41	9.79	1.85
List-Delayed Recall	10.47	2.21	10.56	2.19
Story-1st Recall	4.29	2.64	4.82	2.81
Story-Delayed Recall	4.25	2.57	4.82	2.60
Digits Forward	6.06	1.48	6.12	.86
Digits Backward	4.71	1.21	4.53	1.18
Star Span	4.31	1.14	4.59	.87
Designs-Same/Different	4.00	1.06	4.06	.90
Designs-Multiple Choice	7.94	2.44	7.94	2.41
Drawing 1	2.88	1.11	2.65	.86
Drawing 2	3.44	1.39	3.44	1.43
Names/Faces-2nd Trial	8.76	1.39	8.13	1.92
Names/Faces-Delayed	8.29	1.83	8.81	1.52

[a] Based on percentage correct scores

One limitation concerns subject selection. Cardiac patients who were most seriously ill and in coronary care prior to surgery were excluded from the study because they were unable to submit to psychological testing. Since data were not collected on these patients, how they would have performed is not known, but it is quite possible that they were at greater risk for postoperative memory and CNS problems due to more compromised cardiovascular systems and presumably more generalized health problems. A finding that age was negatively correlated with spatial memory performance following CPB surgery lends indirect support this this inference when it is considered that health problems tend to increase with aging.

A second limitation concerns attrition. Although the amount was not as great as had been reported in most previous studies, at pretesting, cardiac patients who dropped out of the study scored significantly lower than those who completed the study on both VMS verbal and spatial scales. This finding also suggests patients who were already more impaired, and conceivably at greater risk, were excluded from posttesting.

REFERENCES

1. M. Budabin, Neurologic complications of cardiac surgery, in: "Care of the Cardiac Surgical patient," R. Litvak and R. Jurado, eds., Appleton-Century-Crofts, Norwalk, CT (1982).

2. T. Åberg, P. Ahlund, and M. Kihlgren, Intellectual function late after open heart operation, Ann Thorac Surg. 36:680 (1983).

3. T. Åberg, G. Ronquist, H. Tyden, P. Ahlund, and K. Bergstrom, Release of adenylate kinase into cerebrospinal fluid in connection with open heart surgery and its relation to intellectual function, Lancet, 1 (Pt. 2):1139 (1982).

4. R. Carlson, A. J. Lande, B. Landis, B. Rogoz, J. Baster, R. H. Patterson, K. Stenzel, and C. W. Lillehei, The Lande-Edwards membrane oxygenator during heart surgery, J Thorac Cardiovasc Surg. 66:894 (1973).

5. B. Landis, J. Baxter, R. N. Patterson, and C. E. Tauber, Bender-Gestalt evaluation of brain dysfunction following open heart surgery, J Pers Assmt., 38:556 (1974).

6. J. A. Savageau, B. A. Stanton, C. D. Jenkins, and M. D. Klein, Neuropsychological dysfunction following elective cardiac operation. I. Early assessment, J Thorac Cardiovasc Surg. 84:585 (1982).

7. M. D. Lezak, "Neuropsychological Assessment," 2nd ed., Oxford, New York (1983).

8. L. R. Squire, The neuropsychology of memory dysfunction and its assessment, in: "Neuropsychological Assessment on Neuropsychiatric Disorders," I. Grant and K. M. Adams, eds., Oxford, New York (1986).

9. C. Delaney, J. D. Wallace, and S. Egelko, Transient cerebral ischemic attacks and neuropsychological deficit, J Clin Neuropsy. 2:107 (1980).

10. J. L. Ponsford, G. A. Donnan, and K. W. Walsh,
    Disorders of memory in vertebrobasilar disease,
    J Clin Neuropsy. 2:267 (1980).
11. F. B. Wood, L. C. McHenry, and D. A. Stump, Memory and
    related neurobehavioral deficits in TIA patients:
    Behavioral, rCBF, and outcome measures, (NIH
    Research Protocol No. 188-18-8951), Bowman Gray
    School of Medicine, Winston-Salem (1981).
12. R. Kolka and M. Hilberman, Neurological dysfunction
    following cardiac operation with low-flow, low-
    pressure cardiopulmonary bypass, J Thorac
    Cardiovasc Surg. 79:432 (1980).
13. K. M. Taylor, Brain damage during open heart surgery,
    Thorax. 37:873 (1982).
14. A. J. Lewis, "Mechanisms of Neurological Disease,"
    Little, Brown & Co., Boston (1976).
15. M. Little, J. Williams, and C. Long, Clinical memory
    tests and everyday memory, Arch Clin Neuropsy.
    1:323 (1986).
16. J. M. Williams, "The Vermont Memory Scale: Initial
    Studies of Reliability and Validity," Unpublished
    doctoral dissertation, University of Vermont (1983).
17. J. M. Williams, M. W. Little, S. Scates, and N.
    Blockman, Memory complaints and abilities among
    depressed older adults, J Consul & Clin Psy.
    55:595 (1987).

NEUROPSYCHOLOGICAL FINDINGS AND PERSONALITY STRUCTURE ASSOCIATED WITH CORONARY ARTERY BYPASS SURGERY (CABS): AN EIGHT MONTH FOLLOW-UP STUDY

Carl-Erik Mattlar and Lars-Runar Knuts

The Rehabilitation Research Centre of the
Social Insurance Institution
Turku, Finland

Erik Engblom, Esko Vanttinen

Turku University Central Hospital
Turku, Finland

INTRODUCTION

This study addresses the issue of cognitive impairment and personality disturbance, particularly depression, associated with coronary artery bypass surgery (CABS). These data are part of a collaborative study comprising the Turku University Central Hospital (TUCH), where the annual number of operations is about 170, and the Rehabilitation Research Centre (RRC). The RRC has specialized in comprehensive rehabilitation after acute myocardial infarction, and also in quantitative neuropsychological and personality research.

There are a number of studies indicating that both cognitive impairment, and psychiatric and personality disturbances, are associated with valvular surgery, as well as with bypass surgery [1-5]. The cognitive impairment has also been claimed to be reversible [6, 7]. There are, however, studies that question the issue of surgery-related disturbances [8]. There are probably many medical as well as methodological issues which

Impact of Cardiac Surgery on the Quality of Life
Edited by A. E. Willner and G. Rodewald
Plenum Press, New York, 1990

explain the different findings.   In studies investigating
the issue of cognitive impairment the psychodiagnostic
methods are crucial; above all the sensitivity of the
tests [9].   Another major problem is to find relevant
control groups.   We have, for instance, in a population
study found that the Piotrowski Organic Signs criterion
is fulfilled in 24% of 50 year olds and 33% of 60 year
olds who are otherwise healthy.

THE PSYCHODIAGNOSTIC INVESTIGATION

The Aims of the Study

        The aim of this study was to investigate the occurr-
ence of cognitive impairment and personality disturbance
associated with CABS, using primarily robust methods.
(The major goals of the project are to study physical
fitness, return to work, and the change of risk factors
of coronary artery disease.)

Subjects

        The study comprises a total of 228 patients (202
males and 26 females), randomized in a rehabilitation
group (108 males and 15 females), and a hospital group
(94 males and 11 females).   The mean age was 54 years,
and the age-range was 36 - 64 years.   There were five
surgical deaths.   The hospital group was examined with
fewer tests than the rehabilitation group.

        Further, during 1983-1989, the first writer conducted
a series of studies on four random-sample based groups (a
total of 679 subjects) of males and females aged 30 - 70
years, using a number of psychodiagnostic tests and questionnaires.   The results from these studies are used for
comparison purposes.

        In this presentation, data are given for the males
(n = 108) in the rehabilitation group, and for the males
aged 40 - 60 years in the random sample-based studies.

Surgery

        Surgery was performed during a single aortic cross-
clamping, using cold crystalloid cardioplegia, topical
cooling, and moderate hypothermia.   A bubble-oxygenator
with laminar flow was used.

Rehabilitation Measures

The comprehensive rehabilitation program was conducted at the RRC and consisted of three inpatient phases, the first prior to, the second 2 months, and the third 8 months, after surgery.

The Psychodiagnostic Methods

Considering the personnel and time available for the psychodiagnostic examination, the shortage of really parallel test versions, and the fact that not all methods are suitable for retesting, the following approach was used:

1) At all three phases (before, and at 2 months, and at 8 months) the following questionnaires were used: Eysenck Personality Inventory (EPI-C), the Cesarec-Marke Personality Schedule (CMPS), and the Beck Depression Inventory, as well as the Wartegg Projective Method were presented.

2) Preoperative intellectual levels and possible congitive impairment were examined using the Benton-D, and WAIS: Information, Picture Completion and Similarities subtests. Further, the Locus of Control test was presented.

3) Two months postoperatively the whole WAIS and Wechsler Memory Scales and a number of neuropsychodiagnostic tests: Benton-C, Trail Making Test, Stroop, Subtracting Serial Sevens (SSS), Rey-Osterrieth Complex Figure, Word Memory Test of Schultze, Finger Tapping, and the Rorschach were presented.

4) Eight months postoperatively those tests considered suitable for retesting: Benton-D, WAIS (Digit Span, Digit Symbol, Picture Completion, Block Design), Wechsler Memory Scale (Logical Memory, associate learning), SSS and Stroop were presented once more, in addition to the Zulliger.

RESULTS

A visual memory deficit (cf. Table 1) on the Benton was found for about 12% of patients, both preoperatively and at 2 months. On the average, the results for the whole group were worse than for the random sample. At 8 months the patient group did show recovery of function, the results being even better than for the random sample.

TABLE 1.   Mean Results for Visual Memory Function In

	Benton Differences		Rey-Osterreith Differences for Copy Memory	Wechsler Memory Scale - Visual Reproduction
	Correct	Errors		
Pre-op (n=102)	1.6	2.7	--	--
2 Mo. Postop (n=105)	1.5	3.1	13.9	10.1
8 Mo. Postop (n=101)	1.0	1.6	--	--
Random Sample	1.1	2.5	13.8	9.5

The results on the Rey-Osterrieth and the Wechsler Visual
Reproduction were, however, intact at 2 months.

In regard to verbal memory functions (Table 2), at 2
months the Wechsler Memory Scale results for the patient
group were slightly better than for the random sample.
These differences were not significant. For the Schultze
(verbal memory span), however, the results at 2 months
were slightly worse than for the random sample. On the
WMS Logical Memory and Associate Learning, the results
were clearly better at 8 months than at 2 months.

TABLE 2.   Mean Results for Tests of Verbal Function

	2 mo. Postop	8 mo. Postop	Random Sample
WMS lgm	8.4	9.3	8.2
WMS assoc.learn.	15.9	16.7	15.7
WMS DSp	10.2	--	10.0
WMS ret			
- lgm	6.1	7.7	5.1
- assoc.learn.	8.4	9.0	8.0
Schultze			
- memory span	75.7	--	76.5
- 5 min ret.	5.9	--	6.6

TABLE 3.   Mean Results of Neuropsychological Function

	2 mo. Postop	8 mo. Postop	Random Sample
WMS mental control	3.6	--	4.1
WMS, MQ	111	--	108
Stroop, all errors	3.2	2.5	2.8
TMT A	49.6	--	44.3
TMT B	129	--	141
TMT A + B	177	--	185
Tapping, dx	136	--	134
Tapping, sin	124	--	123
SSS	2.1	1.4	2.2

In regard to the most sensitive tests of neuropsychological function, (Table 3) the results were on the same level for the patients as for the random sample. For the Stroop (average for sum errors 3.2 - > 2.5) and the SSS (average for sum errors 2.1 - > 1.4) an improvement was found from 2 months to 8 months.

In regard to the WAIS (Table 4), nearly all results were about 1 SD above the expectancy norms (which were gathered 1956-1962).

In regard to depression, and the Eysenck scales (Table 5), the most important finding was an elevated level of depression (mean value preoperatively 11.2 and at 2 months 11.3) and neuroticism (mean value preoperatively 10.2 and at 2 months 10.6). Also important was that 12% of the patients had Beck scores of ≥ 20, and about 10% revealed a masked depression.

C. E. MATTLAR ET AL.

TABLE 4. Mean Results for the WAIS

	Pre-op (n=104)	2 mo. Postop (n=105)	8 mo. Postop (n=102)
WAIS GI	12.7	--	--
WAIS GC	--	13.7	--
WAIS A	--	11.8	--
WAIS S	14.1	--	--
WAIS DSp	11.6	--	12.0
WAIS V	--	12.3	--
Verbal IQ	112.3	115.1	--
WAIS DSy	--	9.7	10.1
WAIS PC	13.5	--	14.0
WAIS BD	--	11.9	12.4
WAIS PA	--	10.9	--
WAIS OA	--	11.9	--
Perf. IQ	--	111.0	117.2

On the Murray-based scales (the CMPS) only slight differences with respect to the random sample were found, the patients showing less affiliation, but more aggression, defense of status, and dominance. This difference was still observed at 8 months for affiliation and dominance only.

In regard to the Locus of Control (Table 5), the patients preoperatively did show a significantly lower value on internal control, and a higher value on external control, than the randomly selected subjects.

CONCLUSIONS

The results on the Benton, both preoperatively and at 2 months, indicate in some of the patients a deficit.

This also applies both for the Stroop, and the WMS Mental Control at 2 months. These findings might be explained by the higher occurrence of depression (probably also masked depression) immediately before and after surgery, thus being reversible.

TABLE 5. Mean Results for the Beck Depression Inventory, the EPI-C, and the Locus of Control

	Pre-op (n=107)	2 Mo. Postop (n=105)	8 Mo. Postop (n=102)	Random Sample
BDI	11.2	11.3	9.8	7.2
EPI-C, N	10.2	10.6	10.4	8.7
EPI-C, E	9.5	8.7	8.7	10.2
EPI-C, I	5.9	5.6	5.3	7.2
EPI-C, L	2.8	2.7	2.8	2.7
External	12.6	--	--	11.3
Internal	13.8	--	--	15.3
Chance	12.2	--	--	11.6
Weight	6.7	--	--	6.7

On all other measures of cognitive function the results both before, at 2 months and 8 months after surgery were at least at the same level as for a major random-sample based study of the same age and gender, gathered in the same area as the bypass patients. Unfortunately it was not possible to present all the tests of cognitive function preoperatively. If the results of the postoperative tests, which were equivalent to same level as the random samples', represent these patients' "level of impairment," then they must have been outstanding at some earlier time. It is most unlikely that this would be the case. Our conclusion thus is that no impairment has occurred, even for the tests presented only postoperatively.

Particularly important for returning to work as well as for every-day functioning is that verbal memory, and a number of cognitive functions (e.g. remote memory, common-sense reasoning and knowledge of social expectations, ideational discipline, abstract thinking, verbal and visuospatial percept formation, and an ability to grasp the essential) are intact. Data particularly on the WAIS and on the WMS indicate this to be the case.

The need-structure, according to the Murray-based questionnaire (CMPS) was normal - even if the patients were slightly more distant ("detached"), and aggressive, than the normals.

Further, the patients were more dependent (low internal and high external control), and in particular more neurotic and depressed than the subjects in the random sample. Both before, and 2 months after surgery about 12% revealed a conscious depression of a level of $\geq$ 20 on the BDI, indicating a need for psychiatric counselling. An additional 10% revealed a probably serious masked depression.

REFERENCES

1. K. A. Sotaniemi, A. Juolasmaa, and E. T. Hokkanen, Neuropsychologic outcome after open-heart surgery, Arch Neurol. 38: 2-8 (1981).
2. S. Slogoff, K. Z. Girgis, and A. S. Keats, Etiologic factors in neuropsychiatric complications associated with cardiopulmonary bypass, Anesth Analg. 61: 903 - 911 (1982).
3. A. Gilston, Permanent brain damage after cardiac surgery, Lancet I: 216 (1987).
4. S. Newman, P. Smith, T. Treasure, P. Joseph, P. Ell, and M. Harrison, Acute neuropsychological consequences of coronary artery bypass surgery, Curr Psychol Res & Rev. 6: 115 - 124 (1987).
5. P. C. Chandarana, A. J. Cooper, M. M. Goldbach, J. C. Coles, and M. A. Vesely, Perceptual and cognitive deficit following coronary artery bypass surgery, Stress Med. 4: 163 - 171 (1988).
6. J. A. Savageau, B-A. Stanton, C. D. Jenkins, and R. W. M. Frater, Neuropsychological dysfunction following elective cardiac operation. II. A six-month reassessment, J Thorac Cardiovasc Surg. 84: 595 - 600 (1982).

7. M. Raymond, C. Conklin, J. Schaeffer, G. Newstedt, J. Matloff, and R. J. Gray, Coping with transient intellectual dysfunction after coronary bypass surgery, Heart & Lung. 13: 531 - 539 (1984).
8. C. M. C. Allen, Cabbages and CABG, BMJ. 297: 1485 - 1486 (1988).
9. Anon, Brain damage after open-heart surgery, Lancet. I: 1161 - 1163 (1982).

PREDICTING MEMORY OUTCOME FROM MEDICAL VARIABLES AFTER CARDIAC SURGERY WITH CARDIOPULMONARY BYPASS

Gregory W. Harter

Arkansas Rehabilitation Institute
Little Rock, AR

J. Michael Williams,

Hahnemann University
Philadelphia, PA

Wilborn George

Methodist Hospital
Memphis, TN

Murry Mutchnick, Ivan Torres

Memphis State University
Memphis, TN

Because the incidence of complications in CNS functioning is reportedly higher in cardiac surgeries requiring CPB than in other types of thoracic surgery without CPB assistance [1], the identification of risk factors has been of major concern in efforts to improve cerebral protection. A review of Barash [2] identified several factors that have been predictive of CNS complications in one or more studies: prolonged hypotension during CPB, overall duration of CPB, age of patient, previous neurological conditions, type and severity of heart disease, and specific components of the CPB process such as pulsatile versus nonpulsatile flow, type of oxygenator, degree and duration of hypothermia, and the use of filters in the circuit.

Impact of Cardiac Surgery on the Quality of Life
Edited by A. E. Willner and G. Rodewald
Plenum Press, New York, 1990

The current study, part of a larger investigation on memory functioning after CPB-assisted cardiac functioning, focused on medical variables that might prove predictive of memory outcome. It was hypothesized that structures mediating memory functions might be especially at risk for ischemic-based changes since one of the suspected mechanisms for changes in brain function after CPB is inadequate cerebral perfusion due to low arterial pressures and (or) blood gas irregularities [3, 4]. In particular, the hippocampus, a structure critical to memory consolidation processes, because of its location in a boundary zone between the supply areas of the major cerebral arteries, appears to be selectively vulnerable to partial ischemia [5].

METHOD

Subjects

Thirty-eight cardiac surgery patients completed the study out of a group of 47 patients who were randomly recruited between December 1986 and March 1988, at Methodist Hospital in Memphis. All potential subjects were briefed as to the purpose of the study, and those agreeing to participate signed informed consent forms. All patients in this group underwent elective coronary artery bypass graft (CABG) surgery, and three patients received additional heart surgery procedures as well. All of these procedures required cardiopulmonary bypass (CPB). Cardiac surgery cases which did not involve CPB were excluded from the study, as were pediatric heart surgery cases (CA < 20) and emergency cardiac surgery patients. Demographics and elective surgical procedures for each of the 38 cardiac patients are summarized in Table 1.

Procedure

Monitoring during surgery. In addition to monitoring vital signs and anesthesia levels for both groups, data were collected during cardiac surgery from the CPB machine on blood gas tensions, hematocrit levels, arterial pressure, blood flow rate, and temperature. The basic CPB equipment used included a Sarns 5000 pump with a BOS CM50 membrane oxygenator and a Pall arterial line filter. Total time on the machine, total time in surgery, the number of blood units transfused, the amount of Heparin administered, and the number of grafts performed were recorded in perfusionist and surgeon reports, which also noted perioperative complications.

TABLE 1. Cardiac Patient Characteristics

Pt#	Age	Sex	Race	Ed[a]	Surgical Procedure[b]
01	63	F	W	12	CABG X 2
02	39	F	W	12	CABG X 5
03	77	M	W	12	CABG X 4
04	53	M	W	19	CABG X 3
05	47	F	W	12	CABG X 1, AOR V
06	75	M	B	20	CABG X 4
07	61	M	W	13	CABG X2
08	49	M	W	14	CABG X 3
09	50	M	W	12	CABG X4
10	44	M	B	12	CABG X 3
11	48	M	W	14	CABG X4
12	70	F	W	12	CABG X 2
13	68	F	W	10	CABG X 3
14	62	M	W	12	CABG X4
15	50	M	W	15	CABG X 4
16	40	F	W	12	CABG X 3
17	35	F	B	6	CABG X 3
18	57	F	W	11	CABG X 2
19	60	M	W	12	CABG X 4
20	71	M	W	12	CABG X 5
21	45	M	W	15	CABG X 4
22	69	F	W	6	CABG X 3
23	53	M	W	12	CABG X 5
24	70	M	W	10	CABG X 4
25	56	M	W	8	CABG X 3
26	43	M	W	12	CABG X 5
27	47	F	W	13	CABG X 2
28	72	F	W	17	CABG X 2
29	61	M	W	16	CABG X 1, V ANEUR
30	50	M	W	14	CABG X 5
31	66	M	W	14	CABG X 4
32	50	M	W	16	CABG X 4
33	61	M	W	12	CABG X 3
34	59	M	W	10	CABG X 4,THROM
35	66	M	W	10	CABG X 3
36	60	M	W	16	CABG X 3
37	58	M	W	12	CABG X 4
38	71	M	W	3	CABG X 4

[a]Highest Grade Completed. [b]CABG=Coronary Artery Bypass Graft; AOR V=Aortic Valve Replacement; V ANEURYSM= Ventricular Aneurysm Resection; THROM-Thrombectomy

Coronary care monitoring. Cardiac surgery patients
typically spent three to five days in coronary care
following surgery. During this period, nursing staff
continued to monitor patients on parameters of heart
function, post-operative complications, response to
treatment, and overall physical condition. They also
made hourly ratings of patients' neurobehavioral functioning in such areas as level of consciousness, size and
symmetry of pupils, conjugate eye movement, lateralized
body weaknesses or asymmetries, quality of speech,
orientation (to person, place, and time), and presence of
anxiety, depression, or uncooperative behavior.

Post-surgery. Six to eight weeks after their hospitalization, patients were tested in their own homes
on the Vermont Memory Scale (VMS). This comprehensive
memory scale contains subtests which measure list
learning ability, story recall, digit span, recognition
of geometric designs, reproduction of geometric designs
from memory, and a names-faces recognition task [6].
Based on percentage of correct scores, composite scores
for verbal memory and spatial memory were computed. A
previous investigation of the verbal and spatial subscales
found alternate forms and test-retest reliabilities that
ranged from .62 to .88. In a validity study using
discriminant analysis, the VMS was found to classify 95
per cent of organically amnestic patients (n = 12) and
normal subjects (n = 62) as compared to an 88 per cent
classification rate for the Wechsler Memory Scale [7].

Medical data collection. The hospital records for
all patients in the study were accessed blindly (i.e.,
without knowledge of memory test results) to obtain
demographic and medical history data (e.g., duration of
symptoms, previous heart surgeries, pre-existing neurological conditions). Cardiac risk factors such as
smoking, high cholesterol, diabetes, peripheral vascular
disease, hypertension, chronic obstructive pulmonary
disease, and family history of heart disease were
additionally recorded. Also at this time, cardiological
(e.g., left ventricular ejection fraction), CPB, and
surgical data, as well as coronary care nurses' ratings,
were collected. All of these data were obtained for
entry into subsequent statistical analyses.

Statistical Analyses

Pearson correlations were computed to determine the
relationship of demographics, medical history data, CPB

and perioperative measures, and nurses' neurobehavioral ratings, with VMS summary scores. Multiple regressions were performed to determine which variables are the best predictors of memory performance after CPB-assisted surgery.

RESULTS AND DISCUSSION

Memory Outcome

As a group, the cardiac patients scored in the average range on all VMS measures [7, 8] with no significant clinical findings. Descriptive data are summarized in Table 2. In general, higher scores signified better performances, except on the Screening Test, in which the opposite pattern held.

Relationship Between Memory Outcome and Medical Variables

Medical variables were subdivided according to medical history, cardiology and perioperative measures (chiefly pertaining to CPB), and nurses' neurobehavioral ratings from the days 2-5 of the postoperative period. Descriptive data for these variables are presented in Table 3. Pearson correlations between medical data and outcome measures are listed in Table 4. Every cardiac patient had complete, or at least 90 per cent complete, medical data.

Medical history. Among medical history variables, a significant positive relationship was obtained between absence of diabetes and the VMS verbal score. Likewise, the absence of cardiac arrhythmias and fibrillations was positively correlated with the VMS spatial score. There are no other significant correlations between medical history and outcome measures.

Cardiac and CPB measures. This category had 15 variables. None of them were found to correlate significantly with any of the outcome measures.

Neurobehavioral ratings. From nurses' neuro-behavioral ratings collected during the early post-operative recovery period, three correlations obtained significance. Absence of disorientation problems after day one of the postoperative period, and absence of depression, were positively correlated with VMS verbal outcome. Absence of disorientation problems was also positively correlated with VMS spatial outcome.

TABLE 2.   Means and Standard Deviations for the Cardiac
           Group

Measures	Mean	S.D.
VMS Composite Scores[a]		
Immediate Verbal	.63	.13
Delayed Verbal	.68	.16
Verbal Summary	.66	.14
Immediate Spatial	.72	.17
Delayed Spatial	.67	.17
Spatial Summary	.70	.14
VMS Selected Subtests		
Screening (No. wrong)	1.11	1.27
List-Direct Recall	9.32	2.78
List-Cued Recall	9.59	2.68
List-Delayed Recall	10.11	2.82
Story-1st Recall	5.05	1.75
Story-Delayed Recall	4.73	1.61
Digits Forward	6.47	1.13
Digits Backward	4.47	1.16
Star Span	4.97	.88
Designs-Same/Different	4.16	.83
Designs-Multiple Choice	8.27	2.13
Drawing 1	2.56	1.40
Drawing 2	3.07	1.54
Names/Faces-2nd Trial	8.24	1.83
Names/Faces-Delayed	8.00	2.01

[a]Based on percentage correct scores

Prediction of Memory Performance after CPB-Assisted Cardiac Surgery

Multiple regression analyses were done for the VMS
outcome scores to determine if memory performance at six
to eight weeks postsurgery could be predicted from
medical data. Variables entered into stepwise derived
equations were selected on the basis of their association
with the outcome scores or with neuropsychological
findings in previous studies. The results of the VMS
regression analyses are summarized in Table 5.

TABLE 3.   Means and Standard Deviations on Medical
           Variables

Measures	Mean	S.D.
Medical History		
Duration Symptons (mos.)	7.18	15.02
Smoking (Pack yrs.)	21.76	21.21
Chronic Obstr. Pulmonary Disease*	1.84	.44
Obesity*	1.58	.50
Hyperlipodemia/Hypercholesterolemia*	1.49	.51
Hypertension*	1.71	.46
Cardiac Arrhythmias, Fibrillations*	1.87	.34
History of Myocardial Infarction*	1.55	.50
Previous Cardiac Surgery*	1.89	.31
Family Hx Cardiovascular Disease*	1.24	.43
Peripheral Vascular disease*	1.97	.16
Diabetes*	1.87	.34
Renal Disease*	1.97	.16
Hx Carotid Disease/Endarterectomy*	1.87	.34
Hx Neurological Disease*	1.84	.37
Cardiology & Perioperative Variables		
Left Ventricular Ejection Fraction	.56	.13
Left Main Coronary Artery Disease*	1.89	.31
# of Bypass Grafts	3.37	1.08
Time in Surgery (min.)	264.95	52.38
Time on CPB (min.)	100.53	27.34
Total Heparin Administered (mg)	425.08	112.03
Lowest Level Hypothermia (^{o}C)	24.53	2.72
Mean CPB Flow Rate (ml/min.)	4061.21	510.78
Mean Arterial Pressure (mm Hg)	63.60	6.09
Hematocrit Level (ml/100 ml)	24.20	4.58
pCO_2 (mm Hg)	34.96	4.18
pO_2 (mm Hg)	227.90	53.78
Nurses' Neurobehavioral Ratings		
Disturbed Level of Consciousness*	1.89	.31
Pupil Asymmetries*	1.97	.16
Disconjugate Eye Movement*	2.00	0.00
Lateralized Weakness in Extremities*	1.97	.16
Stimulus Response Deficits*	2.00	0.00
Speech Problems*	1.89	.31
Disoriented: Person, Place or Time*	1.87	.34
Anxiety*	1.82	.39
Depression*	1.95	.23
Uncooperativeness*	1.97	.16

*Dichotomous Measure: 1=Presence   2=Absence

TABLE 4. Relationship Between Medical Measures and VMS
          Summary Scores

Measures	Verbal	Spatial
Medical History		
Duration Symptoms (mos.)	-.029	-.110
Smoking (Pack yrs.)	.247	.294
Chronic Obstr. Pulmonary Disease	.097	-.019
Obesity	.118	.064
Hyperlipodemia/Hypercholesterolemia	-.001	-.202
Hypertension	-.112	-.139
Cardiac Arrhythmias, Fibrillations	.162	.486*
History of Myocardial Infarction	.168	.235
Previous Cardiac Surgery	.046	-.106
Family Hx Cardiovascular Disease	-.261	-.214
Peripheral Vascular Disease	-.121	-.016
Diabetes	.392*	.360
Renal Disease	.038	-.160
Hx Carotid Disease/Endarterectomy	.229	.103
Hx Neurological Disease	.152	.078
Cardiology & Perioperative Variables		
Left Ventricular Ejection Fraction	-.087	.159
Left Main Coronary Artery Disease	-.118	.158
# of Bypass Grafts	.029	.029
Time in Surgery (min.)	-.001	.267
Time on CPB (min.)	.022	.127
Total Heparin Administered (mg)	-.271	-.222
Lowest Level Hypothermia ($^{\circ}$C)	.292	.352
Mean CPB Flow Rate (ml/min.)	-.120	-.096
Mean Arterial Pressure (mm Hg)	.059	-.019
Hematrocrit Level (ml/100 ml)	.320	.040
pCO_2 (mm Hg)	.084	.101
pO_2 (mm Hg)	.032	.233
Nurses' Neurobehavioral Ratings[a]		
Disturbed Level of Consciousness	-.039	.243
Pupil Asymmetries	.009	.244
Lateralized Weakness in Extremities	.009	.244
Speech Problems	.127	.329
Disoriented: Person, Place, or Time	.512**	.403*
Anxiety	.351	.012
Depression	.418*	.251
Uncooperativeness	.231	.136

[a]Constant values precluded computation of rs for certain
neurobehavioral ratings. * p < .01   ** p < 001

TABLE 5.   Prediction from Medical Variables of Memory
            Outcome

Outcome	Step	R	R^2-Change	Predictor
VMS Verbal[a]	1	.51	.26	Disorientation Early Postop.
VMS Spatial[b]	1	.49	.24	Hx Arrhythmias, Fibrillations
	2	.61	.13	Disorientation Early Postop.

[a]Variables not accepted in equation: Age, Hx. Diabetes,
Depression in Early Postoperative Period, Time on CPB,
Lowest Level of Hypothermia, Time Arterial Pressure < 50
mm Hg, Hx. Neurological Problems, & Perioperative
Complications.

[b]Variables not accepted in equation: Age, Time on CPB,
Lowest Level of Hypothermia, Time Arterial Pressure < 50
mm Hg, Hx. Neurological Problems, & Perioperative
Complications.

When the VMS verbal outcome measure was regressed on
a series of medical variables, only one of these variables, disorientation problems during the early postoperative period, reached significance for entry into the
equation. By itself, this variable accounted for 26 per
cent of the variance in VMS verbal outcome. Two variables, history of cardiac arrhythmias and fibrillations,
and disorientation problems during the early postoperative period, were predictive of VMS spatial outcome.
Together, they accounted for 37 per cent of the variance
in VMS spatial outcome. For all three predictors, the
absence of these problems was associated with better VMS
memory performance 6-8 weeks later.

Unlike findings in earlier studies [2], CPB measures
and perioperative factors were not predictive of outcome
from surgery. This current finding may simply reflect
differences in focus and outcome measures since earlier
studies did not typically assess memory comprehensively.
This finding may also suggest that current cardiac

surgical and CPB procedures are doing an increasingly
better job of protecting the brain.   The identification
of disorientation problems in the early postoperative
course (days 2-5) as a predictor of both verbal and
spatial memory outcome several weeks later suggests that
this is a critical area to monitor after surgery.

REFERENCES

1. M. Budabin, Neurologic complications of cardiac
   surgery, in: "Care of the Cardiac Surgical
   Patient," R. Litvak and R. Jurado, eds.,
   Appleton-Century-Crofts, Norwalk, CT (1982).
2. P. G. Barash, Cardiopulmonary bypass and postoperative
   neurologic dysfunction, Amer Heart J., 99:675
   (1980).
3. R. Kolka, M. Hilberman, Neurological dysfunction
   following cardiac operation with low-flow,
   low-pressure, cardiopulmonary bypass, J. Thorac
   Cardiovasc Surg., 79:432 (1980).
4. K. M. Taylor, Brain damage during open heart surgery,
   Thorax, 37:873 (1982).
5. A. J. Lewis, "Mechanisms of Neurological Disease,"
   Little, Brown & Co., Boston (1976).
6. M. Little, J. M. Williams, C.J. Long, Clinical memory
   tests and everyday memory, Arch Clin Neuropsy.,
   1:323 (1986).
7. J. M. Williams, "The Vermont Memory Scale: Initial
   Studies of Reliability and Validity," Unpublished
   doctoral dissertation, University of Vermont
   (1983).
8. J. M. Williams, M. Little, S. Scates, N. Blockman,
   Memory complaints and abilities among depressed
   older adults, J Consul & Clin Psy., 55:595 (1987).

NEUROPSYCHOLOGICAL IMPAIRMENT IN CANDIDATES FOR

CARDIAC TRANSPLANTATION

R. Bornstein, D. Hammer, R. Starling,
J. Stang, R. Lewis, R. Magorien

Departments of Psychiatry and Cardiology
The Ohio State University
Columbus, Ohio 43210

INTRODUCTION

Several studies have considered the question of neurobehavioral impairment in patients with cardiac disease. In most cases these studies have focused on patients who were undergoing surgical intervention such as valve replacement (open heart) or coronary artery bypass procedures. To date there have been no studies of neuropsychological function in patients who undergo heart transplantation. This procedure is being performed more frequently due in large part to improvements in surgical technique and in prevention of complications (e.g. tissue rejection). In view of the increasing number of patients who are evaluated for this procedure, it was of interest to examine the possibility of neuropsychological impairment in a sample of patients who were candidates for cardiac transplantation. In view of the fact that the etiology and nature of cardiac pathology was somewhat different than in previously reported cardiac disease samples, the nature and extent of neuropsychological deficits may also be different.

The total sample included 53 patients who underwent a neuropsychological examination as part of the routine pre-transplant evaluation. This therefore represents a consecutive series (except for those who were too ill to be assessed). The mean age of the sample was 45.1 years (SD = 10.8, range = 23-64). The mean educational level

Impact of Cardiac Surgery on the Quality of Life
Edited by A. E. Willner and G. Rodewald
Plenum Press, New York, 1990

was 12.1 years (SD = 3.3).   There were 42 males and 11
females.   The majority of patients had either ischemic
(n = 24) or dilated (n = 21) cardiomyopathy.   For the
purposes of data analysis, only these patient groups were
considered.

The neuropsychological test battery included the
WAIS-R, Wechsler Memory Scale Revised, and an expanded
Halstead Reitan Neuropsychological Test Battery.   All
patients were inpatients at the time of assessment.   In
some cases the examination was conducted over several
sessions because of patient fatigue.   The patients with
ischemic disease were slightly older (t = 2.53, p < .02)
and better educated (t = 1.96, p < .06) than the patients
with dilated disease.   The data were analyzed by analysis
of covariance (with age as the covariate).   Data were
also analyzed to determine possible differences in the
incidence of impaired performance on the various tasks.

RESULTS

In regard to mean performance there were relatively
few differences between the groups.   The ischemic group
was significantly more impaired than the dilated group on
the Figural Memory subtest from the Wechsler Memory Scale
Revised, and on the Knox Cube Test.   For the Figural
Memory test the difference was (t = 2.35, p < .025) and
for the Knox Cube Test the difference was (t = 1.75,
p < .03).   From the Halstead Reitan measures the ischemic
group was also significantly worse than the dilated group
on the Location score from the Tactual Performance Test
(t = 2.14, p < .05) and approached significance on the
Seashore Rhythm Test (t = 1.75, p < .10).   The groups did
not differ on an Impairment Index (p > .15) which was a
summary variable indicating the percentage of measures
falling in the impaired range for each patient.

In addition to the mean scores, the percentage of
patients in the two groups with impaired performance was
examined for each of the variables.   It was found that
the ischemic patients had a higher percentage, with
impaired scores on the proportional recall scores for the
Visual Reproduction subtest from the Wechsler Memory
Scale, and the Time and Location scores from the Tactual
Performance Test.   Finally, the distributions of test
performance in the two groups was examined.   There was a
clear pattern for the ischemic group to have a higher
percentage of impaired scores.   It was decided to examine

the number of measures in which the proportion of impaired scores in the two groups differed by 10% or more. There were nine variables that met this criterion, and in eight of the nine the ischemic patients had a higher percentage of impaired scores. In additon, eight of the nine measures were tests of memory or concentration.

In addition to the neurospychological test battery, the patients also completed the MMPI. The mean score on the Depression scale was 67 (SD = 12.4). The mean score on the Psychasthenia (anxiety) scale was 59 (SD = 9.8). Thirty-eight percent of the sample had a T score of 70 or more on the Depression Scale, and 13% had scores above 70 on the Psychasthenia scale. The summary neuropsychological impairment rating was significantly correlated with the Depression scale, but not with the Psychasthenia scale.

DISCUSSION

These results indicate a high incidence of impaired performance in patients who are candidates for cardiac transplantation. Among these patients, there was consistent evidence that patients with ischemic disease have a greater degree of impairment on several tasks, and also show a higher incidence of impaired performance. This pattern is observed most clearly in tests of memory and concentration.

The etiology of these deficits is unclear, although several mechanisms might be proposed. It is possible that these deficits may simply reflect fatigue or decreased energy, and thus may not reflect impaired cerebral function. This possibility seems unlikely because rest breaks in the testing were given ad lib, and several patients were actually examined in their rooms. In addition, the examiners who administered the tests are trained to be sensitive to patient fatigue and to offer breaks when the need arises.

If these deficits are, in fact, not an artifact of patient fatigue, then they may well represent impaired cerebral function. This could be due to diminished cardiac output and secondary cerebral hypoxia. Alternatively, these deficits could be the sequelae of cerebral hypoxia subsequent to myocardial infarction. The likelihood of this explanation would appear to be

supported by the fact that the patients with ischemic
disease had somewhat greater neuropsychological impairment. In addition to these explanations, medication
effects would have influenced test performance since
these patients are typically on extensive medication
regimens.

It is also possible that emotional factors may have
played some role in neuropsychological deficits in these
patients. There was a significant relationship between
depression and impairment, although anxiety did not
appear to be related to test performance. A relationship
between depression and test performance is not unexpected
since these patients are all acutely ill with life
threatening illnesses, and may have been preoccupied with
their physical condition. It was unclear whether the
depression or neuropsychological deficit was related to
severity of cardiac disease, but this clearly could have
been a mediating factor.

The nature and pattern of deficits observed in this
sample of cardiac transplant patients is similar to those
reported in studies of patients undergoing other types of
cardiac surgery (1). The high incidence of memory and
concentration problems in these patients (regardless of
etiology) raises certain implications for the clinical
management of these patients. The fact that this was
essentially a consecutive series underscores the importance of these findings because these patients were not
referred for symptomatic complaints. This suggests that
these patients (or those caring for them) may not be
aware of diminished memory or attentional skills. This
subtle deficit in memory or concentration could influence
a patient's understanding of treatment decisions, and
could also affect their ability to comply with treatment
protocols. This, therefore, supports the screening of
patients, (even those without obvious deficits) with
measures of attention and concentration to identify
difficulties that may not be apparent without sensitive
neuropsychological assessment.

Finally, it is not clear that these deficits are
permanent in all cases. Reversible cognitive deficits
could occur in response to improved cerebral oxygenation
(due to increased cardiac output following transplantation), or could also occur related to decreased medication, decreased fatigue, or improved emotional state. It
would be of interest to examine patients with a similar
battery before and after surgery, and to examine the

relationship between changes in test performance with
various cardiac variables. This would help determine
the factors related to improvement in neuropsychological
status, and would provide information about the
permanence of the neuropsychological deficits.

REFERENCE

1. R. Becker, J. Katz, M. J. Polonius, H. Speidel,
    "Psycholopathological and Neurological
    Dysfunctions Following Open-Heart Surgery,"
    Springer-Verlag, Berlin (1982).

MEDICAL/SURGICAL DATA

THE SURGEON'S DESCRIPTION OF THE PATIENT POPULATION

D. E. Birnbaum

Department of Cardiovascular Surgery
Rehabilitation Center
7812 Bad Krozingen, West Germany

INTRODUCTION

Performing cardiac surgery in a Rehabilitation
Center has the advantage of permitting a close follow-up
for a long postsurgical period. Thus, we typically dealt
with obvious signs of inadequate functioning of vital
organs and/or subjective complaints of patients and
relatives. This increased our interest in patients'
morbidity after surgery with the aim of beneficial
effects in their quality of life. We did this instead of
increasing the quantity of surgical procedures which
would have been far more popular with those who measure
surgery by the number of cases done. So we were happy to
join and support this multicenter study. We hoped to
enhance our understanding of the patholophysiology of
postoperative disease after cardiac-surgical intervention and its possible hazardous side-effects. It
became my task to present a description of the patient
cohort available to date.

PATIENT POPULATION

Age Distribution

The patient population consisted of 498 patients at
seven participating centers. Eighty-one percent were
male. Two centers contributed 20 patients, one about 50
patients, and all the others had more than 80 patients
with a maximum of 121 patients in one center. The mean
age was 56.3, (std. dev. 9.6% ranging from 41 to 83

Impact of Cardiac Surgery on the Quality of Life
Edited by A. E. Willner and G. Rodewald
Plenum Press, New York, 1990

years). Fig. 1 shows the age distribution in decades, as
well as the mean age for each center. In the United
States in this population, more cardiac surgery is performed in elderly patients while the youngest patients
were in Sao Paulo. Among a total of 340 non-U.S.
patients, almost 75% were 50 years or younger.

Figure 1 shows that there is much heterogeneity of
patients in regards to age among the different centers.
This implies that one should consider the limitations
when attempting to correlate pathophysiology of natural
aging with that of cardiac surgery.

Patients Past History

Previous medical history that is considered
important in regard to neuropsychological outcome is
listed in Table 1. Among those patients with previous
operative procedures, there are only 30 patients for
coronary bypass grafting. Seventeen patients had cardiac
surgery previously two or more times.

Angina pectoris was found in 380 patients out of
a total of 451 patients undergoing coronary bypass
grafting. It is said that postsurgical morbidity in
bypass graft patients depends on whether angina is stable
or unstable. Therefore Table 3 was compiled.

Surgical Procedure

The kind of operative procedure is listed in Table
4. In the major portion of the patients, coronary artery

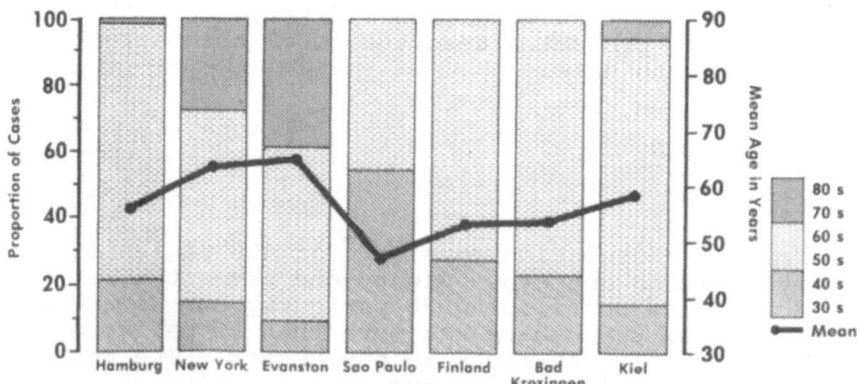

Fig. 1.   Age distribution by Center.

TABLE 1

PAST HISTORY

	N of patients with abnormal history	N of patients with complete data	% of patients with abnormal history
Myocardial infarction	258	398	65.2
Hypertension	153	428	35.7
Diabetes	61	498	12.2
Cerebro-vasc. disease	32	498	6.4
Previous surg. procedures	97	498	19.4

The pathology of the 6.4% of the patients with cerebrovascular disease is listed in Table 2.

TABLE 2

CEREBRO-VASCULAR DISEASE IN PAST HISTORY

Previous stroke	8
Cerebral embolus	8
TIA	8
Asymptomatic bruit	10
Total findings in 32 patients	34

[Total = 32 pts. out of 498 (6.4%)]

bypass grafts were implanted. Some patients with valve disease had reconstructive surgery. In 45% of the bypass patients the internal thoracic artery was used, mostly combined with saphenous graft; however, an isolated arterial replacement was used in only 15% of the cases. An average of 3.1 peripheral coronary anastomoses were performed (std. dev. 0.4, min 1, max 8 anastomoses). In 46 cases (10%) an endarterectomy was carried out.

TABLE 3

ANGINA PAST HISTORY

Chronic stable angina	224	59.0%
Recent onset	16	4.2%
Progressive	85	22.4%
Unstable	55	14.5%
Unstable categories total =	156	(41%)

TABLE 4

OPERATIVE PROCEDURE

Coronary artery bypass	435	88%
CAB and valve surgery	16	3%
Valve surgery alone	42	9%
Other	1	-

The surgical procedure was accomplished by use of cardioplegia in 457 cases; preferably by use of crystalloid solutions (Table 5). For practical reasons, in most cases the cardioplegic solution was drained into the circulation; only 15% of surgeons sucked the fluid away when arriving at the coronary sinus.

TABLE 5

CARDIOPLEGIA (n = 457)

	n	%
Cristalloid	307	67
Blood	99	22
Other	51	11

Patients' Status at Surgery and Clinical Outcome

Of the whole population, 488 patients left the hospital, which reflects a mortality rate of 2%. There were 3 deaths (0.6%) recorded which happened during surgery for technical reasons; one of these was declared as equipment failure.

The cardio-circulatory status in the vast majority was declared as stable (Table 6). A total of 45 patho-physiological events were seen in 33 patients (6.6% of the whole population). Most common is hypertension and low cardiac output syndrome which often results in dificulty weaning off pump (Table 7).

TABLE 6

STATUS AT END OF PROCEDURE

Stable	388	78.0%
Inotropic support	104	21.0%
IABP	3	0.6%
Other	2	0.4%

TABLE 7

INTRAOPERATIVE PATHOPHYSIOLOGICAL EVENTS

Complication	n (events)
Hypotension	11
Difficult pump weaning	10
L.C.O. syndrome	8
Severe arrhythmias	8
Cardiac arrest post-pump	5
Allergic reactions	2
Coagulopathy	1

During the treatment after surgery on the intensive care unit, 413 adverse events occurred in 47% of the patients (see Table 8). Seventy percent of the adverse events were related to abnormal hemodynamic conditions. The most common reason for reopening the chest was, as might be expected, abnormal blood loss (17 cases out of 24).

TABLE 8
ICU EVENTS

Hemodynamics:	Hypotension	113
	Hypertension	78
	L.C.O. Syndrome	57
	Myocardial infarction	22
	Cardioversion	17
	Cardiac Arrest	6
	IABP	6
Operation:	Abnormal blood loss	29
	Re-sternotomy	24
	Cardiac Tamponade	4
Other:	Gas exchange disturbance	49
	Acute renal failure	3
	Cerebral embolism	3
	Sepsis	2

Figure 2 shows how long patients stay in the intensive care unit (ICU) after cardiac surgery in the different centers. Approximately 60% of all patients left the ICU on the second day. More that half of the remainder were treated for at least 3 days on ICU and they were contributed by the groups of New York and

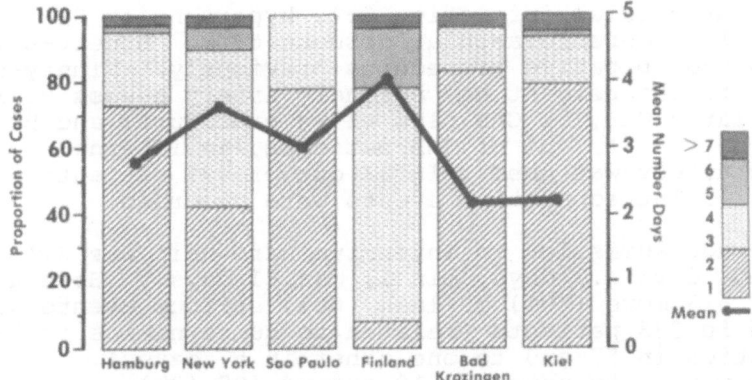

Fig. 2.   Number of days in ICU.

Finland. In the New York patient groups the advanced
average age of the patient cohort may be responsible for
the prolonged ICU treatment. However, subjective consideration, habits, tradition, conviction, and internal
hospital strategies may also contribute to the decision
for discharge.

In my opinion the ICU per se represents an appreci-
able morbidity risk. This may limit interpretations when
one attempts to attribute diminished quality of life
solely to cardiac surgery.

DISCUSSION

The demonstrated population characteristics show
vast variation among participating centers. Obviously
there is a selection of patients on an unknown basis.
This may support the impression that the patients studied
may be less ill than the average cardiac surgical population. Physicians are not standardised. Because the
protocols of some participating centers were incomplete,
considerable effort was required to make them more
complete.

SUMMARY

A total of 498 patients from seven centers are
included in the study to date. Eighty-one percent were
men. Mean age was 56.3, std. dev. 9.6 years (min 41, max
83 years). The following past historical events were

listed: Myocardial infarction 65%, hypertension 36%, diabetes 12%, cerebrovascular disease 6.4%.   Ninety-seven patients had operative procedures previously.   Ninety-one and five tenths percent had coronary artery bypass grafts (88% isolated CAB, 3% CAB plus valve procedure) and 9% valve surgery.   In 45% of CAB-patients, an internal thoracic artery was used.   In 33 out of 497 patients a total of 45 intraoperative events were recorded.

Average admission to intensive care unit was 3.1 days (std. dev. 4.3 days, min 1, max 61 days).   Here a total of 413 more (40%) or less (60%) serious events were observed in 233 patients (related to hemodynamics in 299, to operation in 57 and to one other in 57 cases). Hospital mortality rate was 10 out of 498 (2%).

These data reflect that the patient population in this study is different from that usually seen in many centers today because these patients are selected for a prospective study (see H. -J. Meffert's paper, Comparison of In-Hospital Conditions for International Study and Non-Study Patients).

A STUDY OF EQUIPMENT FOR AND PERFORMANCE OF

EXTRACORPOREAL CIRCULATION

H. Pokar

University of Hamburg
Federal Republic of Germany

Extracorporeal Circulation (ECC), and for that matter, the type of equipment employed and its performance play a central role in any study designed to assess neurological and psychological reactions to cardiac surgery. Accordingly, the data-collecting questionnaires used contain a great many complex questions, of which just the cardinal points will be discussed. The aim of this presentation is to provide information and a general survey for better orientation and critical appraisal of the actual results of this international multicenter study. The patient sample is the same just mentioned in the chapter by Prof. Birnbaum - 498 cases from seven centers.

Equipment for the ECC

The central item of the ECC is the oxygenator. Two different types of oxygenators were used in the study: Bubble and membrane oxygenators. In 225 operations, i.e. in 46%, bubble oxygenators were used, and in 273 operations (54%), membrane oxygenators were employed. The membrane group included a few more membrane-sheet than hollow-fibre oxygenators (29% vs. 24%). Only 2% were membrane-silicone oxygenators. The protocol of the study did not stipulate the number of bubble or membrane oxygenators to be used. The fact that bubblers were used in nearly half the cases indicates that not all cardiac surgeons were convinced of the superiority of membrane

Impact of Cardiac Surgery on the Quality of Life
Edited by A. E. Willner and G. Rodewald
Plenum Press, New York, 1990

247

oxygenators, although the advantages of the membranes are emphasized in the literature.

Eight different models of bubble oxygenators from seven manufacturers were included in this study. The use of individual models varies between 2 and 28% of the total of 225 bubblers. The differing numbers for the individual models reflect differences in the number of operations in the respective centers and do not necessarily show that a particular oxygenator is favored. With regard to differences in the quality of bubble oxygenators, there is a wide range of opinions.

Membrane oxygenators were employed in only four of the seven centers. Four different models of membrane-sheet oxygenators were used in a total of 144 cases and three models of hollow-fibre oxygenators in 120 cases. The silicone-membrane oxygenator was hardly used at all (9 cases). Two models were employed in two centers exclusively. The other five models were distributed among the other two centers. Just as with the bubble oxygenators, the number of individual models of membrane oxygenators employed does not reflect quality or superiority. Practical criteria, such as rapid and safe handling or service of the supplying companies rather than criteria, such as complement activating properties or permeability for gas bubbles, seem to guide the choice of a particular oxygenator in a given center. This is because our knowledge of quality of this device is not yet good enough.

Table 1 depicts the types of oxygenators used by the individual centers. Three of the seven centers used

Table 1. Proportion of oxygenator type per center.

Proportion of Oxygenator Type per Center				
Center		Bubble	Oxygenator Type Membrane	Hollow Fiber
	(n)	%	%	%
Kiel	(55)	100	-	-
Bad Krozingen	(79)	79	15	6
Finland	(101)	3	56	41
Sao Paulo	(29)	100	-	-
Evanston	(22)	100	-	-
New York	(91)	15	2	83
Hamburg	(121)	34	65	1

bubblers exclusively - Kiel, Sao Paulo and Evanston, and
in Bad Krozingen it was 79%. Oulu (Finland), New York
and Hamburg used membranes predominantly, actually in
Hamburg membrane-sheets, in New York hollow-fibres and in
Finland both. For reasons of clarity only, the three
general types of oxygenators are depicted, but in fact 15
different models of oxygenators were used. This great
variety will considerably complicate the final evaluation
of the influence of the type of oxygenator on the central
nervous system.

Another crucial point in ECC is the arterial line
filters. They are used to prevent micro gas bubbles and
corpuscular aggregates from entering the arterial circulation of a patient and thus preventing micro emboli from
travelling to the central organs. Micro bubbles not only
leave bubble oxygenators in the absence of adequate
defoaming, but also appear in membrane oxygenators for
other reasons.

In the study four different arterial line filters
were used. It appears that the use of such filters is
not universally accepted, since in a total of 130 cases
or 26%, none were used. In 36% of all ECCs a filter
model with a pore size of 25 microns was used. It is a
screen filter with a mesh made of nylon. The next most
frequently used was employed in 23%. In contrast, it is
made of polyester with a pore size of 40 microns. This
situation with the arterial line filters again reflects
our uncertain knowledge in ECC. The best material of
which the filter mesh is made (nylon or polyester), and
its optimal pore size and even whether we need filters at
all, remains unresolved.

Table 2 depicts which arterial line filter is used
by which center. The parentheses indicate the total
number of cases in each center. In the next column can
be found the percentage of filters used in relation to
the total number of cases in each center. Two centers -
Finland and Sao Paulo - did not use filters at all; in
Kiel and Hamburg, No. 4 was used - a 25 micron nylon
filter; in New York and Evanston No. 20, a 40 micron
polyester, and in Bad Krozingen a 40 micron filter made
of nylon, was used.

Another important component of the ECC is the cardiotomy reservoir (CTR). All of the cardiotomy suction
is collected here. This collection of blood from the
pericardium is loaded with fat-globuli, tissue debris,
cell aggregates, etc. As such, in all modern equipment,

Table 2. Proportion of arterial line filter by center.

Proportion of Arterial Line Filter per Center					
			Filter Type by Code No.		
Center	none	4	14	20	30
(n)	%	%	%	%	%
Kiel (55)	–	100	–	–	–
Bad Kroz. (79)	–	3	77	–	20
Finland (101)	100	–	–	–	–
Sao Paulo (29)	100	–	–	–	–
Evanston (22)	–	–	–	100	–
New York (91)	–	–	–	100	–
Hamburg (121)	–	100	–	–	–

a 20-40 micron filter is an integral part of the CTR. At
the seven centers 14 different CTR-models were used. The
number of CTR-models employed in a center varied from one
to seven. One can imagine the difficulties for the final
evaluation arising from this variety of CTRs. The
apparent reason for the multiplicity of CTR-models
involved seems to be that the user may not be in the
proper position to judge the quality.

     In all centers the ECC was in general non-pulsatile,
the pulsatile roller pump being rarely used. Only in
four cases a centrifugal instead of a roller pump was
employed.

Performance of the ECC

     It is rather simple to get reliable data on the
equipment used. It seems to be nearly impossible to get
detailed data on the actual performance of ECC. This
however should be the prerequisite for any correlation of
these data with the psycho-neurological disturbances in
terms of cause and effect. The difficulty is the documentation of the performance data with a large enough
number of data points. A central question would be what
is the effect of time with respect to blood pressure,
blood flow rate, body temperature, hematocrit, PO_2, PCO_2
and pH on the patient's cerebral function? Sampling the
data at least at 15 minute intervals would appear to be a
minimal requirement. However, this would result in a
huge amount of data and surpass our logistic and financial
capability. Therefore, the study design only called for
single average values of those time dependent measures.

The most reliable data on ECC performance are the bypass times. Only 9% of all bypass times were shorter than 60 minutes, despite the fact that nearly 90% of all operations were isolated CAB-procedures which often don't require very much time. Fifty percent of all bypasses lasted from one to two hours, 30% were between two and three hours, and the last 10% were more than three hours. This 10% of long lasting perfusions might be caused by special surgical events, or by special conditions in a center.

Table 3 gives the bypass times by center. In Finland perfusion times were three hours or longer in 41% of 101 cases. That means the majority of these bypass times can't be caused by special events, but represent more or less routine cases. Nearly 60% of their perfusions lasted two to three hours and only a few cases were less than two hours. In contrast to Finland are the times in Kiel. Only 5% of their perfusions were longer than two hours, 71% lasted one to two hours and nearly 25% were even below one hour. This huge difference in times between Finland and Kiel might give us the opportunity to clarify the question of whether a long lasting ECC really produces more psycho-neurological and other disturbances. The bypass times of New York and Hamburg were more or less equal, about 40% of their perfusions lasted longer than two hours. In the remaining three centers, Bad Krozingen, Evanston and Sao Paulo, this percentage was only about 20%.

As regards the percentage of systemic blood flow rates during hypothermia, almost half of all patients were perfused with 2.1-2.5 $1/min/m^2$ BSA. In 14% the flow

Table 3. Proportion of bypass time per center.

Proportion of Bypass Time per Center							
				Bypass Time (min)			
Center		Lo-60	61-90	91-120	121-150	151-180	181-210	211-Hi
	(n)	%	%	%	%	%	%	%
Finland	(101)	–	1	2	25	31	26	15
New York	(91)	8	24	28	23	11	4	2
Hamburg	(121)	7	23	33	24	8	3	2
Bad Kroz.	(79)	9	42	33	13	2	–	1
Evanston	(22)	5	36	37	18	4	–	–
Sao Paulo	(29)	14	29	39	14	–	–	4
Kiel	(55)	24	40	31	3	–	2	–

rates were even higher than 2.5 1/min/m^{2}BSA. Normally
these high rates are more in accordance with normothermia.

Thirty-one percent of all flow rates are in the interval
from 1.6 - 2.0 1/min/m^2, which is in the range of the so
called "low flow perfusion," (the use of blood flows less
than 1.8 1/min/m^2). These flow rates are discussed in
the literature as being more adequate in hypothermia.

Figure 1 depicts the percentage of the mean blood
pressure during perfusion. The study questionnaire asked
for the predominant pressure. So we have only one estimated mean pressure independent of the duration of the
ECC. This problem was mentioned before. The two intervals from 60 - 69 and 70 - 79 mmHg included 80% of all
pressures. Only in two percent of the cases was the
blood pressure predominantly below 50 mmHg. Under these
circumstances it might be difficult to answer the question whether low blood pressure during ECC can lead to
psychic disorders or central nervous system impairments.

Almost all patients were operated in hypothermia but
their temperatures showed a wide range, from below 24°C
up to 32°C. Actually the range from 27°C to 29°C seemed
to be preferred with 39% of the cases, but the range
below (24-26°C) and above (30-32°C) included a fair
amount of cases, 22% and 26% respectively. Thirteen
percent were cooled below 24°C. With few exceptions
these patients all were operated in Oulu (Finland), 57%
of their sample. In contrast to Finland, in Bad Krozingen
the temperature was 30-32°C in 80% of the cases.

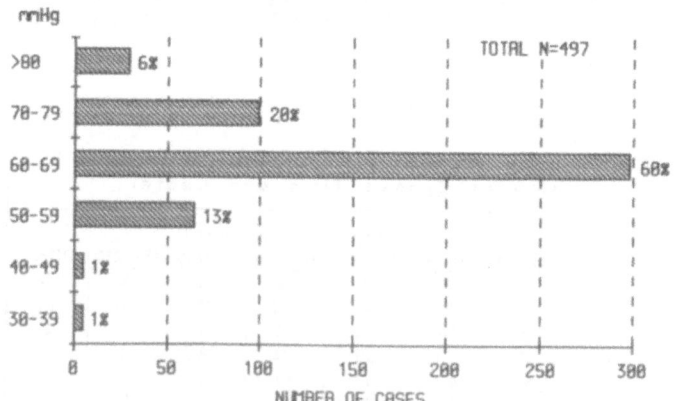

Fig. 1.   Percentage of mean blood pressure during
          perfusion.

A further important detail in performance of ECC is the hematocrit value, because oxygen transfer depends on the product of the blood flow rate, hematocrit and oxygen saturation. During recent years a tendency to lower hematocrit values arose in order to save as much blood as possible to avoid infections with AIDS and hepatitis. Despite many years of experience with hemodilution and discussion of how far hematocrit can be reduced, the question of where a safe limit resides arose again. There are centers not involved in this study which are unafraid to run a hematocrit clearly below 20%.

Among the participating seven centers there was no surgeon who trusted hematocrits in the range of 20% and lower. A clear majority (53%) of hematocrits were between 21% and 25%. This range seems more or less accepted as a safe one. But nevertheless a considerable number (44%) were in the range from 26% to 35% which reflects some disagreement in the discussion of how far hemodilution is possible without any impairment of the oxygen supply.

Closely connected with the problem of a sufficient oxygen supply for the organism is central venous oxygen saturation. In case of low saturation the pump flow has to be increased. But again, it is hard to say which value would be too low. It depends very much on the time the low saturation lasts.

Figure 2 depicts the distribution of the lowest central venous oxygen saturation. We obtained this value from those perfusions where the pump flow was corrected

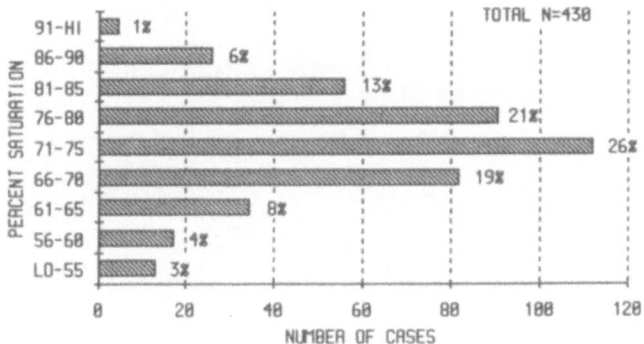

Fig. 2.   Lowest venous O_2 saturation.

to venous saturation, a total of 430 or 86% of the cases.
This means probably only in 14% was the ECC performed on
the basis of precalculated flows. The venous saturation
included values from more than 90% to less than 55%.
This very wide range can be explained by the fact that in
most centers the saturation is measured discontinuously
every 20 or 30 minutes. In the meantime the saturation
can deviate to undesired values. If we assume a good
tolerable range for the saturation is from 66 to 85
percent, almost 80 percent of all values are in that
range.

        Now some data on the arterial blood gases: In 25%
of the cases the PO_2 was in a range from 100 - 200 mmHg,
75% were between 200 and 400 mmHg. Almost 50% of the
arterial PCO_2-values were above 35 mmHg; the others were
below this value. Only for 386 of all 498 cases do we
know whether the gas analyses were corrected for temperature or not. Seventy-two percent of the hypothermic
perfusions were performed with gas analyses not corrected
for temperature. The autoregulation of cerebral perfusion
is better maintained if gas analyses are not corrected
for temperature. But until now it has not been proven
that cerebral outcome is better if one does so. Perhaps
this study will be able to show this advantage. In all,
we have 464 data entries concerning the arterial pump
occlusion adjustment. The pump was adjusted just
occlusively (no drop per minute) in almost 50% of the
cases. In 146 cases, that is 31%, the drop was one inch
per minute and in 20% the drop was greater than one inch
per minute. These differences in handling pump technique
indicate that even after 35 years of using ECC there is a
disagreement in such a basic item. In 99% of all patients
the site of arterial canulation was the aorta. At least
a unanimous opinion exists in this item.

CEREBRAL PROTECTION DURING CARDIOPULMONARY BYPASS:

DEVICES AND TECHNIQUES TO PREVENT AIR EMBOLISM

Mark Kurusz and Vincent R. Conti

Division of Cardiothoracic Surgery
The University of Texas Medical Branch
Galveston, Texas, USA

INTRODUCTION

The subject of optimum cerebral protection during cardiopulmonary bypass is far from resolved [1]. However, in recent years important strides have been made in understanding which devices and techniques protect best. Air, or gas embolism (massive or micro) from the extracorporeal circuit has been implicated in neurologic dysfunction in patients following cardiopulmonary bypass (CPB). Prevention of air embolism has been the focus of surgeons and perfusionists since the advent of open-heart surgery in the 1950s. The dangers and consequences of air embolism, however, have been reported in the literature many centuries prior to the advent of open-heart surgery. The manifestations may be subtle or gross, transient or permanent, depending on several factors including volume and type of gas, rate of infusion, and methods of treatment used when air embolism is recognized. Technique considerations for minimizing gaseous microemboli include choice of circuit components and methods of their operation. Use of arterial filters and membrane oxygenators has been suggested for decreasing gaseous microemboli. In cases of air embolism, safety devices on the CPB circuit may limit the extent of patient injury.

Impact of Cardiac Surgery on the Quality of Life
Edited by A. E. Willner and G. Rodewald
Plenum Press, New York, 1990

MATERIALS & METHODS

On November 1, 1985, 1366 ten-page perfusion accident questionnaires were mailed to perfusionists in the United States and Canada [2]. The mailing list was comprised of all identifiable, active clinical perfusionists. Stamped, self-addressed envelopes were provided to facilitate return of completed questionnaires. An accompanying cover letter stated the purpose of the survey, requested information limited to the perfusionist's direct knowledge, and assured respondents of confidentiality. Provision was made for two or more perfusionists to report their experience on a single questionnaire, and names and addresses of active perfusionists who did not receive a questionnaire were solicited. All questionnaires were numbered for identification purposes to permit follow-up mailings to nonrespondents.

The questionnaire consisted of 110 questions divided into sections that included hematology, hemodynamics, pharmacology, gas embolism, myocardial protection, equipment, and perfusion techniques. A miscellaneous section asked questions on prevention and requested either actual or estimated total caseload experience for the three years between October 1982 and October 1985. When specific accidents were reported, information on patient outcome ("No injury," "Permanent injury," or "Death") was requested. Additionally, clarification of the circumstances of the accidents was requested by asking for specific details. All such questions also had one selection entitled "other" with a request for the respondent to explain if they had information that fell outside the format on the questionnaire.

The questionnaire was coded for keypunching purposes to allow data entry onto an IBM model 3081 mainframe computer (IBM, Inc., Armonk, NY). Six weeks after the initial mailing a planned, follow-up mailing was made to all nonrespondents (See Fig. 1.) Data are represented as percent frequencies of respondents or responses and numbers of cases.

RESULTS

A total of 608 completed questionnaires, or 44% of the target sample group, were returned during the study period. Two hundred of these respondents noted that their returned questionnaire represented the experience of two or more perfusionists. The total caseload experience for

the three-year period reported by the respondents was
573,785 procedures which consisted of 193,001 actual cases
on 217 questionnaires and 380,784 estimated cases on 370
questionnaires.   An additional 198 questionnaires were
returned by the postal service marked "Non Deliverable."
Forty-two questionnaires were returned but were not
included in the survey because the respondents noted that
they had reported their experience on another questionnaire or they had retired or were inactive. Fourteen were
received after the 12-week study period, and four were
incomplete. Geographically, the sampling distribution was
good, with responses from perfusionists in 47 states in
the United States and seven Canadian provinces.

     Regarding gas embolism, an arterial line gas embolism
during CPB considered serious enough to be life-threatening
was observed by 21.5% of the perfusionists in 200 cases.
Permanent injury or death was the patient outcome in 33 of
the cases.   Inattention to the extracorporeal reservoir
level was the cause of this accident in 104 cases, most
often when using a bubble oxygenator. Other reported
causes were ruptured arterial pumphead tubing (16 cases)
or unnoticed rotation of the arterial pumphead (14 cases).
The type of tubing in use during cases of arterial pumphead tubing rupture was reported as polyvinyl chloride
(PVC) in nine cases and silicone rubber in three cases. A
significant number of cases (54) were noted in the "other"
category and were most often described as an "acute drop
in venous return," "air in arterial cannula pre or post
CPB," "improper priming of the arterial line filter," or
"during circulatory arrest with opened aorta." (See Fig.
2.)   Other types of life-threatening gas embolism were
reported by 21.3% in 258 cases, and the outcome was permanent injury or death in 36 patients. Causes were: aortic
root air from cardioplegic solution administration (82
cases); unexpected resumption of heart beat (27 cases);
reversed left ventricular vent line (26 cases); or
pressurized cardiotomy reservoir (15 cases). Eighty-six
cases were reported in the "other" category which most
often were described as "other vent problems during
insertion, use, or removal," "inadequate deairing of the
heart, especially following valvular operations," "IV
lines from anesthesia," or "monitoring lines." (See Fig.
3.)

     Questions regarding prevention revealed percent usage
of the following safety devices: 81.1%, arterial line
filter; 69.9%, low-level alarm; 47.9%, air bubble
detector; and 35.4%, one-way, pressure relief valve in
the left ventricular line. Less than five percent used an

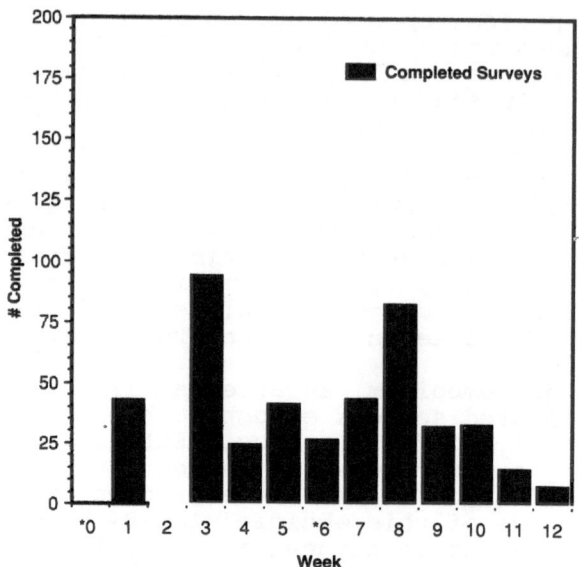

Fig. 1   Perfusion accident survey weekly returns. The
          asterisk at 0 indicates the initial mailing on
          November 1, 1985, and the asterisk at week six
          indicates when a followup mailing was made.
          Total number of usable returned questionnaires
          was 608.

arterial line bubble trap (without filter media), an
arterial in-line ball check valve, or an oxygenator weight
arm servo-regulated to the arterial pump. Sixty-eight
respondents, or 11.2% of the total group, noted they used
"other" safety devices such as a "one-way valved filter
purge line," a "soft bag venous reservoir," or a "vortex
arterial pump." Seventeen respondents, or 2.8% of the
total group, reported that no safety devices were used.
For those who use a low-level alarm, it is used in the
manual mode routinely by 64% and the automatic, pump
shut-off mode by 36%.

     One question allowed for hand-written comments
regarding the perfusionists' experience with safety
devices. Specifically, they were asked to note if such
devices were in use (during reported accidents), whether
they failed, or whether they functioned properly and
prevented patient injury. One-fourth of the question-

naires had comments, and while this method of survey is
statistically less precise, tabulation of the available
comments revealed that when an arterial line filter or an
air bubble detector were in use, they were effective in
the majority of cases. However, a low-level alarm was
effective only about one-half of the time, and a one-way
pressure relief valve in the left ventricular vent line
was noted to fail to prevent patient injury more often
than not. Such information should be qualifed by the fact
that there were a small number of responses on specific
devices. Also important were the comments made by many
respondents that such safety devices were ineffective if
they were turned off or if gas was introduced distal to
placement of the device on the extracorporeal circuit.
Two other questions in the section on gas embolism asked
about the use of vents and the availability of a hyperbaric chamber for treatment. Thirty-seven percent of the
perfusionists noted that the left ventricular vent was
checked under water or blood prior to use in the heart to
verify proper function, and 62.4% reported that it was
not. If a massive gas embolism occurred, 41.4% noted that
a hyperbaric chamber was available for treatment and 58.6%
noted one was not available.

DISCUSSION

     Air embolism during cardiopulmonary bypass is still a
rare occurrence, but did rank third overall (out of 15
types of pefusion accidents) for a patient outcome of
permanent injury or death. When incidence rates were
calculated from the respondents' total caseload experience, gas embolism occurred once every 8000 cases in the
current survey versus once every 2500 cases in the 1980
survey by Stoney et al. [3]. This decreased incidence may
be due to the fact that more perfusionists use a low-level
alarm (70% now versus 42% earlier). Fewer now, however,
operate such an alarm in the automatic, or pump shut-off,
mode (36% versus 48% in the earlier survey). The availability of another safety device, the air bubble detector
which, when activated, shuts off the pump nearly instant-
aneously if a gas bolus greater than one cubic centimeter
in volume is detected, is used by nearly one-half of the
respondents and may explain why fewer use the low-level
alarm in the automatic, pump shut-off mode.

     Based on the handwritten responses, low-level alarms
were reportedly less reliable than the air bubble detector
or arterial filter in preventing gas embolism. This may
be because low-level alarms require user placement and

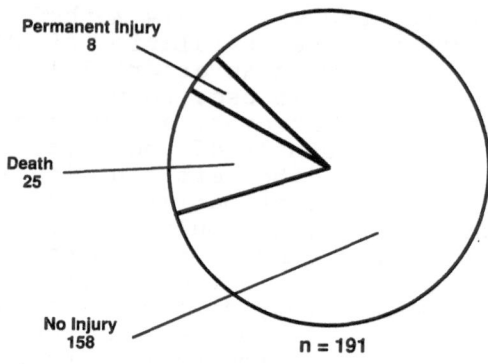

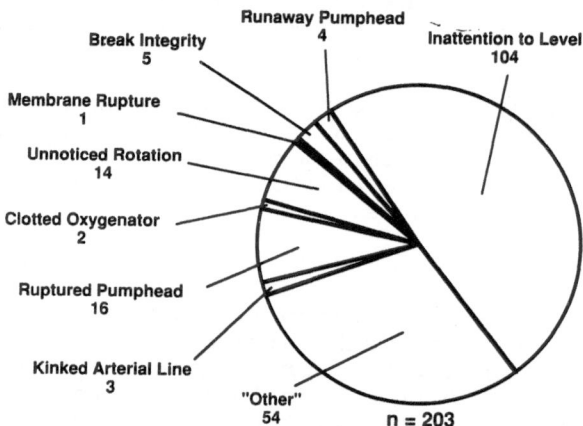

Fig. 2.   Arterial line gas embolism. Cases with reported
           patient outcomes are shown at the top and causes
           at the bottom.

sensitivity adjustment, and most types can be affected by
ambient room light. Use of redundant safety devices such
as the air bubble detector, arterial filter, and one-way
pressure relief valve in the left ventricular vent line
also may reduce the odds of such a catastrophic accident.
The use of membrane oxygenators, most of which incorporate
a soft bag venous reservoir, has increased, and usage of
membranes according to the survey respondents slightly
exceeds that of bubble oxygenators (51.4% versus 48.6%).
Also, this fact may have had a positive impact on the
decreased numbers of massive gas embolism cases. A new
and surprisingly significant cause of such an accident is
air administered into the aortic root at the time of
cardioplegic solution administration. Crystalloid or

blood cardioplegia can be administered several different
ways, and many teams also use the administration line for
aortic root venting which may predispose air entry into
the aortic root unless precise control over direction of
flow and negative pressure is maintained.

Other techniques to reduce the incidence of air
embolism include: 1) Prebypass checklist. Three-quarters
of the respondents use a prebypass checklist to ensure
that the circuit and equipment are ready for CPB; 2) Test
vents. Two-thirds did not report this simple technique
first reported by Mills and Ochsner in 1980 [4] to verify
proper operation of the vent prior to placement in the

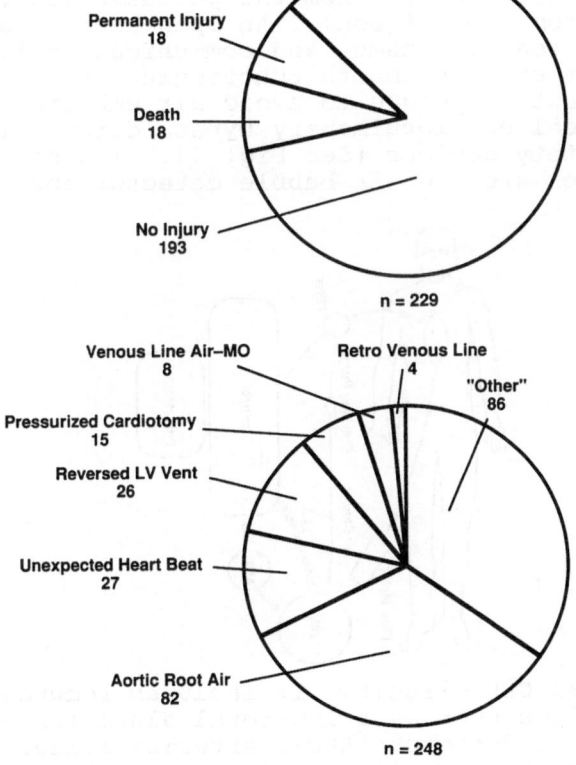

Fig. 3.   Other gas embolism. Cases with reported patient
           outcomes are shown at the top and causes at the
           bottom.

heart or vessels;   3) Gas scavenging. Anesthetic gas
scavenge lines must be unobstructed to avoid pressuriza-
tion of the oxygenator;   4) Temperature gradients.
Judicious (< 10° C) cooling and rewarming gradients can
prevent gaseous microemboli when inducing or reversing
hypothermia [5];   5) Watch level. This is a cardinal rule
taught to perfusion students and is one of the most
important safety techniques during CPB;   6) Communication/
Teamwork. An often cited need during CPB is verbal
communication among surgeon, perfusionist and anesthesiologist [6]. Some independent actions by any one
team member, if performed without the others' knowledge,
can cause an air embolism accident.

     In summary, the types of air embolism may be classi-
fied according to their sources by those on the open-heart
team. There are three basic types: anesthetic (from the
anesthesiologist), pump (from the perfusionist), and
operative (from the surgeon). An open-heart team may be
considered a team of teams, and communication is the
hallmark that ensures smooth functioning of the team and
is an important technique to avoid air embolism during
CPB. The ideal cardiopulmonary bypass circuit incorporates
redundant safety devices (See Fig. 4). The best currently
available ones are the air bubble detector and the

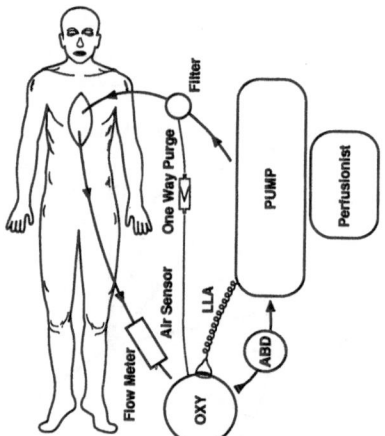

Fig. 4.   Ideal CPB circuit. It includes redundant safety
          devices such as a low-level alarm (LLA), air
          bubble detector (ABD), arterial filter with
          one-way purge line, and a venous line flowmeter/
          air sensor (not commercially available).
          NOTE: OXY-oxygenator; blood flow is in
          direction of arrows.

arterial line filter. A new device consisting of a combination flow meter/air sensor on the venous line using
Doppler technology could further reduce the incidence of
an air embolism when using conventional CPB. In this
manner, an early warning of decreased venous return or air
in the venous line would alert the perfusionist of these
conditions.

In closing, the finer aspects of cerebral protection
during open-heart surgery can be negated nearly instanta-
neously if an air embolism accident occurs. Use of safety
devices by a well-disciplined team can decrease the risk
of this complication.

REFERENCES

1. M. Kurusz, Cerebral protection and cardiopulmonary
    bypass: A review, Proceed Am Acad Cardiovasc
    Perfusion. 7:115 (1986).
2. M. Kurusz, V. R. Conti, J. F. Arens, J. P. Brown,
    S. C. Faulkner and J. V. Manning Jr., Perfusion
    accident survey, Proceed Am Acad Cardiovasc
    Perfusion. 7:57 (1986).
3. W. S. Stoney, W. C. Alford Jr., G. R. Burrus, D. M.
    Glassford Jr. and C. S. Thomas Jr., Air Embolism
    and other accidents using pump oxygenators, Ann
    Thorac Surg. 29:336 (1980).
4. N. L. Mills and J. L. Ochsner, Massive air embolism
    during cardiopulmonary bypass; Causes, prevention,
    and management, J Thorac Cardiovasc Surg. 80:708
    (1980).
5. M. Kurusz, Gaseous microemboli: Sources, causes and
    clinical considerations, Med. Instrument. 19:73
    (1985).
6. M. Kurusz and D. R. Wheeldon, Perfusion safety,
    Perfusion. 3:97 (1988).

CEREBRAL BLOOD FLOW DECLINES INDEPENDENTLY OF

METABOLISM DURING HYPOTHERMIC CARDIOPULMONARY BYPASS

David A. Stump, Anne T. Rogers,
Donald S. Prough, and A. S. Hudspeth

Depts. of Anesthesia, Neurology and Surgery
(Section on Cardiothoracic)
Wake Forest University Medical Center
Winston-Salem, NC, USA 27103

Although neurologic sequelae are common [1, 2] following nonpulsatile hypothermic cardiopulmonary bypass (CPB), the etiology of neurologic dysfunctions in this setting are still unclear because of the difficulty of monitoring cerebral blood flow (CBF) and cerebral metabolism during the operative procedure. We have used the Xe-133 desaturation method to measure CBF in over 200 patients during CPB to define the cerebrovascular response to a variety of physiological conditions, such as changes in pump flow [3], acid-base management [4, 5], hypercarbia [6], anesthetics [7], and to evaluate the effects of age and cerebrovascular disease [8, 9, 10]. Our studies have demonstrated a spontaneous decline in regional CBF (rCBF) during hypothermic CPB that is independent of the cerebral metabolic rate.

There are four possible mechanisms for the observed decline in CBF: 1) a decrease in cerebral metabolic rate for oxygen $CMRO_2$; 2) cerebral microcirculatory obstructions; 3) pathological vasoconstriction; and 4) measurement error.

We have begun a systematic series of experiments to determine the cause of this unexplained change in CBF. The first priority was to confirm the validity of the methodology.

Impact of Cardiac Surgery on the Quality of Life
Edited by A. E. Willner and G. Rodewald
Plenum Press, New York, 1990

Two independent studies using different methods of
estimating CBF were initiated to confirm the rate and
degree of the decline on CBF over time. 1) The Xe-133
method, which gives quantitative results, was used to
acquire data in 12 patients, at two intervals, 20 to 30
minutes apart and 2) Transcranial Doppler, which provides
a qualitative result, was used to continuously monitor
changes in middle cerebral artery Flow Velocity (FV)
throughout the operative period in another 8 patients.

Methods

After approval by our IRB, 20 patients scheduled for
elective coronary artery bypass grafting (CABG) were
enrolled and gave informed written consent. Preoperative
exclusion criteria included uncontrolled arterial hypertension and clinical evidence of cerebrovascular disease.
After premedication with oral lorazepam and morphine im,
fentanyl 75 mg/kg was used for narcosis, while pancuronium
0.1 mg/kg facilitated endotracheal intubation. No additional agents other than oxygen were administered until
all measurements were completed.

All patients underwent nonpulsatile CPB through an
ascending aortic cannula, with induction of hypothermia to
approximately 28° C. A membrane oxygenator, an arterial
line filter, and a crystalloid priming solution were used
in each case. During CPB the perfusionist maintained
within narrow limits each patient's nasopharyngeal temperature (NPT), $PaCO_2$, pump flow, and hematocrit.

The 12 subjects monitored via the Xe-133 desaturation
method were randomized into one of two groups according to
acid-base management. In Group I the mean $PaCO_2$, uncorrected for temperature, was held at approximately 40
mmHg by varying fresh gas flow into the membrane oxygenator,
whereas in Group II an average uncorrected $PaCO_2$ of 57
mmHg (which is equal to 40 mmHg when corrected for the
patient's temperature of 27°) was achieved by adding
carbon dioxide to the inflow gas. Baseline CBF measurements were obtained after the aorta had been cross clamped
and CPB conditions, including body temperature, had
stabilized for at least 5 minutes. A second CBF measurement was obtained after an interval of 20-30 minutes
without changing any of the controlled variables or using
pharmacologic intervention. Time intervals, varying among
patients, were a function of individual clinical settings.

CBF was measured in both hemispheres using a portable
regional cerebral blood flow system developed at our

institution, which uses 16 miniature cadmium telluride gamma ray detectors positioned in a helmet around the patient's head. The real time uptake and clearance of the Xe-133 is observed on a dedicated Microvax computer and terminal located as far as 30 feet from the subject. Initial results are available within 4 minutes of injection and a complete analysis within 2 minutes after the 11 minute monitoring period. CBF measurements were obtained by injecting 3-5 mCi of Xe-133 dissolved in sterile saline into the arterial tubing of the pump circuit, proximal to the filter.

An additional 8 subjects were evaluated via Transcranial Doppler to provide a continuous record of CBF changes. Mean flow velocity (FV), in cm/sec, was measured in the middle cerebral artery (MCA) with a Carolina Medical Electronics TCD-64b instrument. The Doppler probe was hand held over the temporal region. FV was monitored continuously but was analyzed for statistical purposes at 10-minute intervals from the onset of CPB until normothermic CPB following rewarming.

Results

Table 1 demonstrates that there was very little difference in the controlled variables for the 2 groups of patients studied with Xe-133, except for experimental variation in $PaCO_2$. Further, these variables remained constant across the 2 measurement intervals. Figure 1 shows the effect of time on the individual CBF measure-

Table 1

	Group I		Group II	
	Baseline	Second	Baseline	Second
MAP (mmHg)	68 ± 11	71 ± 10	67 ± 4	71 ± 13
NPT (°C)	26.5 ± 0.8	26.6 ± 0.8	27.3 ± 1.5	27.3 ± 1.4
Hct (%)	22.3 ± 3.4	22.7 ± 2.7	23.3 ± 2.9	22.3 ± 3.2
Q ($l \cdot min^{-1} \cdot m^{-2}$)	1.9 ± 0.1	1.8 ± 0.1	1.9 ± 0.2	1.9 ± 0.2
P_aCO_2 (mmHg) [+]	41 ± 3	40 ± 4	58 ± 4	60 ± 6
ET (min)	-	30 ± 20	-	20 ± 4
CBF ($ml \cdot 100g^{-1} \cdot min^{-1}$)	16 ± 4	13 ± 2 [*]	27 ± 7	27 ± 7 [*]

[*] = p<0.05; MAP = mean arterial pressure; NPT = nasopharyngeal temperature; Hct = hematocrit; [+] = uncorrected for body temperature; Q = pump oxygenator flow rate; ET = elapsed time between measurements; CBF = cerebral blood flow. (Modified with permission from Anesthesiology 1988;69:547-551)

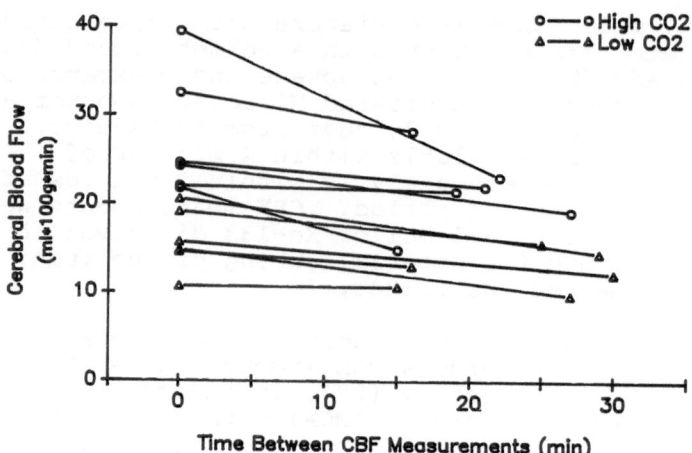

Fig. 1   Effect of time on CBF measurements during CPB.

ments during CPB.   All subjects showed a decrease over
time.   The low CO_2 group (Group I) showed an average
decline of $0.7 \pm 0.5\%/min$.   The high CO_2 group (Group II)
averaged a $1.0 \pm 0.8\%/min$ decrease.   There was no difference in the rate of decline between the groups.

Table 2 displays the $PaCO_2$ mean arterial pressure
(MAP), pump flow, and hematocrit (Hct) for the duration of
the study.   FV decreased to 67% of the initial value by

Table 2

	P_aCO_2 (mmHg) [†]	MAP (mmHg)	Q (l·min^{-1}·m^{-2})	Hct (%)
Normothermia	39 ± 3	75 ± 15	-	30 ± 8
Cool	40 ± 3	62 ± 11	2.3 ± 0.4	29 ± 7
Cross-Clamp	40 ± 3	66 ± 11	2.0 ± 0.5	27 ± 7
10	40 ± 3	64 ± 11	1.8 ± 0.5	26 ± 7
20	40 ± 2	65 ± 11	1.7 ± 0.2	25 ± 6
30	40 ± 3	65 ± 9	1.7 ± 0.2	22 ± 4
40	39 ± 4	63 ± 8	2.0 ± 0.5	23 ± 4
Warm Perfusion	37 ± 5	63 ± 7	2.8 ± 0.3	23 ± 4
Post Bypass	38 ± 3	69 ± 10	-	24 ± 2

MAP = mean arterial pressure; Q = pump oxygenator flow rate; Hct = hematocrit; and
[†] = uncorrected for body temperature.

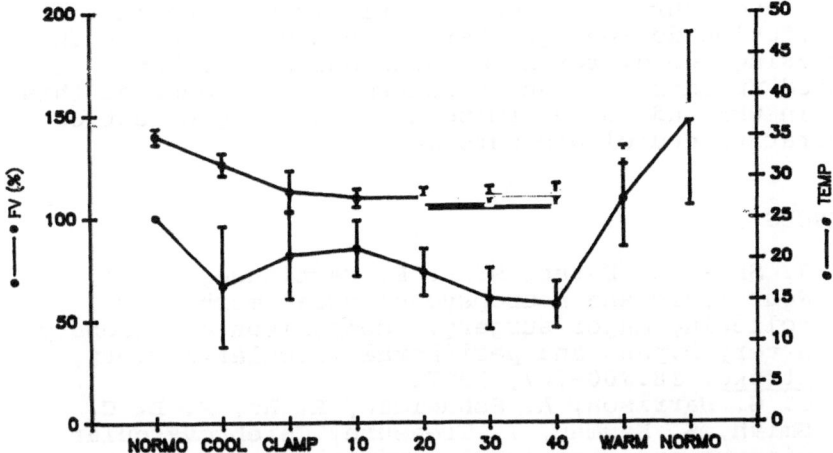

Fig. 2. Flow Velocity (FV) expressed as a percent of
the normothermic baseline compared to the
nasopharyngeal temperature.

the time of aortic cross clamp and to 58% by 40 minutes
post cross clamp (p>.01) (Fig. 2). The greatest change in
FV took place during the initial cooling phase and between
10 and 30 minutes post-clamp, although FV continued to
fall throughout the CPB period. FV increased progressively
during the rewarming period, eventually exceeding the
initial value by almost 40%.

Discussion

The results of these studies indicate that CBF
declines an average of approximately 1% per minute during
CPB, with the largest changes occurring during the cooling
phase and then again 10 to 20 minutes after cross clamp.
FV continues to decline throughout the entire CPB period
and begins a rapid increase during rewarming to overshoot
the pre-CPB flow values. The effect of temperature and
reduced hematocrit are the most probable explanation for
the large increase seen during rewarming. The possible
mechanisms for the decline in CBF include differential
cooling rates for the brain or a progressive decline
related to the cerebrovascular effects of non-pulsatile
perfusion.

We have confirmed a characteristic decline in cerebral perfusion during hypothermic, nonpulsatile CPB in humans using two different methodologies. We have initiated further studies to determine the cause of this change in CBF and to determine if it has any effect on postoperative neurologic outcome.

REFERENCES

1. P. J. Shaw, D. Bates, N. E. F. Cartlidge, et al, Neurologic and neuropsychological morbidity following major surgery; comparison of coronary artery bypass and peripheral vascular surgery, Stroke, 18:700-707, 1987.

2. M. J. G. Harrison, A. Schneidau, R. Ho, P. L. C. Smith, S. Newman, T. Treasure, Cerebrovascular disease and functional outcome after coronary artery bypass surgery, Stroke. 20:235-237, 1989.

3. D. S. Prough, D. A. Stump, A. T. Rogers, J. Phipps, L. Hinshelwood, Effects of pump flow reduction on cerebral blood flow during hypothermic cardiopulmonary bypass, Anesthesiology. 67 (suppl):A11, 1987.

4. D. S. Prough, D. A. Stump, R. C. Roy, G. P. Gravlee, T. Williams, S. A. Mills, L. Hinshelwood, G. Howard, Response of cerebral blood flow to changes in carbon dioxide tension during hypothermic cardiopulmonary bypass. Anesthesiology. 64:576-581, 1986.

5. A. T. Rogers, D. A. Stump, G. P. Gravlee, D. S. Prough, et al., Response of cerebral blood flow to phenylephrine infusion during hypothermic cardiopulmonary bypass: influence of $PaCO_2$ management, Anesthesiology. 69:547-551, 1988.

6. D. S. Prough, A. T. Rogers, D. A. Stump, S. A. Mills, A. R. Cordell, G. P. Gravlee, J. Phipps, D. Charles, Hypercarbia depresses cerebral oxygen consumption during cardiopulmonary bypass, Stroke, in press.

7. A. T. Rogers, D. S. Prough, D. A. Stump, G. P. Gravlee, K. C. Angert, R. C. Roy, S. A. Mills, L. Hinshelwood, Cerebral blood flow does not change following sodium nitroprusside infusion during hypothermic cardiopulmonary bypass, Anesth Analg. 68:122-126, 1989.

8. G. P. Gravlee, R. C. Roy, D. A. Stump, A. S. Hudspeth, A. T. Rogers, D. S. Prough, Regional cerebrovascular reactivity to carbon dioxide during CPB in patients with cerebrovascular disease, J Thorac Cardiovasc Surg, in press.

9.   F. G. Brusino, J. G. Reves, D. S. Prough, D. A. Stump,
      The effect of age on cerebral blood flow auto-
      regulation during hypothermic cardiopulmonary
      bypass, J Thorac Cardiovasc Surg. 97:541-547, 1989.
10. F. G. Brusino, J. G. Reves, D. S. Prough, D. A. Stump,
      Cerebral blood flow during cardiopulmonary bypass
      in a patient with occlusive cerebrovascular
      disease, J Cardiothorac Anesth. 3:87-90, 1989.

EMISSION OF MICRO-BUBBLES IN BUBBLE (BO) AND

MEMBRANE-OXYGENATORS (MO): A COMPARATIVE INVESTIGATION

C. Grefe, K. Ayisi and J.-J. Krebber

University of Hamburg
Hamburg, Federal Republic of Germany

SUMMARY

By means of Doppler-sonography, the emission of
gas-bubbles in the arterial line was investigated in 10
in-vitro and 30 in-vivo experiments employing as
oxygenators, two bubble (BOI + BOII), and two membrane
oxygenators (MOI + MOII). It became evident that the
occurrence of micro-bubbles was more frequent and greater
in bubble oxygenators during extracorporeal circulation
than in membrane oxygenators. Lowering blood levels and
increasing gas-perfusion rates in the oxygenator reser-
voirs resulted in increased registration of micro-bubbles
in the bubble oxygenators. When these parameters were
similarly changed in the membrane oxygenators, there were
no micro-bubbles produced, due to the absence of direct
blood/gas contact. Observation of micro-bubbles in the
arterial line of membrane oxygenators occurred during
simultaneous injection of fluids into the venous line and
during increased cardiotomy suction as was the case in
MOII, meaning bubbles escaped through the membrane oxygenator. Just as in MOII, the membrane in MOI is not a
perfect gas-filter. Prevention of gas-emboli could be
achieved through insertion of a de-foamer and additional
filters. By keeping blood volume at safe levels as
prescribed by the producer, we observed no micro-bubbles
in the arterial-line during this investigation.

INTRODUCTION

The development of cerebral dysfunction and behavioral
disorders after open heart bypass surgery are not uncommon

Impact of Cardiac Surgery on the Quality of Life
Edited by A. E. Willner and G. Rodewald
Plenum Press, New York, 1990

273

and may be influenced by factors such as the duration of
extracorporeal circulation (ECC), the level of pCO_2, the
patient's age, as well as history of previous neurological
and cardiac diseases. Important etiological factors in
cerebral dysfunction, underlined by many studies, include:
(1) inadequate cerebral perfusion resulting from hypotensive pressures during ECC; (2) extremely high venous
and intracranial pressures, and (3) low-output syndrome
before and after ECC.

In most cases, however, micro-emboli, either gas or
corpuscular, may well be responsible [1, 2]. A major
source of the gas-emboli is the oxygenator or the venous
line [3, 4]. In most cases where the membrane oxygenator
was employed, registration of micro-bubbles both in the
arterial-line and in the arteria cerebri media was
extremely low [1, 3].

In this study, the sizes of the gas-bubbles were
categorized into 4 groups according to average amplitude
of the echo at intervals of 10 sec. Similarly, there were
4 groupings of bubble-densities according to the rate of
appearance at intervals of 10 sec., e.g. occasional,
regular, irregular, or regular with high density. In
order to keep the sonic angle of $45°$ constantly aligned to
the direction of blood flow in each investigation, the
transducer-head was fixed in a block. In each investigation, only one parameter was varied at a time while the
others were kept constant.

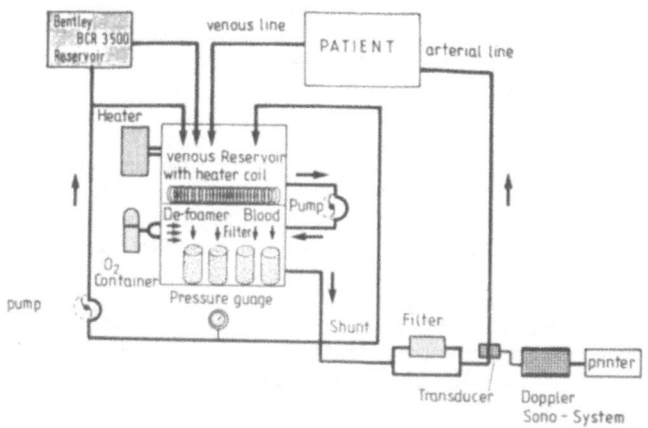

Fig. 1.   Diagrammatic Set-up of the Cobe Membrane
           Oxygenator.

Fig. 1 shows the set-up of the in-vitro experiments. Additionally, massive bubbles were purposely produced in order to test the effectiveness of the different oxygenators for extreme conditions.

Method and materials

Gas-bubble activity, which is a product of bubble size and bubble density, was measured by means of an ultrasonic Doppler gas bubble detector from Polystan A/S, bK-2730 Herlev. In the in-vivo experiments, the production of micro-bubbles was continuously registered from the start to the end of cardio-pulmonary bypass, paying particular attention to the frequency of production and the conditions under which they are produced. The average rates of bubble production in each study and the number of gas-bubbles per 100 min of extracorporeal circulation were registered for each in-vivo tested oxygenator.

Results

Higher perfusion rates, intensified cardiotomy suction, as well as declining blood levels in the tested bubble-oxygenators led to increased bubble activity. The same phenomenon was observed at higher gas/perfusion ratio rates. Furthermore, bubble activity was registered even after inserting hemofilters and by applying vibration to the oxygenators and tubing systems at the re-start of the heart-lung machine after a short pause.

The temperature of the blood had no significant influence on the production of micro-bubbles. High emission of gas-bubbles was observed in bubble oxygenators after breakdown of the shunt circulatory system, during intensive coronary suction of air and with blood levels below the minimum permitted level. Under such conditions, bubble production was higher in the Polystan venotherm oxygenator than in the Bentley.

As shown in Fig. 2, the BO produces not only bigger but also more frequent bubbles than the MO. The MO of 3M produced even fewer bubbles than the better of the two tested BOs. Bubbles were seldom detected in the Cobe MO.

In the membrane oxygenators there is no direct blood/ gas contact. As a result, the O_2-Insufflation, the perfusion rate and lowering of the blood level in the reservoir do not play a role in the production of micro-bubbles.

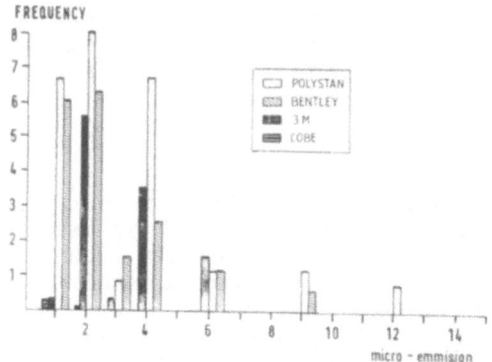

Fig. 2.   Micro-Emission in the Tested Oxygenators (in vivo).

Gas-bubbles developed in 3-M MO (as a result of cardiotomy suction (Fig. 3b), injection of fluids into the venous line (Fig. 3a), and turbulence in the venous reservoir) escaped through the membrane and were detected in the arterial line.   Fig. 3a shows gas-bubbles before and after leaving the membrane with corresponding changes in bubble size and rate of activity.   The insertion of a de-foamer and additional filters as well as keeping within the prescribed safety levels of reservoir blood prevented gas-emboli.   In the in-vivo and in-vitro studies, only in cases where blood volumes were allowed to fall below the minimum levels did we detect bubble activity in the arterial line (Fig. 3c).   At very high bubble activity both in vivo and in vitro, we still observed micro-bubbles beyond the arterial filter (pore: 25 um+40um) (Fig.3a).

Discussion

Our work shows that production of gas-bubbles is significantly lower in MO than in BO.   The membrane oxygenators are characterised not only by minimal production of micro-bubbles but also by factors such as low hemolysis, less thrombo- and leukocyte damage and protein denaturation, as well as minimal complement activation [5].

The use of hemofilters in the arterial line is advisable when using MO as long as the recommended minimum blood level is kept.   It is imperative, however, on the basis of our experimental results, to use hemofilters when employing bubble oxygenators in the heart-lung machine.

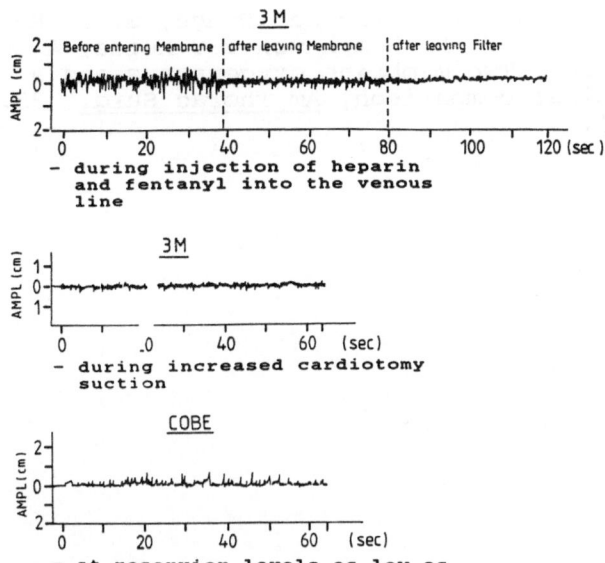

Fig. 3.   Echo-signals of Bubbles During in Vivo
          Measurements.

REFERENCES

1. P. B. Deverall, T. S. Padayachee, S. Parsons, R.
    Theobold, S. A. Battistessa, Ultrasound detection
    of micro-emboli in the middle cerebral artery
    during cardiopulmonary bypass surgery from the
    departments of: Radiological Sciences,
    Anaesthetics, Cardiothoracic Surgery, Guys
    Hospital, London, and Chief Perfusionist, London
    Bridge Hospital, London (1988).
2. D. T. Pearson, B. G. Watson, P. S. Waterhouse, An
    ultrasonic analysis of the comparative efficiency
    of various cardiotomy reservoirs and micropore
    blood filters.   Thorax. 33:352 (1978).
3. D. T. Pearson, R. F. Carter, H. B. Hammo, P. S.
    Waterhouse, Gaseous microemboli during open heart
    surgery, in: "Toward safer cardiac surgery," D. B.
    Longmore, ed., MTP Press, Lancaster (1980).
4. T. H. Pedersen, H. M. Karlsen, G. Semb, K. Hatteland,
    Comparison of bubble release from various types of
    oxygenators, Scand J Thorac Cardiovasc. Surg. 21:73
    (1987).

5.   M. Boers, T. J. A. M. van den Dunge, G. F. Karliczek,
     U. Breuken, J. N. Homan von der Heide, A. R. H.
     Wildevuur, Two membrane oxygenators and a bubbler:
     A clinical comparison, <u>Am Thorac Surg.</u>   35:455
     (1983).

COMPARISON OF IN-HOSPITAL CONDITIONS FOR "INTERNATIONAL

STUDY" AND "NON-STUDY" PATIENTS

H. J. Meffert

Department of Cardiovascular Surgery and
Experimental Cardiology
University Hospital
Hamburg-Eppendorf, FRG

U. Lamparter

Department of Psychosomatic Medicine and
Psychotherapy
University Hospital
Hamburg-Eppendorf, FRG

A. Boll

Rehabilitation Center
Bad Segeberg, FRG

This article reports observations about the
comparability of "International Study" and "Non-Study"
patients at the Department of Cardiovascular Surgery of
the University Hospital, Hamburg, FRG. "International
Study" patients are those cardiac surgery patients who
were investigated according to the International Study
protocol while "Non-Study" patients are all those cardiac
surgery patients who are not included in the International Study but were operated on during the same
period of time.

Both groups are undoubtedly comparable over all with
respect to basic criteria such as age, sex, work-status,
surgical procedure, equipment, performance of extracorporeal circulation, perfusion techniques, oxygenators,
filters, and methods of anaesthesia, etc. This is more

Impact of Cardiac Surgery on the Quality of Life
Edited by A. E. Willner and G. Rodewald
Plenum Press, New York, 1990

doubtful for psychological variables. Because the
patients' perioperative psychopathology and neurology are
one focus of this research program, their preoperative
psychopathology, including such variables as anxiety,
depression, attitudes and behavior in the hospital
situation, and social environment had to be investigated
and compared, too. In order to study and to measure the
patients' psychology there is no other way than to interview them. This interview, of course, changes the patient,
for example, the level of pre- and postoperative anxiety
varies, depending upon the intensity of perioperative care,
quality of information and the in-hospital situation.
Anxiety can even vanish after talking about it. This
phenomenon is well known but rarely accepted in science and
research. In order to stress the importance of such effects,
this article deals with the influence of the International
Study on the "Study" patients, which means it describes the
differences between "Study" and "Non-study" patients,
instead of their common aspects.

Considering the performance of the "International
Study" in Hamburg, the fact is that the "Study" patients'
course through surgery and their in-hospital situation
differed in a number of aspects from "Non-Study" patients.
And, it became a common observation of the researchers
involved in the study, as well as of the clinical staff not
involved and of "Non-study" patients, that these differences
in fact turned out to be privileges for the "Study"
patients, although this was not intended. On the contrary,
the intention was to handle this study in the most uncomplicated and most comfortable way for the patients and the
clinicians involved. The study required special organisa-
tional arrangements which the Hamburg Cardiovascular
Surgery Department normally cannot provide:

Due to the shortage of beds and operating facilities, instead of the necessary 6 patients per day, only
3 to 4 are operated on. Therefore the routine cardiac
patient in Hamburg has to wait about 3 to 4 months for
his heart surgery. One or two days before the scheduled
date of operation he is admitted (either from home or from
any hospital in or around Hamburg or from different cardiac
rehabilitation centers outside Hamburg) to the Cardiovascular Surgery Department or to one of 6 different intern
wards of the University Hospital. The postoperative situation is comparably complicated. As long as no serious
complications require a special timetable, the patients
leave the ICU on the first or second postoperative day,
spend another 3 to 5 days in the open ward and are then

transferred forward, not necessarily to the ward or hospital they came from. There they stay for another fortnight before they leave for a rehabilitation clinic.

This description shows the normal unsatisfying situation for the patients; it furthermore makes clear that under these circumstances the study could not have been carried out.

To get the study under way, an arrangement was made with the Rehabiliation Center in Bad Segeberg, about 40 miles outside Hamburg. This is an important clinic for cardiac and neurological diseases, providing many physical and psychological diagnostic as well as rehabilitative facilities.

Physicians and psychologists of that center selected two patients per week, who met the study inclusion criteria, informed them about the International Study and offered them participation. These two patients came to the Hamburg Cardiovascular Surgery Department on Mondays, underwent preoperative study - and routine check-up, were operated on Friday and were discharged "home" to the Bad Segeberg Rehabilitation Clinic after the postoperative study investigation on the 8th postoperative day, Saturday of the next week. This cooperation was of mutual interest for both institutions. The staff of the Segeberg clinic was glad to get a weekly operation day for two of their surgical patients, and the Hamburg investigators were glad to be released from organizational problems and to deal with well-informed and prepared patients.

The effects of this arrangement for the patients were:

1. The waiting time for the operation for study patients was about two weeks, instead of the usual 3 to 4 months.

2. The course through surgery was clear from the first moment: it was like a journey, following an exact time-table and ending at a well-known destination. That means a solid, postitive structure, which the patients could absolutely rely on, while the usual patient has only a vague idea about timetable, course and destination. Such a structure is especially important for coronary patients, who normally are very structured people.

3. From the moment the patient decided on participation in the study, he was embedded in a network of psycho-

social and psychological care. This consisted of
preparatory talks in the rehabilitation clinic and pre-
and postoperative diagnostic talks with psychologists and
psychiatrists in the Cardiovascular Surgery Department
for study reasons, covering private problems, personality
attitudes, actual moods and behavior, family and social
life. The fact that, in addition to the normal talks
with ward physicians, surgeon, anaesthetist, another four
physicians and psychologists showed interest in the
patient and repeatedly gave him the chance to talk
about his situation and problems provided very unusual
stabilizing care, which the ordinary patients very
rarely get.

    4. The two study patients per week came together
(they normally knew each other from the rehabilitation
clinic), they stayed together in the Hamburg department
and normally left together after surgery. In many
respects these two patients supported each other. This
was not intended, but again proved to have a positive
stabilizing psychological effect, which was called
"Tandem-effect."

    5. Because the first author was coordinating the
study in Hamburg, he presented himself to the patients
as a contact person for all questions arising. So he
accompanied the patients along the two weeks of their stay
from their arrival on the open ward through the ICU to the
open ward again until discharge. Many of the patients'
questions turned out to be more concerned with personal
problems than with lack of information and he also tried to
help with these problems. Few of the non-study patients
got this chance.

    The stabilizing effects on the patients also
stabilized the study process, which increasingly developed
spontaneous dynamics:

    1. After the patients' return from Hamburg to the
rehabilitation clinic they told fellow preoperative
patients about their experiences, which obviously in
general were not too bad. The good news spread around
that an attractive study program was going on in Hamburg
and more and more patients applied to become study
patients.

    2. During the two years of the study the physicians
and psychologists at the rehabilitation clinic changed
their study patient selection criteria. While they were

full of scepticism in the beginning and preferentially sent the physically stable uncomplicated cases, they later on, impressed by the positive reports of the returned patients and their objective physical stability, more and more selected the psychically complicated and physically urgent cases for the study.

3. In the Hamburg Cardiovascular Surgery Department, too, during the two study-years the study patients increasingly in the physicians' and ward staff's eyes gained the reputation of being unproblematic, easy to handle, and easygoing patients, despite the patients' objectively increasing physical and psychical problems.

It should be repeated that these effects were neither intended nor foreseen.

Concerning the comparison of the "Study" and "Non-Study Patients" the following conclusions can be drawn:

From a statistical point of view it is difficult to judge the differences between the groups because this was not a comparative study. Some indications nevertheless support the general impression, that the "Study" patients coped psychically better with the operation and with adjustments after surgery:

The official statistics of the Hamburg Cardio-vascular Surgery Department for 1987, excluding emergencies, counts 11.6% so-called "psychoses," which means only obvious severe psychic, mostly psycho-organic symptoms. Divided into "Non-Study" and "Study" patients, the figures result in 13% for "Non-Study" and 7% for "Study" patients, about a two to one ratio.

Two years after the operation the first 45 Study patients who underwent follow-up investigation did so well physically and psychically that study-independent physicians as well as the study-investigators and the patients themselves were surprised.

What do these observations mean for the "International Study?"

1. From a researcher's standpoint the Hamburg Center acted against the study intention, because the study arrangement in Hamburg probably reduced the number of psychopathological disturbances in the study group

compared to the realistic number of psychopathological
disturbances in the usual population of cardiac surgery
patients in Hamburg.

    2. On the other hand the carrying out of the Study in
Hamburg should be regarded as having a value of its own,
meaning that its typical environmental variables, e.g.
solid information, social network and reliable escort
through surgery result in stabilizing therapeutic effects.

    For many reasons the development of the study was a
delightful surprise. In the eyes of most patients, they
were fortunate to participate and in the authors' eyes this
article should have the title which they thought of when
they first planned it: "The positive impact of the
International Study on the patients' quality of life."

WEIGHT GAIN AND THE DEVELOPMENT OF SLEEP APNEA

FOLLOWING HEART TRANSPLANTATION

Mark F. Leveaux, Susan Hook

Department of Psychiatry
Kaiser Medical Center
4700 Sunset Blvd.
Los Angeles, CA   90027

INTRODUCTION

Cardiac transplantation has increasingly become a more routine procedure. Successful transplantation requires subsequent chronic immunosuppression to prevent rejection of the donor organ. Immunosuppression of patients using cyclosporine, azathioprine, and prednisone and other glucocorticoids, has multiple physical and neuropsychiatric side effects as recently reviewed by Lough [1]. Progressive post transplant weight gain contributing to hyperlipidemia, which is thought to cause an acceleration of coronary artery disease in the donor heart, has recently been demonstrated [2,3]. Prednisone's positive side effects on appetite and weight gain are presumed to be the cause of heart transplant recipients' weight gain, and this is supported by Renlund [4] who reported substantially less weight gain in a subgroup of transplant recipients who could tolerate glucocorticoids (including prednisone) being eliminated from their immunosuppressive regime.

The sleep apnea syndromes, as recently reviewed by Ingbar [5], are a group of sleep disorders associated with paroxysmal episodes of apnea during sleep, resulting in frequent awakenings and lack of restful sleep. Patients with sleep apnea frequently complain of insomnia, excessive daytime sleepiness, cognitive impairment, and affective symptoms, but are actually unaware of their

Impact of Cardiac Surgery on the Quality of Life
Edited by A. E. Willner and G. Rodewald
Plenum Press, New York, 1990

apneic episodes. Observations of bed partners are often helpful in raising the possibility of sleep apnea, and polysomnography is diagnostic. Severe sleep apnea is associated with pulmonary hypertension, cor pulmonale, arrhythmias, and nocturnal sudden death. Sedative drugs and alcohol are contraindicated for patients with sleep apnea. Though sleep apnea frequently occurs in non-obese individuals, severe obesity, and associated increase in upper airway resistance are considered to be contributory, and weight reduction is an initial intervention in obese individuals with sleep apnea.

A thorough review of the literature has to this point revealed no reports of sleep apnea in organ transplant recipients or populations chronically immunosuppressed on glucocorticoids.

CASE REPORT

In the context of the preceding, psychiatric evaluation was requested on a 43 year old, white, married male, who was 36 months post cardiac transplant. The patient's chief complaints were insomnia, depression, tearfulness, and lack of libido. The patient requested a "stronger" sedative for sleep, having found flurazepam, 30 mg. p.o. q.h.s. ineffective. The patient's medication regimen included cyclosporin, 250 mg. b.i.d., prednisone, 7.5 mg. b.i.d., azathioprine, 150 mg. b.i.d., enalapril, 10 mg. b.i.d., cimetidine, 400 mg. q.d., furosemide, 75 mg., b.i.d., chlortrimazole, 70 mg. b.i.d., and flurazepam, 30 mg. q.h.s. Recent laboratory evaluation including electrolytes, CBC, renal function tests, liver function test, and EKG were unremarkable.

Further history from the patient and his wife revealed loud snoring, excessive daytime sleepiness, frequent night-time awakening, and severe post transplant weight gain. Examination revealed severe obesity with the patient weighing 330 pounds (219% of his ideal weight by New York Life's standards). Subsequently, the diagnosis of sleep apnea was made by polysomnography which revealed the patient had frequent episodes of obstructive sleep apnea and hypopnea with average durations of 10-15 seconds during sleep. The patient's baseline oxygen saturation of 99% fell to as low as 71% during these episodes. The patient responded well to continuous positive airway pressure (CPAP) with improved mood and energy, and a modest weight loss (15 pounds). Polysomnography during CPAP showed a minimum saturation of 93%.

SURVEY OF CARDIAC TRANSPLANT RECIPIENTS FOR WEIGHT GAIN
AND SYMPTOMS OF SLEEP APNEA

Because of the issues raised by the preceding information, the writer reviewed clinical records and conducted
a brief telephone survey of the 13 cardiac transplant
recipients followed at our Medical Center. It is of note
that as a large group model HMO, pretransplant and post
transplant care is provided to our subscribers at our
Medical Center, but the actual transplant procedure and
immediate postoperative care is performed at other medical
centers in California. Fourteen of our subscribers have
been transplanted in the 40 months preceding this report,
and one is deceased secondary to immediate postoperative
complications. The time period post transplant in this
group ranged from three to 40 months. All transplant
recipients have been maintained chronically on immunosuppressive regimen including cyclosporine, azathioprine,
and prednisone.

Figure 1 reviews the average percent ideal weight
based on New York Life standards over time following
transplantation in these recipients. It is of note that
only one recipient was below ideal body weight (96% of
ideal body weight). This data supports the findings of
Keogh [2] and Grady [3] that substantial weight gain above
ideal body weight is a significant problem for cardiac
transplant recipients.

Table 1 reviews the results of a simple survey of the
13 cardiac transplant recipients for symptoms of sleep

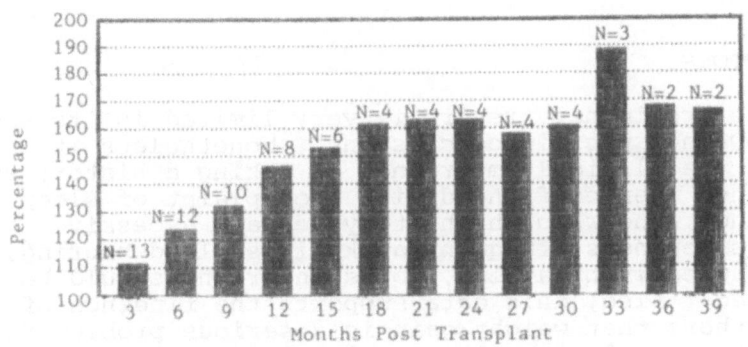

Figure 1.   Mean percent ideal weight (New York Life
           Standards), cardiac transplant patients

Table 1.   Telephone Survey of 13 Post Cardiac Transplant
           Patients

Symptom	Postive N	Response %
Tendency to Gain Excessive Weight	8	(62)
Difficulty Falling Asleep	2	(16)
Early Morning Awakening	2	(16)
Snoring Reported by Bed Partner	9	(69)
Frequent Nighttime Awakenings[a]	7	(54)
Excessive Daytime Sleepiness	7	(54)

[a] Four patients related this to need
    to urinate due to diuretic.

apnea. Of note is that this data includes the case described above and since these symptoms are not specific,
polysomnography is planned for the affected group.

IMPLICATIONS

     This preliminary report is very limited in its scope,
and allows no specific conclusions. Nonetheless it
supports the clinical importance of taking a history for
sleep apnea when confronted with a complaint of sleep
disturbance, and when the history reveals excessive
daytime sleepiness, frequent awakenings, loud snoring,
and/or pauses in breathing, polysomnography should be
considered. Also, this data supports the findings of
other authors that weight gain is a serious problem for
many post transplant patients maintained on glucocorticoids. The need for behavioral and dietary
interventions in this area, as well as research to find
immunosuppressive regimens that minimize the use of
glucocorticoids is further supported.

Finally, the discovery of sleep apnea in one heart transplant recipient in the context of severe weight gain and symptom reports consistent with this disorder in other recipients is of interest. Further research on the prevalence of this disorder using polysomnography in transplant populations and study of its relationship to glucocorticoid administration and/or glucocorticoid associated weight gain should be considered.

REFERENCES

1. M. E. Lough, A. M. Lindsey, J. A. Shinn, and N. A. Stotts, Impact of symptom frequency and symptom distress on self-reported quality of life in transplant recipients, Heart & Lung. 16:193 (1987).
2. A. Keogh, L. Simons, P. Spratt, et al., Hyperlipidemia after heart transplantation, J. Heart Transplant. 7:171 (1988).
3. K. Grady and L. Herold, Comparison of nutritional status in patients before and after heart transplantation, J. Heart Transplant. 7:123 (1988).
4. D. Renlund, J. O'Connell, E. Gilbert, et al., Feasibility of discontinuation of corticosteroid maintenance therapy in heart transplantation, J. Heart Transplant. 6:71 (1987).
5. D. H. Ingbar and J. B. L. Gee, Pathophysiology and treatment of sleep apnea, Ann. Rev. Med. 36:369 (1985).

CORRELATIONS BETWEEN MEDICAL/SURGICAL DATA AND
POSTOPERATIVE PSYCHIATRIC, NEUROLOGICAL AND
PSYCHOMETRIC CONDITION

DEMOGRAPHICS OF THE MULTI-CENTER SAMPLE

Michael Borenstein
Allen E. Willner

Hillside Hospital
Long Island Jewish Medical Center
Glen Oaks, NY

Georg Rodewald

University Hospital Hamburg - Eppendorf
Hamburg, Federal Republic of Germany

A number of papers included in this volume are based on analyses conducted on the multi-center study sample. The present paper includes a brief overview of the mechanics of data analysis utilized in the study and describes the demographic characteristics of this sample.

Data from all centers were forwarded to New York (Long Island Jewish Medical Center) where they were collated and then entered into a series of PC class machines running SPSS/DE. This data then underwent an extensive verification procedure during which the record for each patient was checked for missing data and for logical errors. During an iterative procedure that continued for twelve months, the staff at the New York center maintained contact with persons at the various other centers, obtaining whatever data was missing from the files and correcting the identified errors.

The steering committee met in New York for several days in mid-1988 to discuss plans for the analyses which were then carried out in New York over the following eight months. The analyses were executed on PC's

Impact of Cardiac Surgery on the Quality of Life
Edited by A. E. Willner and G. Rodewald
Plenum Press, New York, 1990

293

running such programs as SPSS/PC and BMDP/PC.   These
machines were also used to create graphs which were made
into slides in anticipation of the conference.

Since data continued to arrive on a steady basis, a
decision was made to limit the current set of analyses
to data that had been received as of the end of 1988.   A
substantial amount of data received after that time has
been added to the data base and will be included in the
next round of analyses.

The current sample included a total of 498 cases,
including patients from Hamburg, New York, Evanston, Sao
Paulo, Finland, Bad Krozingen, and Kiel.   The precise
number (and proportion) of cases from each center is
reported in Table 1.

TABLE 1.   Cases Included in the Current Analyses

	Frequency	Percent
Hamburg	121	24.3
New York	91	18.3
Evanston	22	4.4
Sao Paulo	29	5.8
Oulu, Finland	101	20.3
Bad Krozingen	79	15.9
Kiel	55	11.0

The procedures were classified as either bypass
(86.5%), valve replacement (8.0%), or both (3.2%).

Overall, 81.2% of the cases were male, but the
proportion of males varied from one center to the next.
In Hamburg 83% of the cases were male; in New York, 65%;
in Evanston, 81%; in Sao Paulo, 64%; in Finland, 91%; in
Bad Krozingen, 92%; and in Kiel, 80% of the cases were
male.

The age of the patients varied from 31 to 83 years,
with a mean of 56 (SD of 10) and a median of 56 years.
The ages varied substantially between centers.   Table 2
presents the mean age for each of the centers separately.

   The specific procedures employed in the analyses
are described in the individual papers. As a general
rule, procedures such as multiple regression and
Analysis of Variance were employed to enable us to
simultaneously account for the impact of multiple
variables and the possibility of interactions between
them.

TABLE 2. Age by Center

Group	Count	Mean	Standard Deviation	Standard Error	Range
Hamburg	121	55.35	7.91	.71	36-74
New York	91	63.09	11.25	1.17	31-83
Evanston	21	64.42	9.31	2.03	43-76
Sao Paulo	22	47.00	11.37	2.42	31-63
Finland	101	52.91	7.09	.70	34-65
Bad Krozingen	78	53.50	6.26	.70	37-65
Kiel	52	58.38	8.81	1.22	34-74
Total	486	56.33	9.63	.43	31-83

TYPE OF OXYGENATOR, TYPE OF ARTERIAL FILTER, AND BYPASS TIME, IN RELATION TO OUTCOME

Georg Rodewald

University Hospital
Hamburg - Eppendorf
Federal Republic of Germany

Allen E. Willner
Michael Borenstein

Department of Psychiatry
Hillside Hospital
Glen Oaks, NY

A whole clinical spectrum of neurological complications has been reported after cardiac surgery, ranging from: fatal cerebral injury, impairment of conscious level, stroke, ophthalmological complications, seizures, spinal cord injury to "miscellaneous CNS abnormalities," Shaw [1]. Aberg and his colleagues [2-5] found substantial neuropsychological abnormality early on and documented declining rates of abnormality as the performance of perfusion and surgery improved. Recently, several studies have related postoperative neuropsychological changes to such factors as retinal microembolisation, preoperative cerebrovascular disease and bypass time [6-10].

This paper describes analyses which were performed to identify whether type of oxygenator, type of arterial filter, and/or bypass time were related to outcome. The analyses reported are based on the multi-center sample of 498 patients for which demographic data have been presented elsewhere in this volume. However, patients were included in the present analyses only if (a) the procedure was performed with one of the eight combinations of oxygenator

Impact of Cardiac Surgery on the Quality of Life
Edited by A. E. Willner and G. Rodewald
Plenum Press, New York, 1990

297

and arterial filter which occurred with substantial
frequency, and (b) the patient was assessed for cognitive
functioning both prior to and following the operation. A
total of 356 patients met these criteria.

Identifying Patients Who Suffered a Drop in Cognitive Functioning During Surgery

The purpose of the analyses was to determine whether
patients treated with a particular combination of
materials (filter type/oxygenator type/bypass time) were
at higher risk of poor outcome than other patients.
Therefore, the outcome measure had to address the change
that occurred during surgery.

Patients' cognitive functioning was assessed by
various psychometric measures during the days just prior
to the operation, and a few days after the operation,
prior to discharge from the hospital. Three measures were
included in this classification system: The CLAT, the
WAIS Digit Symbol test, and the WAIS Block Design test.
The three measures provided a more comprehensive measure
than any one of these tests could have on its own. Specifically, the CLAT measures a fairly complex level of
reasoning ability while the WAIS sub-tests are sensitive
to a more basic type of cognitive function. By including
the three tests in this battery, we were able to identify
patients whose cognitive functioning had dropped, regardless of their initial level. (For a more detailed discussion of these measures and the outcome criteria, see
other papers in this volume). A patient was classified as
having a drop in cognitive functioning if his/her score on
any of the tests dropped by one standard deviation or
more, and was classified as stable otherwise. By this
criterion, 274 (77.0%) of the patients remained stable and
82 (23.0%) dropped in cognitive functioning.

Bypass Time

Bypass times ranged from 19 to 480 minutes with a
mean of 122 minutes, standard deviation of 53 minutes, and
a median of 113 minutes (Figure 1). Bypass time differed
from one center to the next: Table 1 shows the proportion
of cases in each center with bypass times in the range of
30-60 minutes, 60-120 minutes, 120-180 minutes, and over
180 minutes.

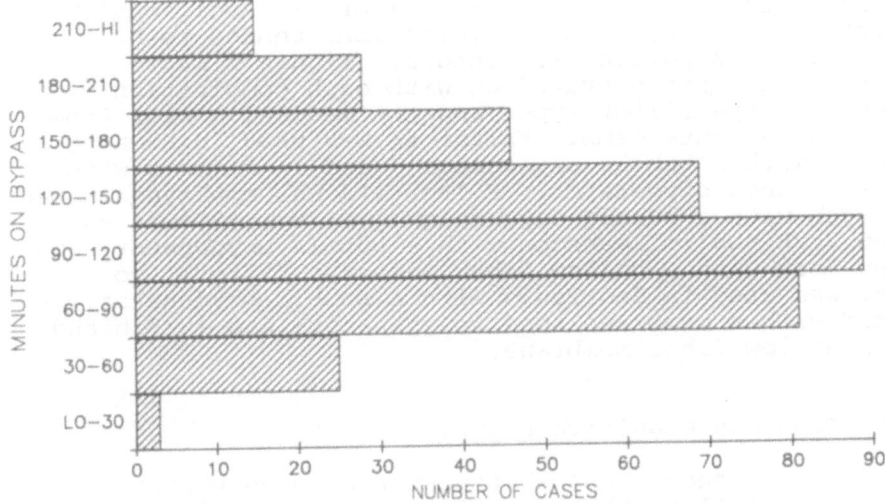

Fig. 1. Distribution of bypass time.

TABLE 1. Distribution of Bypass Times at the Various Centers (N=356)

		Under 60	61-120	121-180	Over 180	Mean (SD)
Hamburg	(N=94)	5.3%	56.4%	33.0%	5.3%	115 (41)
New York	(N=55)	9.1%	52.7%	32.7%	5.5%	112 (40)
Evanston	(N=16)	6.3%	68.8%	25.0%	0.0%	98 (28)
Sao Paulo	(N=24)	16.7%	66.7%	16.7%	0.0%	89 (27)
Finland	(N=89)	0.0%	3.4%	57.3%	39.3%	176 (43)
Bad Krozingen	(N=48)	8.3%	79.2%	12.5%	0.0%	93 (27)
Kiel	(N=30)	30.0%	66.7%	3.3%	0.0%	78 (23)
Total	(N=356)	7.9%	47.8%	32.3%	12.1%	121 (50)

Selection of Surgical Equipment

The nature of the study did not allow for patients to be assigned at random to particular types of equipment. Therefore, specific oxygenators were consistently paired

300   G. RODEWALD ET AL.

with specific types of arterial filters.   Additionally,
specific filter/oxygenator combinations tended to be
concentrated in particular centers.   Figure 2 shows the
number of patients operated on with each combination of
oxygenator type/filter type, and the medical center from
which the patients came.   Filter #4 was used in Hamburg
and Kiel with a bubble oxygenator;   and in Hamburg with a
membrane sheet oxygenator.   Filter #14 was employed in Bad
Krozingen with a bubble oxygenator.   Filter #20 was used
in New York and in Evanston with a bubble oxygenator; and
in New York with a hollow fiber membrane filter.   No
filter was used in Sao Paulo with a bubble oxygenator; in
Finland with a membrane sheet oxygenator; and in Finland
with a hollow fiber membrane.

Bypass Time and Cognitive Functioning

Figure 3 shows the relationship between bypass times
and the probability that a patient would experience a drop
in cognitive functioning.   The probability of a drop
increases from 11% when bypass time is on the order of 60
minutes, to about 36% when bypass time is on the order of
240 minutes.   (Note these values are relative to each
other, rather than absolute.   The absolute values depend
on a host of other factors such as hematocrit level,
saturation level, and, as discussed below, on the filter
and oxygenator combination).

	FILTER 4	FILTER 14	FILTER 20	NO FILTER
BUBBLE OXYGENATOR	HAMBURG KIEL (64)	BAD KROZ (46)	NEW YORK EVANSTON (26)	SAO PAULO (27)
MEMBRANE SHEET	HAMBURG (62)			FINLAND (49))
HOLLOW FIBER			NEW YORK (45)	FINLAND (37)

Fig. 2.   Combinations of oxygenator/arterial filter type.

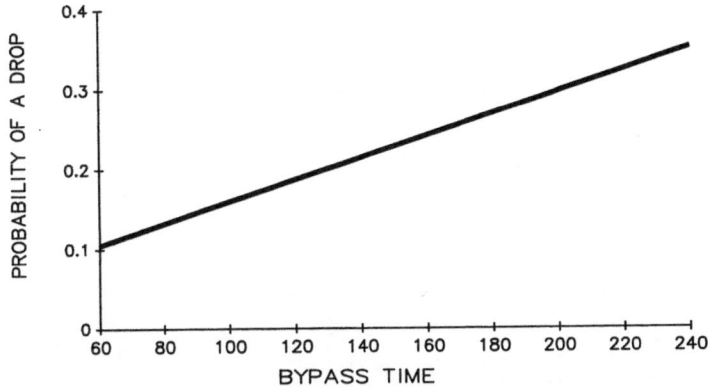

Fig. 3.   Impact of bypass time on drop in CLAT/WAIS
          (assumes hematocrit = 28).

Perfusion Equipment and Cognitive Functioning

Figure 4 shows how outcome varied as a function of
oxygenator type/arterial filter type. The rows and
columns in this figure correspond to the rows and columns
in Figure 2. Each cell contains a bar graph showing the
combination of filters and oxygenators specified, in
addition to the proportion of cases that experienced a
drop in cognitive functioning. The proportion of cases in
which functioning dropped varied from 15% to 34%. This
amount of dispersion is not significant (by Oneway ANOVA,
p=.25), i.e. there is no evidence that some treatment
combinations of oxygenators and filters are associated
with worse outcomes than others.

Interaction of Perfusion Equipment and Bypass Time as Predictor of Cognitive Functioning

A very different picture emerges when bypass times
and oxygenator/filter are considered simultaneously
(Figure 5). The cells in this figure correspond to the
cells in the previous figure. In this case, however,
within each cell, the bar graph shows the proportion of
cases with decreased functioning for cases with low bypass
time separately from cases with high bypass time. (The
distinction between short and long bypass time is defined
as 100 minutes for all centers except Finland. In
Finland, virtually all cases had bypass times exceeding
100 minutes, and so the line was drawn at 180 minutes).

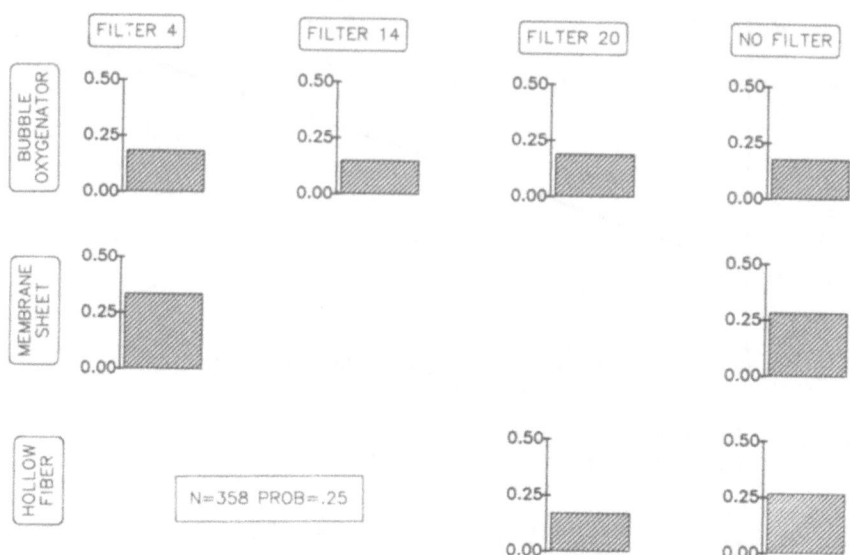

Fig 4.   Drop on CLAT/WAIS as a function of
          oxygenator/filter.

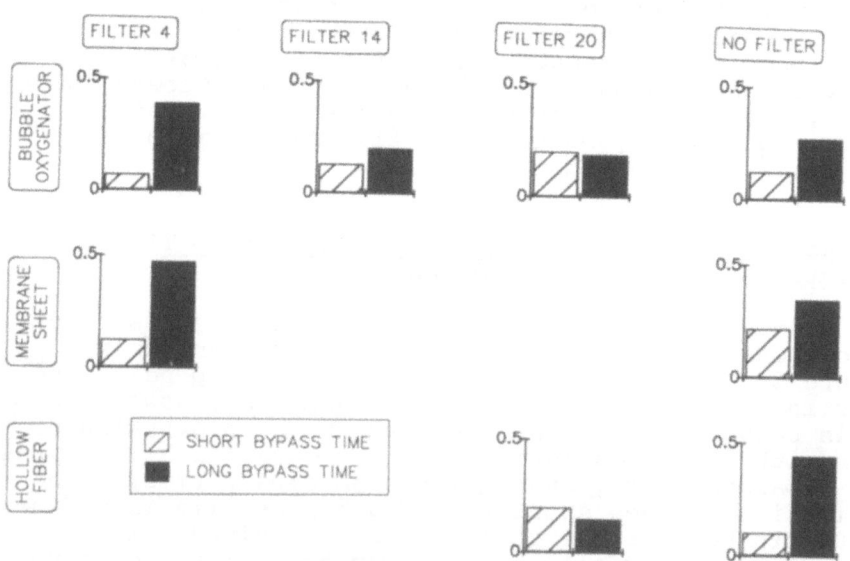

Fig. 5.   Drop on CLAT/WAIS as a function of oxygenator/
           filter/bypass time.

Cells in Which Bypass Time is Related to Cognitive Deficit

In three cells, patients with a short bypass time had only a small probability of a drop in cognitive functioning whereas those with long bypass times had a substantially higher probability of a drop. Specifically, for Bubble oxygenator/Filter #4, the probability of a cognitive drop was 7% for short bypass time vs 39% for long bypass time. For membrane sheet/Filter #4 these figures are 13% vs 47%. Finally for No filter/Hollow fiber membrane the figures are 11% vs 47%.

The data from one of these cells (Filter 4 with bubble oxygenator) have been graphed from another perspective in Figure 6. The 64 cases in this cell are plotted as 64 circles. The 12 cases which did suffer a drop are plotted at the top of the graph while the 37 cases which did not show a drop in functioning are plotted at the bottom. The horizontal axis represents bypass time: The further to the right a case is plotted, the longer the bypass time for that case. A vertical line separates the cases with bypass times under 100 minutes from those over 100 minutes.

There are a total of 41 cases with short bypass times (i.e. to the left of the vertical line). Of these, 3 are plotted at the top (dropped) while 38 are shown at the bottom (stable). Thus 3/41 or 7% of the cases with short bypass times suffered a cognitive drop.

There are a total of 23 cases with long bypass times (i.e. to the right of the vertical line). Of these, 9 are plotted at the top (dropped) while 14 are shown at the bottom (stable). Thus 9/23 or 39% of the cases with long bypass times suffered a cognitive drop.

The proportion of cases suffering a cognitive drop is thus 7.3% for short bypas time vs 39.1% for long bypass time. This corresponds also to the two columns in the corresponding cell of Figure 5.

Cells in Which Bypass Time is Not Related to Cognitive Deficit

In five cells the probability that the patient would experience a drop in functioning was comparable for short bypass time and long bypass time. Specifically, for the combination of Filter 14 plus bubble oxygenator the probability of a cognitive deficit was 13% for short

bypass time and 20% for long bypass time; for Filter 20
with bubble oxygenator the figures are 20% vs 19%; for
Filter 20 with hollow fiber the probability of a drop is
20% vs 15%; For no filter with bubble oxygenator the
figures are 13% vs 27%; and for No filter with membrane
sheet the figures are 22% vs 35%.)

Again, one of these cells (Filter 14 with Bubble
Oxygenator) is graphed more in detail in Figure 7. Here,
13% of the cases in the short bypass time range suffered
cognitive drop, whereas 20% of the cases with long bypass
time had a cognitive drop. The proportions suffering a
drop in the two bypass ranges (20% vs 13%) correspond to
the two columns in the corresponding cell in Figure 5. In
this case the two proportions are comparable: There is no
indication that increased bypass time is associated with
increased risk of a cognitive deficit.

DISCUSSION

For certain combinations of filter/oxygenator, the
probability that the patient will experience a cognitive
deficit increases as a function of bypass time. A patient
whose operation requires a lengthy bypass time and was
treated with one of these units would be at increased risk

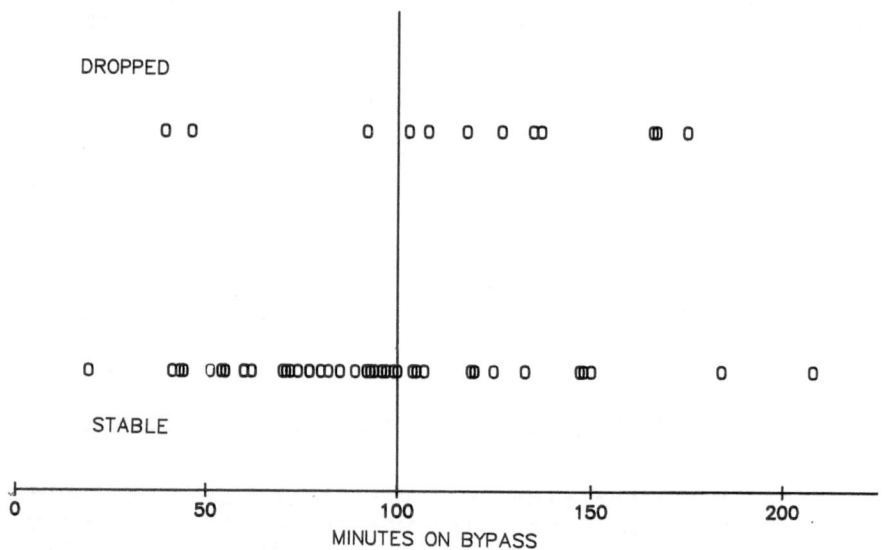

Fig. 6.   Filter Type 4/Bubble Oxygenator.

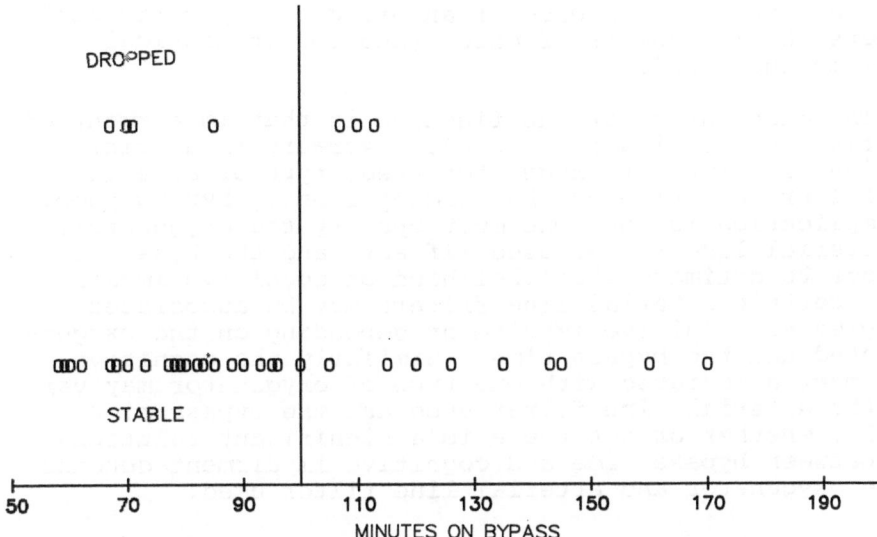

Fig. 7.   Filter type 14/Bubble Oxygenator.

for a cognitive deficit. No such relationship was found
for the other treatment units, which suggests that in
these units any drop that occurs is likely to occur within
the first 30 minutes of bypass time; increased bypass time
was not found to substantially increase the probability of
a cognitive drop.

This may explain the fact that some studies had
reported that longer bypass times were associated with
poor prognosis while other studies failed to find such an
association. The former would be expected if a study used
a combination of filter and oxygenator in which bypass
time is related to outcome; the latter would be consistent
with our findings for certain other combinations of filter
and oxygenator.

It is important to note that the absence of a significant effect in some cells implies only that we lack
evidence that bypass time is related to outcome in these
cells; it does not indicate that bypass time is unrelated
to outcome in these cells. The distinction is a vital
one; it is entirely possible that increased bypass time
does yield a higher probability of a cognitive drop in all

cases, and that the absence of an effect in specific cells
reflects the low number of cases (and low statistical
power) in these cells.

The main thrust of the findings is that impairment of
cognitive functioning after cardiac surgery is a joint
function of: type of oxygenator used, type of arterial
line filter, and time on the cardiopulmonary bypass pump.
The implication is that one must specify the oxygenator,
the arterial line filter used (if any) and the bypass time
in order to estimate the likelihood of cognitive impairment. Certain arterial line filters may be associated
with greater cognitive impairment depending on the oxygenator used and the bypass time. Similarly the cognitive
impairment associated with one type of oxygenator may vary
with the arterial line filter used and the bypass time.
Finally, whether or not there is a significant relationship between bypass time and cognitive impairment depends
on the oxygenator and arterial line filter used.

REFERENCES

1. P. J. Shaw, The incidence and nature of neurological
    morbidity following cardiac surgery: A review,
    Perfusion. 4:83-91 (1989).
2. T. Åberg, M. Kihlgren, Cerebral protection during open
    heart surgery, Thorax. 17:748-753 (1977).
3. T. Åberg, M. Kihlgren, K. Jonsson, et al., Improved
    cerebral protection during open heart surgery, a
    psychometric investigation on 339 patients, in:
    "Psychopathological and Neurological Dysfunctions
    Following Open-Heart Surgery," Becker, Katz,
    Polonius, H. Speidel, eds., Springer Verlag, Berlin
    (1982).
4. T. Åberg, G. Ronquist, H. Tyden, et al., Adverse
    effects on the brain in cardiac operations as
    assessed by biochemical, psychometric and
    radiologic methods, J Thorac Cardiovasc Surg.
    87:99-105 (1984).
5. T. Åberg, M. Kihlgren, Effect of open-heart surgery on
    intellectual functioning, Scand J Thorac Cardiovasc
    Surg. Suppl. 15 (1974).
6. S. Newman, P. Smith, T. Treasure, P. Joseph, P. Ell,
    M. Harrison, Acute neuropsychological consequences
    of coronary artery bypass surgery, Carr Psych Res
    Rev. 6:115-24 (1987).

7. W. Pugsley, L. Klinger, C. Pascalis, S. Newman,
        M. Harrison, T. Treasure, Do microemboli contribute
        to bypass related cerebral impairment? J Cardiovas
        Surg. 29:81 (1988).
8. G. E. Venn, L. Klinger, S. Newman, M. Harrison, P. Ell,
        T. Treasure, The neuropsychological sequelae of
        bypass 12 months following coronary artery surgery,
        Br Heart Journal.   57:564 (1987).
9. M. Harrison, A. Schneidau, R. Ho, P. Smith. S. Newman,
        T. Treasure, Role of cerebrovascular disease in the
        development of neuropsychological impairment after
        coronary artery bypass surgery (CABS), Stroke.
        20:235-237 (1989).
10.   S. Newman, The incidence and nature of neuropsycho-
        logical morbidity following cardiac surgery,
        Perfusion. 4:93-100 (1989).

SEVERAL PARAMETERS OF EXTRACORPOREAL CIRCULATION

AND OUTCOME

Georg Rodewald

University Hospital
Hamburg, Federal Republic of Germany

Allen E. Willner

Hillside Hospital
Glen Oaks, New York

The aim of cardiopulmonary bypass is the maintenance of peripheral gas exchange and nutrition by adequate tissue perfusion during open heart surgery. At first sight, the present low hospital mortality rate at least in elective cases - in our International Study 2% of 500 cases so far - seems to demonstrate that extracorporeal circulation generally meets this demand. However, according to authors like Wheatley [1], we have to question whether cardiopulmonary bypass guarantees a complete restoration of organ function after surgery.

As far as cerebral function is concerned, as was shown in the preceding chapter, there is indeed an impairment in a certain percentage of patients after open heart surgery. In the same patient population post-operative disturbance of other organs like lung and kidney was almost never observed. This is in sharp contrast to the experience during the early years of open heart surgery where almost all major organs showed more or less severe dysfunction postoperatively.

The fact that the brain is more often disturbed today than that of other organs indicates clearly that the brain is the most vulnerable organ at least to perfusion. This

Impact of Cardiac Surgery on the Quality of Life
Edited by A. E. Willner and G. Rodewald
Plenum Press, New York, 1990

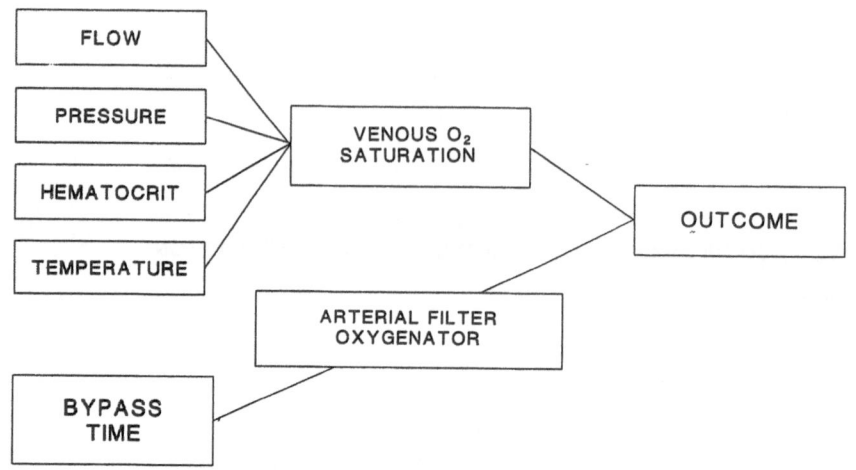

Fig. 1.   Factors Affecting Outcome

vulnerability is reflected by the fact that the brain has the lowest tolerance of any organ to ischemia.

Fig. 1 shows several factors evaluated so far which may be among those relevant for cerebral perfusion. As far as physiological parameters are concerned, the percentage of oxygen saturation of mixed venous blood - subsequently called venous saturation - seems to be a very important determinant for outcome. Provided the arterial oxygen saturation was normal, as was the case in this study, venous saturation mainly depends on parameters like oxygen consumption, cardiac output and hematocrit. This well known correlation, which applies for normal physiological conditions, does not apply to cardiopulmonary bypass.

Hemodilution is induced in order to: improve tissue perfusion, avoid the homologous blood syndrome, minimize the risk of infections related to donor blood, economize the performance of blood banks, etc. The consequence is a drop of hematocrit and therefore of oxygen capacity.

Body temperature is artificially lowered by 10 or more degrees centigrade thus decreasing oxygen demand in order to compensate for decreased oxygen capacity. Furthermore, it is used to increase tolerance to ischemia in general and especially to provide a safety margin in case of technical accidents. Some even prefer low flow perfusion in order to reduce damage of the perfusate caused by the heart-lung machine.

These profound changes are intended to protect the patient against the drawbacks of cardiopulmonary bypass. However, we should keep in mind that all these alterations are far from normal conditions. In this context I should emphasize that it is erroneous to equate the status of induced hypothermia in warm blooded animals with poikilo-thermia. This term is used to characterize a different species with completely different qualities.

Fig. 1 does not show another important aspect of cardiac surgery, namely the reaction of the patient to extracorporeal circulation imposed upon him, e.g. feedback to nonpulsatile flow, the yet unsolved problem of flow distribution within the body, or peripheral shunting of arterial blood due to increased circulatory resistence induced by hypothermia.

Before going into details we would like to stress some problems with measurement of venous saturation. This value imprecisely reflects the oxygen saturation of the venous blood of the brain. Furthermore, it is difficult to measure this directly and continuously during bypass. Other methods for indirect monitoring of the quality of brain perfusion during bypass, e.g. EEG, evoked potential responses or biochemical markers were not applied in this study. Moreover, this preliminary presentation neglects the influence of temperature on pH and pCO_2 and on the O_2-Dissociation curve. The percentage of oxygen saturation depicted on the vertical axis remains unchanged because these parameters shift the curve along the horizontal axis with a corresponding change of oxygen pressure.

Venous saturation was not monitored continuously. The study protocol asked whether venous saturation was measured, this was the case in 6 of the 9 centers reported here, and if so, what was the lowest venous saturation during perfusion.

Previous reports at this symposium showed impairment of cerebral function after open heart surgery. The main question is which neurological and psychometric investiga-tions correlate to perfusion parameters?

Fig. 2 shows percentage of patients with worse neuro-logical status 2 - 3 days postoperatively as a function of venous saturation after surgery. Range of venous satura-tion and number of patients respectively are depicted horizontally below each bar. As one can see, there is no correlation between lower and higher levels of venous saturation and neurological outcome.

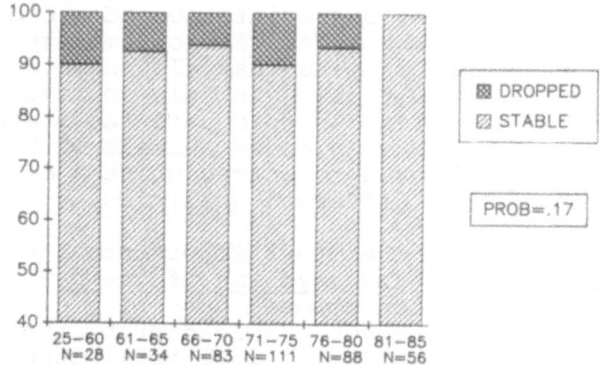

Fig. 2. Drop on Neurological Status as a Function of
         Lowest Saturation

Fig. 3 shows, for the same ranges of venous saturation and for the same numer of patients, the percentage of
those with a drop in cognitive test scores. The CLAT and
WAIS here and in the following figures refer to a battery
of 3 tests: CLAT, WAIS Digit Symbol and WAIS Block
Design. A drop refers to a drop of at least one standard
deviation postoperatively in one or more of these 3 tests
(see preceding chapter). The relationship between venous
saturation and drop in these psychometric test scores is
significant (p=.001).

We conclude that cognitive tests show a high sensitivity for detection of cerebral impairment related to
cardiopulmonary bypass. This finding is not surprising
because these tests are sensitive to higher mental

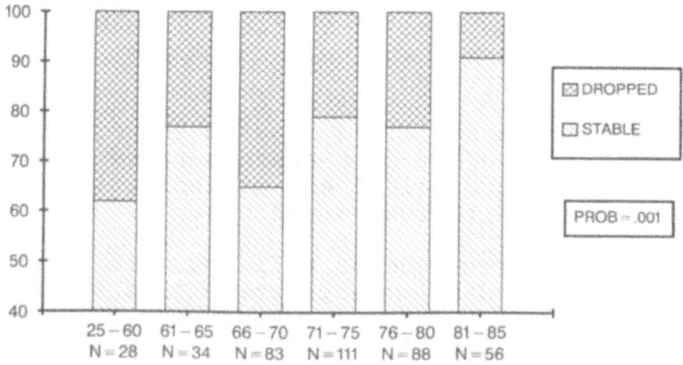

Fig. 3. Drop on CLAT/WAIS as a Function of Lowest
         Saturation

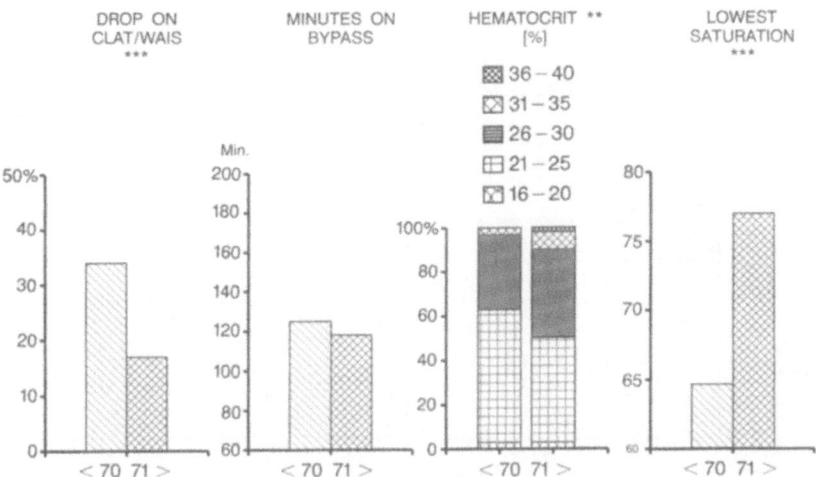

Fig. 4.   Analysis of Saturation: Full Sample

functions.   In the course of evolution these qualities are
the last acquired and the first impaired.

Fig. 4 shows for a sample of 400 patients the relation of venous saturation to other parameters.   On the
horizontal axis below each bar two ranges of venous saturation are shown: through 70% and over 71%.   The mean
values for these two classes are depicted on the right:
65% for the lower range of venous saturation and 78% for
the higher.

The two bars to the left show that 33% of 145
patients in the lower saturation range displayed a postoperative drop on psychometric test scores compared to 17%
of 255 patients in the higher range.

Furthermore, there is a correlation between hematocrit and venous saturation since the lower range group
also has lower hematocrit values and vice versa.   There is
no correlation of venous saturation to bypass time.

Fig. 5 shows factors possibly affecting venous saturation, again evaluated for 400 patients. The patients were
divided in the same two groups as in Fig. 4.   The relation
to hematocrit has already been demonstrated.   The lower
the temperature and the lower the flow, the lower the
venous oxygen saturation.   There is no correlation to
perfusion pressure.

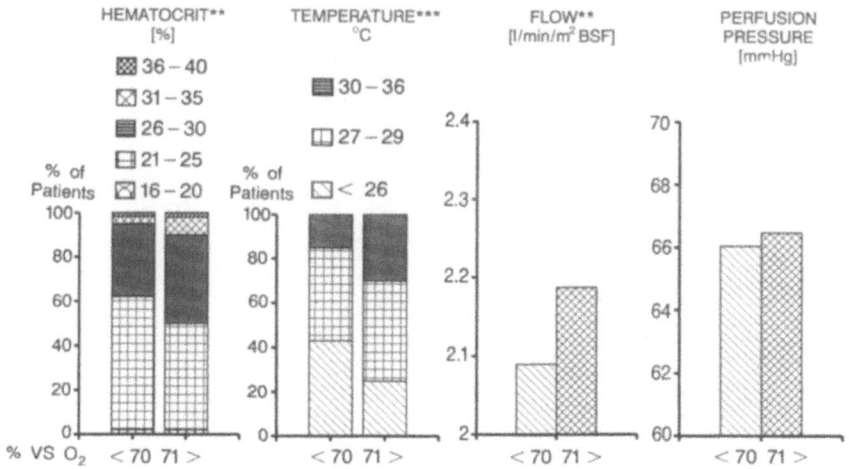

Fig. 5.   Factors Affecting Saturation (N=144/284)

Fig. 6 shows the relation of venous saturation to other parameters but for a sample of 99 patients only. These patients had extracorporeal circulation using a bubble oxygenator and an arterial line filter #4. The correlation between lower and higher ranges of venous saturation, drop in psychometric test score and hematocrit is even more distinct here. Moreover there is a significant correlation to bypass time.

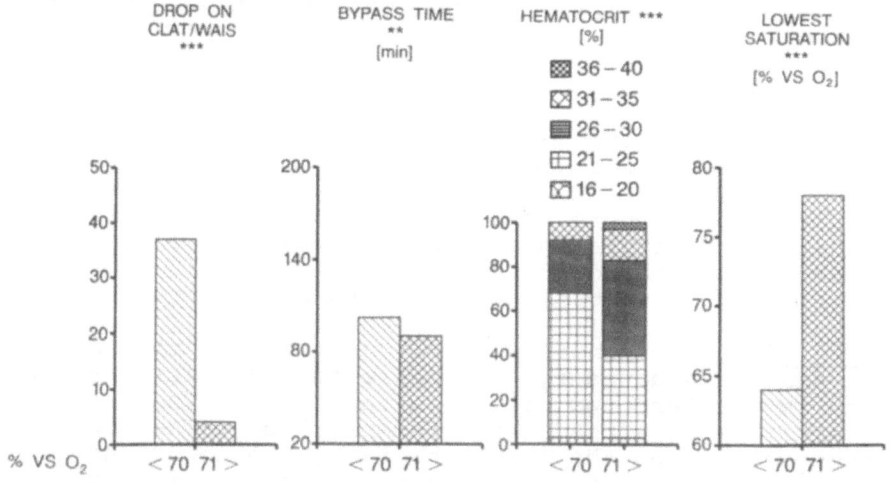

Fig. 6:   Saturation: Bubble Oxygenator/Filter 4, N=99

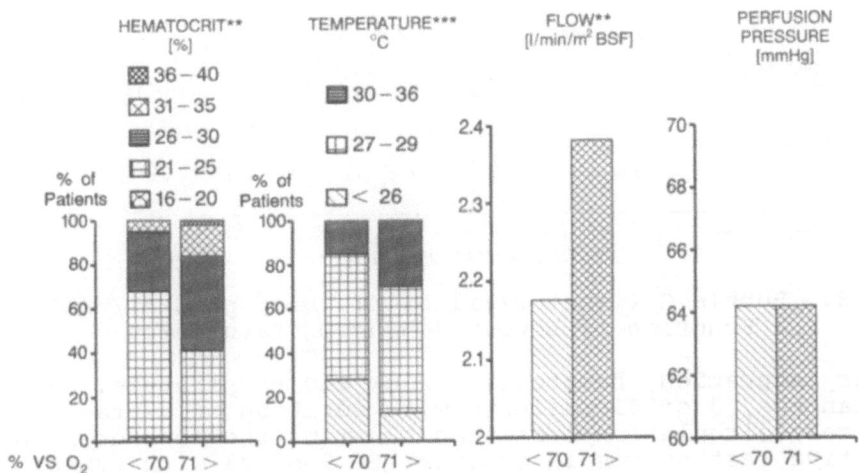

Fig. 7.   Factors Affecting Saturation: Bubble
          Oxygenator/Filter 4 (N=65/34)

In Fig. 7, we analyze other factors affecting venous
saturation in this smaller group of patients. We observe
a similar significant relationship between different
levels of venous saturation and hematocrit, temperature
and flow. Perfusion pressure is equal in both groups.

Fig. 8 shows again the outcome assessed by cognitive
tests in relation to venous saturation. Cardiopulmonary
bypass was performed with a bubble oxygenator and arterial
line filter #4. This analysis is independent of flow,
temperature, hematocrit and bypass time. The horizontal
axis represents venous saturation increasing from left to
right. A vertical line is drawn at 70% venous saturation.
The patients are represented as circles. The number of
circles does not necessarily correspond to the number of
patients because patients with identical values are over-
printed as one circle. Eleven of 29 patients in the lower
venous saturation range showed a postoperative drop,
whereas only one of 35 had such a drop in the group with
venous saturation over 70%.

Fig. 9 is similar to the preceeding except that
instead of venous saturation, bypass time is shown on the
horizontal axis. Here a vertical line is drawn at 100
min. of bypass time. This evaluation is independent of

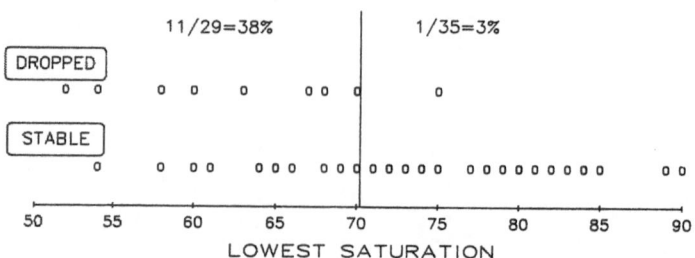

Fig. 8.   Bubble Oxygenator/Filter 4:   Drop on CLAT/WAIS as
a Function of Lowest Venous O_2 Saturation

venous saturation, hematocrit, flow and temperature. As
one can see, 3 of 41 patients with duration of extracorporeal circulation less than 100 min. showed a drop in
cognitive test scores in contrast to 9 of 23 with bypass
times over 100 min.

From these preliminary results we can very cautiously
draw a few conclusions:

1.   In this study cognitive tests seem to be the most
sensitive instrument for detection of cerebral
impairment following open heart surgery.

2.   In contrast to neurological investigations, cognitive
tests show correlations to some variables of cardiopulmonary bypass.

3.   Oxygen saturation of mixed venous blood shows a highly
significant correlation to cognitive outcome.

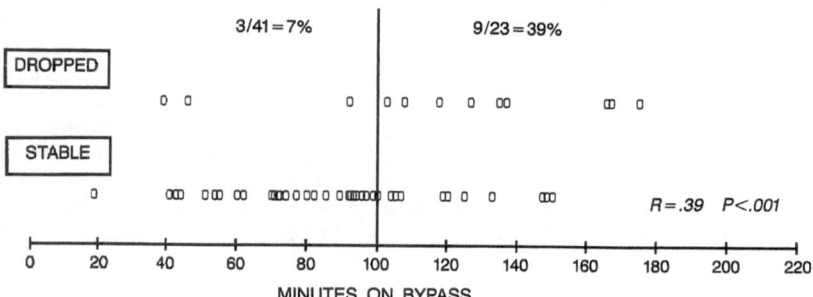

Fig. 9.   Bubble Oxygenator/Filter 4:   Drop on CLAT/WAIS as
a Function of Bypass Time

Whereas these three statements sound reasonable, factors affecting venous oxygen saturation and therefore their relation to outcome present some puzzles: it is difficult to understand why methods generally believed to protect the patient such as lower temperature and lower hematocrit actually correlate with a larger drop in psychometric test scores.

All this seems complicated enough, but it becomes even more complicated when we take into account essential parts of cardiopulmonary bypass, namely oxygenators and arterial line filters.

REFERENCE

1. Wheatley and Chasio, Adequacy of Perfusion: General view, in: "Cardiopulmonary bypass: Principles of Management, K. M. Taylor, ed., Chapman and Howell, London (1988).

ANESTHESIA AND PSYCHOMETRIC TESTS - PROBLEMS IN

PSYCHOLOGICAL ASSESSMENT OF COGNITIVE RECOVERY AFTER

ANESTHESIA

Bernhard Dahme and Hellmut Pokar

University of Hamburg
Hamburg, W. Germany

INTRODUCTION

To get more insight into the development of post-operative psychic disturbances, it would be useful to have more detailed knowledge about the process of cognitive recovery from anesthesia after open heart surgery, i.e., recovery from unconsciousness during surgery through a transient state of sleep and drowsiness to more or less wakefulness. In this regard we are not only concerned with the normal awakening process after any operation, but with recovery from very extreme to normalized physiological conditions. This raises some major unresolved research problems, especially methodological ones.

There are still strong arguments for the assumption that at least some major postoperative psychic disturbances are caused or aggravated by intraoperative factors [1] or physiological abnormalities in the recovery process after surgery (e.g. platelet aggregation) [2]. These factors can interact with anesthesiological factors. It becomes evident that neuropsychological testing as early as possible after awaking from anesthesia is an important prerequisite to understanding this relatively unexplored area of normal and abnormal postoperative psychic recovery.

Impact of Cardiac Surgery on the Quality of Life
Edited by A. E. Willner and G. Rodewald
Plenum Press, New York, 1990

ANESTHESIOLOGICAL AND PSYCHOLOGICAL REQUIREMENTS FOR
EMPIRICAL STUDIES OF POSTOPERATIVE COGNITIVE RECOVERY

Before evaluating methodological attempts made in
former or current research to explore the process of
cognitive recovery from anesthesia, some important
anesthesiological and psychological requirements have to
be stated:

(1)   Most narcotic effects normally will be "washed out"
        no later than the 2nd or 3rd postoperative day, so
        that psychological tests administered at the 3rd day
        or after are too late to reveal after-effects.
        Instead, repeated measurements on the first day after
        awakening from anesthesia are necessary.

(2)   "Paper and pencil" tests demand too much cognitive
        and motor efforts from patients, so they are
        inappropriate to reflect the process of cognitive
        recovery. Special short and comprehensive tests,
        demanding only oral or simple motor responses, are
        preferred.

(3)   Psychological data on cognitive recovery must be
        controlled for considerable interindividual differ-
        ences, e.g. preoperative neuropsychological status,
        intra- and postoperative hemodynamics, liver and
        kidney function, etc.

APPROPRIATE NEUROPSYCHOLOGICAL TESTING

We will try to give a comprehensive survey of tests
or simple procedures that might be appropriate for early
neuropsychological testing after awakening from anesthesia
after cardiotomy. For several reasons (practicality of
tests in the field of anesthesiology, etc.) we restricted
our review of relevant reports to neuropsychological
testing within anesthesiology. For the purpose of this
paper we excluded the following research results or
reports:

(1)   All studies in which postoperative neuropsychological
        data were assessed only after the 3rd postoperative
        day;
(2)   Neuropsychological tests demanding too much effort
        from the patient;

(3)   Neuropsychological tests that have been exclusively
      applied to patients who underwent surgery while
      conscious, with regional anesthesia.

The "Free Operant Technique" of Lindsley et al.

      A very simple, ingenious technique for testing the
process of awakening from anesthesia itself has been
described and applied by Lindsley, et al. [3]. The
technique has been adopted from Skinner's operant
behavioral studies and can be regarded as a so called
"free operant behavior technique." This is the principle
of operant behavior: If a subject operates a lever, switch
or similar reactive device, he is promptly rewarded or
reinforced by the presentation of a rewarding or the withdrawal of an aversive event. The subject is free to
respond at any time.

      This principle has been realized by the following
technique: An intermittent loud tone was delivered
through an earphone to one ear of each patient before,
during, and after anesthesia. The volitional or free-
operant response was that of touching the index finger to
the thumb of the preferred hand. Each response actuated
an electrical apparatus which briefly reduced the intensity
of the tone in the patient's ear. Rapid closing of the
hand reduced the tone intensity below the auditory
threshold and the patient could avoid hearing the tone by
continued responding at a high rate. Slow responding kept
the tone at a moderate intensity. If no responses were
made, the tone rose to and was maintained at its maximum
intensity of 90 decibels. Thus, the patient's rate of
responding directly controlled the intensity of the tone
and he was reinforced for avoiding or escaping aversive
tone intensities.

      Although Lindsley, et al [3] obtained impressive
results by this method, it seems never to have been
applied again in research, perhaps for ethical reasons,
i.e. there is no easily persuasive justification for con-
fronting patients with loud aversive tones during anesthesia and recovery. But one must remember that operant
techniques have two sides: instead of being reinforced by
avoiding or escaping aversive stimulation, patients can be
reinforced by pleasant stimulation, e.g. classical music
in the recovery ward. Such stimulation has often been
applied without being coupled with an operant procedure.
We think that the Lindsley-technique of "free operant
behavior" should be reactivated in a modified version for
research into cognitive recovery from anesthesia.

Simple Tests of Attention and Concentration

Grabow et al. [4] presented some well known simple tests of attention, concentration and even short-term memory to patients after thoracotomy and laparotomy only 2 hours after surgery with repeated measurements 6 and 24 hours after the operation. They used:

- Digit number series ranging from 3 to 9 one-digit numbers that are presented orally by a staff member at a rate of 1 sec. for each digit, for the patient to repeat in the same order.

- Digit number series with backward reproduction. These series ranged from 2 to 8 one-digit numbers.

- Arithmetic: 10 problems of low to moderate difficulty in normal school arithmetic.

- Benton Recognition Test: 10 cards with 1 to 3 simple geometric figures on each card are presented each for 10 seconds. After each display the patient has to recognize a figure on a card also containing 3 similar distractor figures.

All these tests require only an oral response from the patient. The scoring is well defined, making for objective quantification of the patient's performance. For all tests, parallel forms were constructed, making possible repeated measurement, without testing only long term memory.

Another test, similar to the backward-digit-number-series, to assess the state of concentration has been applied by Smith, et al. [5]. Patients had to recite the months of the year backwards. This test has been well standardized, also.

Tests of Orientation in Time and Place

Tests of orientation seem to be important, but have not often been applied. Smith, et al. [5] report a test procedure of 17 questions assessing orientation in time and place with objective scoring of the patient's answers.

Memory Tests

The Benton-Recognition Test mentioned above can be regarded as a memory test as well as a test of attention/

concentration. The Bethune-Williams Test of delayed
recall has been applied in several anesthesiological
investigations [6], plus in the context of open heart
surgery [2]. It can be used for testing short-term memory
but also long term storage and retrieval. Conceptualized
for testing recall from memory, it can also be applied as
a recognition test. Quantification is well established,
allowing assessment of a wide range of memory functions.
Visual stimuli of common objects (drawings of tools,
animals, etc.) are presented to the subject and he is
asked about them after a short and a long term interval.
In the standard instruction, patients are asked to repro-
duce the stimuli by free recall. If free recall fails,
the patient is helped by "prompting" with associative
words that are assumed to facilitate retrieval. If
prompting fails, the subject is then asked to recognize
the relevant stimuli among distractors on a special
recognition card. Performance is scored in terms of
errors, giving low scores to success in recall, higher
scores for prompting and recognition, and highest scores
for complete memory failure of an item. As far as we
know, the Bethune-Williams Test has not been applied prior
to the second postoperative day. A similar but not so
refined visual memory test was applied by Smith, et al.
[5].

CRITICAL EVALUATION

     The number and quality of psychological tests that
have been employed in research on recovery from anesthesia
is rather low. All tests presented here, except the
Bethune-Williams delayed recall test, have not been applied
more than once in recovery research. From a methodological
viewpoint, all these tests have to be considered as ad-hoc
tests, even if they are variations of tests that have been
often used in other research areas (e.g. the Benton or the
digit number series test). Consequently, there are no
standard norms. The effect of age on performance of these
tests remains obscure or contradictory. Grabow, et al.
[4] found that the arithmetic test is strongly, and the
Benton recognition test partially, age-dependant. Smith,
et al. [5] show results concerning mean deficits in
orientation, concentration and visual memory which are
age-related, but even more likely, sex by age interactions
can be inferred. It is unclear from their report whether
these effects are statistically significant.
     When systematic intraindividual pre-/postoperative
comparisons have been performed, all tests were sensitive

enough to reflect significant pre-/post-effects. However,
Grabow, et al. [4] did not make a statistical pre-/post
comparison; they only assessed the tests preoperatively.

The cognitive abilities evaluated by the methods
proposed here are limited to attention/concentration,
orientation, and memory. It is generally agreed that
psychomotor ability is also important in evaluating
cognitive functions, as Gelfman, et al. [7] have demonstrated. They found that even after oral surgery in young
patients (mean age about 23 years), after intravenous
sedation with diazepam-methohexital with or without
fentanyl and naloxane reversal patients appeared to regain
psychomotor skills before perceptual and cognitive
functions.

We think that it should be relatively easy to install
an apparatus for a multiple choice reaction time task with
a finger switch at the patient's bed in the recovery ward.
With this, it would be possible to assess psychomotor
recovery on a very elementary level. Literally, the
Lindsley-free operant technique should be regarded as a
psychomotor task as well.

NEED FOR CONTROL OF OTHER VARIABLES

We have stated that studies collecting data on the
psychological recovery from anesthesia need to incorporate
controls for other important variables that may be responsible for differences between various types of anesthesia
or surgical diagnoses or treatments. These variables
might obscure respective group differences. A minimum
requirement should be that all tests of cognitive recovery
be administered preoperatively, and that these scores be
included in adequate statistical pre-/post comparisons.
An explicit preoperative neuropsychological assessment by
a standardized neuropsychological test battery would be
very useful, because age differences often reflect
different levels of neuropsychological deficits provoked
by age and other factors.

In open heart surgery especially, there is growing
empirical and clinical evidence of the importance of intra-
and post-operative hemodynamics, liver and kidney functioning for cognitive recovery [6]. Smith, et al. [5]
showed that the length of the operation was an important
factor for memory deficits during recovery, finding that
contradictory to what they expected, shorter operation
periods led to greater memory deficits.

OUTLOOK

Even if the psychometric material that we offer for systematic study of cognitive recovery from anesthesia after open heart surgery is very limited and not well established in terms of well proven standard methods, there are some easily applicable tests that can and should be used in research on postoperative psychological recovery. Because parallel forms have been constructed or can easily be arranged, the tests presented here are appropriate for repeated measurements as well.

We hope that our proposal is able to encourage further research about this important and interesting field of cognitive recovery after surgery and anesthesia.

REFERENCES

1. H. Pokar, N. Bleese, H. Fisher-Duesterhoff, P. Goetze, G. Huse-Kleinstoll, J. Koedijk, M.-J. Polonius, K. Pruessmann, V. Tilsner, Use of prostacyclin to prevent postoperative psychic and neurological disturbances after open heart surgery, in: "Psychopathological and Neurological Dysfunctions Following Open Heart Surgery," R. Becker, J. Katz, M. J. Polonius, H. Speidel, eds, Springer, Berlin, Heidelberg, New York, 312 (1982).
2. D. W. Bethune, Focal neurological lesions and diffuse organic brain damage in open heart surgery patients, in: "Psychopathological and Neurological Dysfunctions Following Open Heart Surgery," R. Becker, J. Katz, M. J. Polonius, H. Speidel, eds., Springer, Berlin, Heidelberg, New York, 300 (1982).
3. O. R. Lindsley, J. H. Hobika, B. E. Esten, Operant recovery from anesthesia - a simple test, Anesthesia And Analgesia, 48: 136 (1961).
4. L. Grabow, W. Sachs, L. Zelinka, H. Schlemmer, V. Ehehalt, Leistungspsychologische und blutgasanalytische nersuchungen bei euroleptanalgesien und alothanenarkosen, Anaesthesist, 22: 150 (1973).
5. R. J. Smith, N. M. Roberts, R. J. Rodoers, S. Bennent, Adverse cognitive effects of general anesthesia in young and elderly patients, Internat. Clin. Pharmacology, 1: 253 (1986).
6. D. W. Bethune, Test of delayed memory recall suitable for assessing post-operative amnesia, Anesthesia, 36: 942 (1981).

7.   S. S. Gelfman, R. H. Gracely, E. J. Driscou, P. R.
     Wirdzek, D. P. Butler, J. B. Sweet, Comparison of
     recovery tests after intravenous sedation with
     diazepam-methohexital and diazepam-methohexital and
     fentanyl, Journ. Oral Surgery, 37: 391 (1979).

ARTERIAL LINE FILTRATION REDUCES MICROEMBOLISM AND SIGNIFICANTLY IMPROVES NEUROPSYCHOLOGICAL OUTCOME IN CORONARY ARTERY SURGERY

Tom Treasure, Wilfred Pugsley, Louise Klinger,
Christos Paschalis, B. Aspey, Michael Harrison
and Stanton Newman

The Middlesex Hospital and University College
London

INTRODUCTION

From the earliest days of cardiac surgery there has been acute awareness of the possible damage that might be done to the brain. Henry Souttar was amongst the first to operate on the heart 1] in 1925. He saw the opportunity for surgical help and argued that valvular disease of the heart was "to a large extent mechanical, and as such should already be within the scope of surgery were it not for the extraordinary nature of the conditions under which the problems must be attacked." It was thirty years before the development of the heart/lung machine so he had to operate on the heart while it was closed and beating "in view of the extreme danger to the brain from even the shortest check to its blood supply." In a statement in that paper he showed remarkable foresight when he said: "We are, however, of the opinion that these conditions are mechanical, and that apart from them the heart is as amenable to surgical treatment as any other organ."

It appears that he was ostracised by his colleagues for having the audacity to put a finger inside the human heart, an organ which was then still treated with a reverence which we now reserve for the brain. Cardiac surgery made little major progress until after the second

Impact of Cardiac Surgery on the Quality of Life
Edited by A. E. Willner and G. Rodewald
Plenum Press, New York, 1990

world war. Although surgeons now operate on the heart
routinely and may become lulled into a false sense of
security, we still interfere with the normal perfusion of
the brain and may damage it. As surgical results have
improved, and benefit has become more predictable, the
indications for operation have been extended to include
fitter patients who are operated upon for more marginal
benefits and subtle, and perhaps previously unnoticed,
cerebral changes are no longer acceptable.

Aberg brought the subject back into the forefront of
the British literature in a paper in The Lancet in 1982
in which he described the release of the brain enzyme,
adenylate kinase, into the cerebrospinal fluid during
cardiopulmonary bypass [2]. He believed this was due to
microembolic cerebral damage. At the Middlesex Hospital
we embarked on a systematic study of the effects of
cardiopulmonary bypass on the brain and used a range of
clinical, psychological and imaging techniques to define
the problem [3]. It was Deverall's group at Guy's
Hospital who introduced us to the use of transcranial
Doppler ultrasound to identify microemboli in the
cerebral circulation during cardiac surgery [4]. In this
study we set out to establish if use of a filter would
reduce the number of microemboli reaching the brain, and
if this had any influence on cerebral performance.

PATIENTS AND METHODS

Patients undergoing routine coronary artery bypass
surgery, who gave informed consent, were randomised into
one of two groups. The only difference between the
groups was whether the bypass circuit included a 40u
filter or not. Randomisation ensured that each cohort of
ten patients included equal numbers to permit sequential
analysis but the study continued until 100 patients were
recruited. Patients over 70 years of age, diabetics, and
those operated on urgently, for unstable symptoms or
impending infarction, were excluded as were those whose
English was inadequate to undertake neuropsychological
tests. Otherwise the cases were sequential as far as the
logistics of organising a large clinical research project
would allow.

Before surgery all patients underwent clinical
neurological examination and a standardised neuropsychological assessment. The formal neuropsychological
evaluation was repeated at eight days and again at eight
weeks after surgery. The neuropsychological assessment

involved a battery of ten tests designed to assess short
term memory, visuo-motor skills, reaction time, and
attention span. Three were computer administered which
not only gives very standardised, accurately timed and
impartial results but also avoids some of the inhibitions
experienced when tests are administered in an interview
format. The others were performed with a trained
psychologist.

In this symposium report we will only give the
results of the Rey Auditory Verbal Learning Test which
provides information on immediate memory span, learning
ability and susceptibility to learning interference.
Free recall of 15 words is attempted and the use of an
interpolated list with return to the original provides a
sensitive and discriminating test of memory.

The full battery of tests included non-verbal memory
tests in which checkerboard designs are viewed and
recognised on a VDU screen; a computer administered
version of the Wechsler digit symbol test; a letter
cancellation task; choice reaction time; Wechsler Block
Design test; the Purdue Pegboard and Trail Making tests.
Mood state assessments included the Speilberger State
Inventory for Anxiety and the Beck Depression Inventory.

A standard anesthetic technique was used throughout.
Premedication included diazepam, papaveretum and
hyoscine. Anesthesia was induced with thiopentone and
pancuronium, and was maintained with nitrous oxide,
papaveretum and lorazepam. Arterial pressure and central
venous pressures were measured routinely via indwelling
lines, displayed continuously and stored at 30 second
intervals on an Apple IIe microcomputer after analog to
digital conversion. Perfusion pressure during bypass was
kept between 50 and 100 mmHg, as far as possible, using
phenylephrine and phentolamine which do not independently
alter cerebral blood flow. Nasopharyngeal temperature
and end-tidal PCO2 were monitored continuously.

The cardiopulmonary bypass circuit included a bubble
oxygenator (William Harvey H1700), a Stockard "Multiflow"
roller pump and, where indicated by randomisation, a 40u
(Pall EC-plus) self venting blood filter in the arterial
line. The bypass circuit was primed with 1.5 litres of
Hartman's solution and run at a flow of 2.4 litres/
minute/square meter body surface area and then reduced to
1.8 litres at the target nadir temperature of 28°C.
Coronary artery surgery was performed during a single

period of cardiac arrest, with the myocardium protected
by hyperkalemic cardioplegic solution and hypothermia.

Transcranial Doppler (TC2-64, EME, West Germany)
which uses high intensity pulsed ultrasound, was used to
measure cerebral blood flow velocity and to detect microemboli. The probe is held against the temporal bone,
just above the zygomatic arch and at that point the flow
signal in the middle cerebral artery can be detected
coming towards the probe (Figure 1) by the operator who
wears headphones to aid positioning of the probe. The
surgical team is thus unaware of the flow signal. If the
flow is disturbed by microemboli these are heard as
characteristic 'blips' and seen as high amplitude, short
duration signals on the VDU screen (Figure 2). We have
demonstrated that gaseous microbubbles produce these
signals [5] but the size, exact nature, and exact number
of microemboli cannot be determined so we refer to them
as microembolic events (MEE). The output from the
printer port of the TC2-64 was taken to the Apple IIe
and, with software designed specifically for the task,
averaged over 30 second periods and stored along with a
count of the MEEs for subsequent analysis. The method
has been described in detail previously [5].

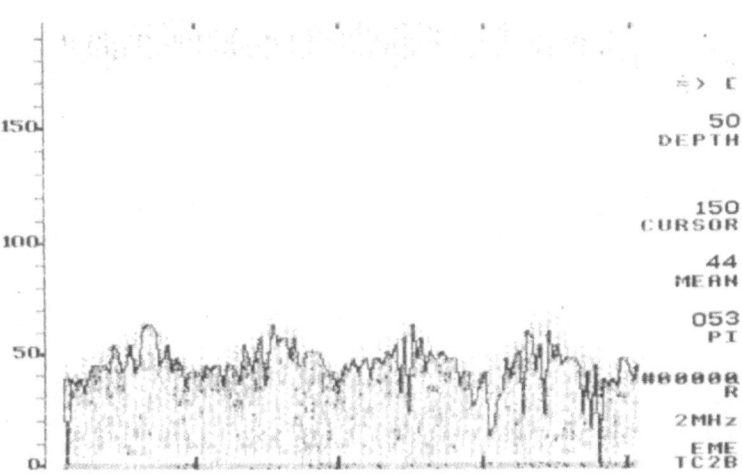

Fig. 1.   Reading from Transcranial Doppler.

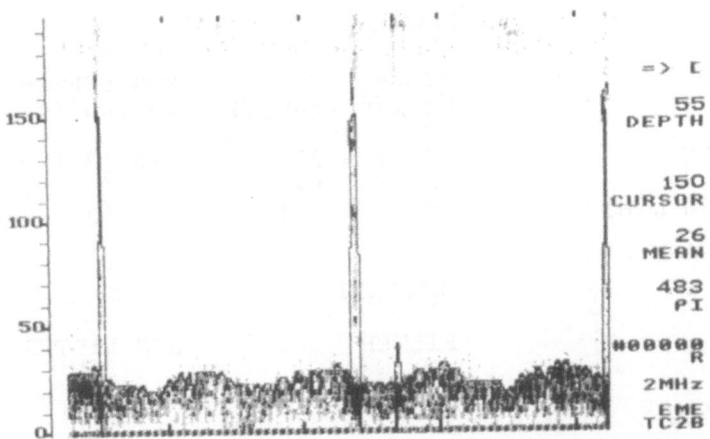

Fig. 2.   Microemboli Appearing on UDU Screen.

RESULTS

We report here on the first 40 patients in this randomised study and confine ourselves to middle cerebral Doppler counts of microembolic events (MEEs), neurological outcome, and the Rey Test of Verbal Memory.

The groups were similar in terms of age and cardiopulmonary bypass time.

There was no difference in the number of MEEs recorded on cannulation or at the inception of cardiopulmonary bypass but there was a marked difference between the two groups once bypass was established.

TABLE I

	FILTER Mean (SD)	NON FILTER Mean (SD)
AGE (years)	57 (6)	54 (9)
CPB Time (mins)	102 (24)	92 (27)

TABLE II

	FILTER Median (range)	NON FILTER Median (range)
CANNULATION	12 (1 - 25)	10 (2 - 20)
INCEPTION	36 (5 - 82)	45 (5 - 100)
CPB (per 30 min)	6 (0 - 10)	243 (30 - 768)

TABLE III

	FILTER	NON FILTER
NORMAL	17	13
'SOFT' SIGNS	3	7

There were no focal neurological signs in either group but fewer patients in the filtered group had 'soft' neurological signs, although this did not reach significance.

In the Rey Test of Verbal Memory there was an overall improvement in the patients who had a filter in the bypass circuit and a deterioration in those who did not. This difference was highly significant (P0.01, Wilcoxon test). (Figure 3)

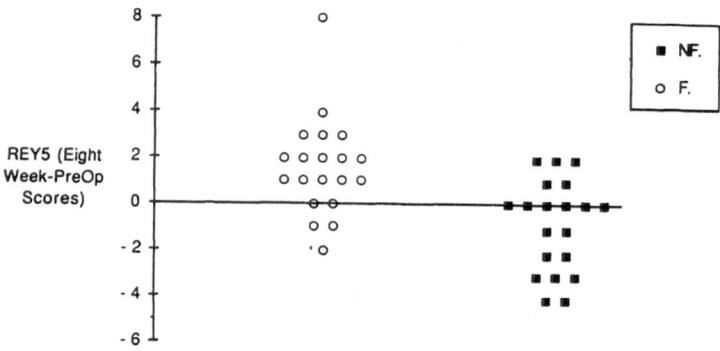

p<0.01, Wilcoxon

Fig. 3.   The change in verbal memory (score at eight weeks, minus preoperative) in 20 patients who had a 40u filter included in the circuit and 20 who had a bubble oxygenator without a filter.

DISCUSSION

Although Åberg believed that microembolism was a cause of the enzyme leakage into the cerebrospinal fluid which occurred during cardiopulmonary bypass [2], his own studies did not include a measurement of microembolism. In a carefully performed study in dogs, Taylor had shown that the level of adenylate kinase in the CSF was influenced by the presence of a 40u filter [6], suggesting that there might be avoidable brain damage being caused by microembolism during cardiopulmonary bypass (CPB). In subsequent work his group have used the eye as a natural window through which they observe the microvascular supply of the central nervous system during CPB and have shown that microvascular occlusions occur in the retina during cardiopulmonary bypass [7], again adding weight to the evidence that microembolism damaged the central nervous system during bypass. However, they were unable to demonstrate that the number and nature of these microvascular occlusions was influenced by the presence or absence of an arterial line filter [8]. Willner addressed the central issue, the effect on the patient's ability to function, in a study of the effect of arterial line filtration on the patients' mental function [9], but the study had a sequential design with historical controls, filters were not only of different size but made of different materials, and the study relied too much on the Conceptual Level Analogy Test (CLAT) for its measure of outcome.

Although the cumulative weight of evidence may suggest that avoidable microembolisation plays a significant part in cerebral malfunction associated with cardiac surgery, the use of an arterial line filter may introduce additional complications. From earlier experience there remains a fear of clotting in the filter, resulting in complete obstruction of the bypass circuit with near certain disaster. Even now, most perfusionists use a filter in parallel with a bypass loop which is normally occluded but can be opened instantly. We have had to use this to save a patient's life. Less dramatic but systematic problems, such as the possibility of creating platelet aggregates on the down stream side of the filter, or increasing the level of complement activation, particularly with a nylon filter, have made some perfusionists reluctant to adopt them. There is also a natural reluctance to avoid additional complexity and expense unless it is seen to be necessary. By the end of the 1970s two thirds of American units were using

arterial line filtration routinely [10], but European
practice was slower to adopt this technique. It is
likely that a difference in wealth, the medico-legal
climate, and innate conservatism accounts for the difference because the scientific evidence was inconclusive.

It was against this background that we undertook a
study of the effects of arterial line filtration [11] and
set out to look both for evidence that we were reducing
the number of microemboli that reached the brain, and
that this influenced the outcome as far as the patient's
cerebral performance was concerned. It required a
prospective randomised trial to do this to our satisfaction. The evidence that a filter reduces the number
of microembolic events seems incontrovertible (Table II).
The difference between the two groups of twenty subjects
reached significance on the tests of verbal memory;
other tests showed better performance in the group with a
filter but with less clear cut differences. On the basis
of these findings we believe that use of an arterial line
filter is good and safe practice.

REFERENCES

1. H. S. Souttar, The surgical treatment of mitral
    stenosis, British Medical Journal, October 3rd 603
    (1925).
2. T. Åberg, G. Ronquist, H. Tyden, P. Ahlund and K.
    Bergstrom, Release of adenylate kinase into
    cerebro-spinal fluid during open heart surgery and
    its relation to postoperative intellectual
    function, Lancet, 1:1139 (1982).
3. P. L. C. Smith, T. Treasure and S. P. Newman, et al,
    Cerebral consequences of cardiopulmonary bypass,
    Lancet, 1:823 (1986).
4. T. S. Padayachee, S. Parson, and R. Theobold, et al,
    The detection of microemboli in the middle
    cerebral artery during cardiopulmonary bypass: A
    transcranial Doppler ultrasound investigation
    using membrane and bubble oxygenators, Ann Thorac
    Surg., 44:298 (1987).
5. W. Pugsley, The use of Doppler ultrasound in the
    assessment of microemboli during cardiac surgery,
    Perfusion, 4:115 (1989).
6. K. M. Taylor, B. J. Devlin, S. M. Mittra, J. G.
    Gillian, J. J. Brannan and J. M. McKenna, Assess-
    ment of cerebral damage during open-heart surgery:
    a new experimental model, Scand J. Thor Cardiovas
    Surg., 14:197 (1980).

7. C. Blauth, J. Arnold, E. M. Kohner, K. M. Taylor,
    Retinal microembolism during cardiopulmonary
    bypass demonstrated by fluorescein angiography,
    Lancet, ii:837 (1986).
8. C. Blauth, J. Arnold, W. E. Schulenberg, A.
    McCartney, K. M. Taylor. Cerebral microembolism
    during cardiopulmonary bypass. Retinal micro-
    vascular studies in vivo with fluorescein
    angiography, J Thorac Cardiovasc Surg., 95:668
    (1988).
9. A. E. Willner, L. L. Caramante, J. W. Garvey, et al,
    The relationship between arterial filtration
    during open-heart surgery and mental abstraction
    ability, Proc Am Acad Cardiovasc Perf., 4:56
    (1983).
10. D. W. Miller, Jr., J. M. Binford, E. A. Hessel,
    Results of a survey of the professional activities
    of 811 cardiopulmonary perfusionists, J. Thorac
    Cardiovasc Surg., 83:385 (1982).
11. T. Treasure, Interventions to reduce cerebral injury
    during cardiac surgery - the effect of arterial
    line filtration, Perfusion, 4:147 (1989).

CEREBRAL MICROEMBOLISM AND NEUROPSYCHOLOGICAL OUTCOME

FOLLOWING CORONARY ARTERY BYPASS SURGERY (CABS) WITH

EITHER A MEMBRANE OR BUBBLE OXYGENATOR

P. L. Smith, C. Blauth, S. Newman,
J. Arnold, F. Siddons, K. M. Taylor

The Royal Postgraduate Medical School
London

INTRODUCTION

With the operative mortality of routine elective cardiac surgery approaching acceptable levels, increasing attention is being focused on the associated morbidities of these procedures [1]. Some of the most important morbidity following cardiac surgery is cerebral in origin. Cerebral dysfunction after cardiac surgery falls into two major categories. First, stroke or focal neurological deficits leading to usually either a hemiplegia or a retinal field defect. This occurs in approximately 5% of patients [2, 3]. Secondly, subtle neuropsychological impairment or change which has been variously documented as occurring in a significant proportion of patients up to at least one year following surgery [4, 5]. This latter form of cerebral impairment is probably due to diffuse cortical damage largely caused by microemboli but also possibly augmented by cerebral hypoperfusion [6]. Microemboli are mainly microbubbles or fibrin platelet aggregates [7].

In an effort to reduce neuropsychological impairment following routine cardiac surgery, a prospective investigation as to the influence of oxygenator type (membrane or bubble) on the genesis of microemboli during cardiopulmonary bypass and subsequent postoperative neuropsychological impairment has been carried out. This is a preliminary report of the initial findings of this study.

Impact of Cardiac Surgery on the Quality of Life
Edited by A. E. Willner and G. Rodewald
Plenum Press, New York, 1990

Cerebral microembolic occurrence was studied with the use of retinal fluorescein angiography as previously developed by this group and reported elsewhere [8, 9]. The neuropsychological status of the patients was investigated with a battery of ten professionally administered neuropsychological tests which have been used in more than 500 patients and also reported extensively elsewhere [10].

PATIENTS AND METHODS

Forty patients undergoing routine elective uncomplicated coronary artery bypass surgery to a standard anaesthetic and surgical protocol have been entered into the study at this time. Those patients suffering from diabetes mellitus and clinically evident cerebrovascular, neurological ophthalmological or psychological disorders were excluded from the study. All patients had pre-operative retinal fluorescein angiography and neuro-psychological testing. Intraoperative retinal fluorescein angiography was performed 5 minutes before the end of cardiopulmonary bypass. After processing the retinal angiograms were projected onto an opaque screen for an assessment with a magnification of approximately x 37 from the retina to the viewing screen. The areas of any perfusion defects were measured by planimetry. Results and measurements were corrected to give an approximation of the area of non-perfusion of the retina in millimetres. The neuropsychological test battery consisted of a battery of tests, as listed below:

1) The Rey Auditory Verbal Learning Test (verbal memory)
2) Two computerised non-verbal memory tests
3) The Trail Making Tests A and B (attention and concentration)
4) A Letter Cancellation Test (attention and concentration)
5) The Purdue Pegboard (perceptuomotor skills)
6) Two choice reaction time tests (attention and concentration)
7) A Symbol Digit Replacement Test (attention and concentration)

These were repeated on the eighth postoperative day. A significant deficit in any one test was judged to be a reduction in the re-test score by a margin of greater than one standard deviation of the mean test of the entire group of coronary artery surgery patients tested. The final neuropsychological index was then taken as the number of tests in which a deficit was recorded.

Cardiopulmonary bypass was carried out with pulsatile perfusion during aortic cross clamping and a 40 micron arterial line filter (EC+, Pall Corporation, Glen Cove, New York) in all cases. A Hartmann's cold crystalloid prime was used and cold cardioplegia was used for myocardial protection. Twenty-three patients underwent cardiopulmonary bypass with a Harvey H1700 bubble oxygenator (Bard Cardiopulmonary, Santa Ana, California) being used. Seventeen patients underwent cardiopulmonary bypass with a Cobe CML flat sheet membrane oxygenator (Cobe Laboratories Inc., Lakewood, Colorado).

The circuit for the membrane oxygenator consisted of a two pump system. Venous return and cardiotomy blood collected in the oxygenator venous reservoir was driven by the venous pump through the membrane oxygenator and into a collapsible arterial reservoir which was not vented. The arterial pump then pumped blood from the arterial reservoir through the arterial line filter into the ascending aorta. The purpose of the second pump was to permit pulsatile perfusion during aortic cross clamping. In the bubble oxygenator group, the mean age of patients was 56.0 years (range 41-67 years) and the mean bypass time was 83.7 minutes (range 29-146 minutes). In the membrane oxygenator group, the mean age was 55.6 years (range 44-67 years), and the mean bypass time was 88.4 minutes (range 57-118 minutes).

RESULTS

Retinal Angiography

23/23 (100%) of the patients in the Harvey H1700 bubble oxygenator group had retinal microvascular occlusions consistent with microembolism compared to 8/17 (47%) in the Cobe CML membrane oxygenator group ($p < 0.001$ Fisher exact test). The mean overall area of retinal non-perfusion per retina in the bubble group was 0.29 mms^2 (range $0.04-1.23$ mms^2), compared to 0.05 mms^2 (range $0-0.49$ mms^2; n=17) in the membrane group, ($p < 0.001$, Mann Whitney U-Test). If only those retinas with occlusions in the membrane group are considered

(n=8), the mean area of non-perfusion was 0.11 mms^2
(range 0.01-0.49 mms^2), and this was significantly less
than in the bubble group (p<0.01, Mann Whitney U-Test).

Neuropsychology

In the bubble group one patient refused the postoperative re-test. Data are available for 22 of 23
patients (95.6%). Five of twenty-two patients (22.7%)
had no measurable neuropsychological impairment and the
overall mean number of tests down was 1.24 (range 0-5).
In the membrane group 4 patients were not re-tested for
logistic reasons and one patient was excluded because of
a prolonged period of hypotension in the immediate postoperative period. Data are therefore only available for
12/17 patients (70.6%). Of these, 4/12 (33.3%) had no
measurable neuropsychological impairment and the overall
mean number of tests down was 0.91 (range 0-2). The
difference between the two groups is not statistically
signficant (p<0.11 Mann Whitney U-Test). There was no
correlation between the area of retinal non-perfusion and
the number of neuropsychological tests done.

DISCUSSION

The purpose of this paper is to report the early
findings of a highly significant reduction in retinal
microembolism which occurred during perfusion with a Cobe
CML membrane oxygenator compared to a Harvey H1700 bubble
oxygenator. Previous studies have shown that membrane
oxygenators generate fewer microemboli than bubble
oxygenators [11]. This has been shown in this study to be
associated with a signficant reduction in the incidence
of retinal vascular perfusion defect during cardiopulmonary bypass in cardiac surgery patients undergoing
coronary artery bypass surgery.

The neuropsychological data suggests a trend of less
impairment after membrane oxygenator and a further examination of these issues will be undertaken on completion
of this study. There is good angiographic and histo-
logical evidence that the retinal perfusion defects
observed after clinical and experimental cardiopulmonary
bypass are consistent with microembolic events but the
method does not identify the nature of the occluding
embolic material. It is likely that the microembolic
phenomena observed in the retina during cardiopulmonary

bypass reflect a mixture of different types of microembolism. In conclusion the Cobe CML flat sheet membrane
oxygenator may confer significant protection against
cerebral vascular microembolism during cardiopulmonary
bypass when compared to the Harvey H1700 bubble oxygenator. Assessment of the neuropsychological consequences,
if any, of the use of a particular oxygenator type for
cardiopulmonary bypass awaits completion of the study.

ACKNOWLEDGMENTS

This study is supported jointly by the Medical
Research Council of Great Britain and the British Heart
Foundation.

REFERENCES

1. Returns of the UK Cardiac Surgical Register. The
    Society of Thoracic and Cardiovascular Surgeons of
    Great Britain and Ireland (1984).
2. A. C. Breuer, A. J. Furlan, N. R. Hanson, et al.
    Central nervous system complications of coronary
    artery bypass graft surgery: prospective analysis
    of 421 patients, Stroke. 14:682-87 (1983).
3. P. Shaw, D. Bates, N. E. F. Cartlidge, et al. Early
    neurological complications of coronary artery
    bypass surgery, Br. Med J. 291:1384-87 (1985).
4. P. L. C. Smith, The cerebral complications of
    coronary artery bypass surgery, Ann Roy Coll Surg
    Engl. 70:212-16 (1988).
5. P. J. Shaw, D. Bates, N. E. F. Cartlidge, J. M.
    French, D. Heaviside, D. G. Julian, D. A. Shaw,
    Early intellectual dysfunction following coronary
    artery bypass surgery, Quart J Med. 58:59-68
    (1986).
6. R. T. Solis, P. S. Kennedy, A. C. Beall, G. P. Noon,
    M. E. DeBakey, Cardiopulmonary bypass. Micro-
    embolism and platelet aggregation, Circulation.
    52:103-08 (1975).
7. R. C. Dutton, L. H. Edmunds, J. C. Hutchinson,
    B. B. Roe, Platelet aggregate emboli produced in
    patients during cardiopulmonary bypass with
    membrane and bubble oxygenators and blood filters,
    J Thorac Cardiovasc Surg. 67:258-65 (1974).
8. C. Blauth, J. Arnold, E. M. Kohner, K. M. Taylor,
    Retinal microembolism during cardiopulmonary
    bypass demonstrated by fluorescein angiography,
    Lancet. ii:837-39 (1986).

9. C. Blauth, J. Arnold, W. E. Schulenberg, A. McCartney,
    K. M. Taylor, Cerebral microembolism during
    cardiopulmonary bypass. Retinal microvascular
    studies in vivo with fluorescein angiography, J
    Thorac Cardiovasc Surg. 95:668-676 (1988).
10. S. Newman, P. Smith, T. Treasure, P. Joseph, P. Ell,
    M. Harrison, Acute neuropsychological consequences
    of coronary artery bypass surgery, Curr Psych Res
    Rev. 6(2):115-24 (1987).
11. R. G. Carleson, A. J. Landé, B. Landis, et al. The
    Landé-Edwards membrane oxygenator during heart
    surgery: oxygen transfer, microembolism counts
    and Bender-Gestalt visual motor scores, J Thorac
    Cardiovasc Surg. 66:894-905 (1973).

EEG MONITORING DURING CARDIOPULMONARY BYPASS PROCEDURES

F. T. Strobl
Minneapolis Clinic
of Neurology
Minneapolis, MN

K. V. Arom
Minneapolis Heart
Institute
Minneapolis, MN

D. E. Cohen
Minneapolis, MN

INTRODUCTION

Severe neurologic complications following heart surgery are less prevalent due to improvements in surgical technique, perioperative care and extracorporeal circulation equipment [1, 2]. However, subtle neurological deficits still occur at rates up to 79% following cardiopulmonary bypass (CPB) [3, 4]. Multiple etiologic factors have been implicated and studied. Included are: equipment related microemboli, intraoperative hypotension, cannula placement and emboli from the surgical field [5, 6, 7]. Not examined are the effects of intraoperative treatment based on concurrent brain activity monitored intraoperatively by electroencephalography (EEG).

EEG has been used successfully for extraoperative assessment of neuronal functioning based on electrical patterns [8, 9]. It is the only direct measurement of neuronal integrity. Normal EEG recordings require adequate cerebral blood flow (CBF). Activity is depressed during ischemia and correlates with EEG changes. If uncorrected, ischemia progresses to irreversible brain damage.

A 2-part study was undertaken to monitor brain activity during hypothermic cardiopulmonary bypass procedures for the purpose of: 1) determining if on-line EEG alterations correlated with neurological outcome, 2) establishing criteria for intraoperative interventions, 3) comparing

Impact of Cardiac Surgery on the Quality of Life
Edited by A. E. Willner and G. Rodewald
Plenum Press, New York, 1990

the postoperative results of a similar group of patients who received intraoperative treatment for global power loss as identified by EEG. Although identification of focal abnormalities was not the focus of this study, they were also treated using the same criteria.

Part I (Group A) consisted of continuous intra-operative monitoring with an easily interpretable computerized EEG (CEEG). Data were analyzed for CEEG power drops greater than the 60% decline accepted for the hypothermic anesthetized patient.

Part II (Group B) consisted of intraoperative treat-ment for sustained CEEG power drops and comparison of global neurological outcomes between the two groups.

METHODS AND MATERIALS (PARTS I & II)

Over a one-year period, 91 unselected patients under-going heart surgery were studied. Approval was granted by the hospital's human studies committee and informed consent was obtained from the participants. Presence or absence of prior neurological symptoms or findings were not selection or exclusion factors. Part I of the study (Group A) consisted of 50 patients. These same 50 patients served as the control group for Part II of the same study.

During Part I of the study, computerized EEG (CEEG) data was collected. Each patient was monitored from anes-thetic induction to the end of surgery by a sixteen channel CEEG monitoring system (CNS Monitor^{TM}, CNS, Inc., Minneapolis, MN). Electrodes were placed according to the international 10-20 system and a standard bipolar anterior-posterior montage was used. Data was then presented on-line in the form of pie charts and bar graphs for easy interpretation. Permanent records were stored on floppy disks for review and analysis. Mean arterial and central venous pressures, pump flow pressures, temperature and blood gas values were also recorded routinely throughout the case. Standard parameters were maintained.

Anesthesia was maintained by a combination of forane, fentanyl and valium unless contraindicated. Hypothermia was maintained in all but one case with body temperature lowered to 28-30 degrees centigrade as indicated by esophageal and rectal temperature probes. Preintervention mean arterial pressures were maintained at 50-60 mmHg on patients in both groups. Extracorporeal circulation was maintained by roller pumps with a membrane oxygenator. A 40 micron filter was used on the cardiotomy suction line. Details of the extracorporeal circuit are described elsewhere [10].

Postoperative CEEG data analysis consisted of examining both frequency and total power. An average total power value was calculated for each channel. A baseline for all channels was determined by averaging the total power from each 20 second update collected from anesthetic induction to the onset of CPB. Total power values in each channel and an average value over all channels (one minute update intervals) from the onset of CPB to the end of the case were compared to the baseline. A global power drop index (PDI) was calculated for intervals with a drop in power of at least 60% using the formula:

PCI = PDI + integer [(40-100 * POWER c/POWER b)/5]
POWERc = Total EEG power in the current sample.
POWERb = Total EEG power in baseline sample.

Both are calculated for each channel.

Data were collected and analyzed by the computer in two second epochs. The EEG frequency bands were color coded and displayed in a pie chart and bar graph format at 20 and 60 second intervals respectively.

A banded average frequency value (AFV) was estimated for each channel using the formula:

AFV = (P(delta) * 2Hz) + (P(theta) * 6Hz) + (P(alpha) * 10 Hz) / P(Total)
(P = Power)

An averaged value was calculated across all channels from induction to the onset of CPB (baseline) and thereafter. A ratio was calculated per patient to detect any frequency shifts. Differences were analyzed using the two sample Student's t-test, Chi Square test and Pearson correlation coefficient.

Three neurological examiantions were performed by a neurologist blinded to all aspects of the study. Exams were performed one day preoperatively and days one (exam 1) and four, five or six (exam 2) postoperatively. They included a standard mental status evaluation of level of consciousness, orientation, attentiveness, memory, calculations, and speech, plus cranial nerve, motor, sensory, coordination and reflex testing. Station and gait were included whenever possible.

Neurologic outcome was classified into three categories: 1) normal, 2) global deficit, and 3) focal deficit. Patients were judged to be normal if there were no neurological changes from their preoperative assessment. Postoperative deficits were further divided by the neurologist into focal and global deficit groups. Patients with a focal deficit in addition to a global deficit were assigned to the global category.

RESULTS: PART I

Of the 50 patients studied, there were no deaths intraoperatively or within the first week postoperatively. There was a statistically significant difference (p <.05) between the diagnostic groups, normal vs. global deficits and their respective drop in EEG power averaged over the whole head (Table 1). This difference was not found to be significant when the normal group was compared with the focal deficit group. The time on the bypass pump was found to be statistically significant (p<.05) when comparison was made between the normal group and the global deficit group. There was also a statistical difference in relation to cerebral perfusion pressure and outcome (p<.01) (Table II).

No significant differences were found in the normal vs. focal deficit group in relation to pump time, surgical procedure, diagnostic groupings or a history of hypertension or prior neurological symptoms.

In summary, the drop in CEEG power (PDI) averaged over the whole head was the most significant EEG correlate with postoperative global neurological deficits. Focal deficits could not be discerned by this indicator alone but they were readily visible on the monitor displays. Further analysis is needed to establish the presence or absence of a positive correlation.

PART II: PURPOSE

Part II consisted of an additional 41 cardiac surgical patients using identical methods and materials described in Part I. Its purpose was to determine if the incidence of global neurologic deficit could be reduced by intraoperative interventions. Using Part I data, correlation of PDI with neurolgical deficits, the following criteria for intraoperative intervention were established.

TABLE I. Correlation of Deficits With PDI: Group A

	PDI (averaged)		AFV estimate (Hz)	
Diagnosis	Exam 1(n)	Exam 2(n)	Exam 1(n)	Exam 2(n)
Normal	107 (18)	154 (32)	1.07 (18)	1.12 (32)
Global Deficit	186 (22)	153 (10)	1.16 (22)	1.15 (10)
Focal Deficit	115 (10)	89 (8)	1.13 (10)	1.11 (8)

TABLE II. Mean Cerebral Perfusion Pressures: Group A (n)

Diagnosis	Exam 1	Exam 2
Normal	64.4 (18)	62.6 (32)
Global Deficit	59.0 (22)	58.2 (10)
Focal Deficit	62.2 (10)	61.5 (8)

Criteria for Intervention:

1) A drop in power to 25% of baseline activity during
   the first five minutes of the pump run or later
   during the pump run.
2) A steady drop in power to 30-35% of baseline
   sustained for 10 minutes.
3) An asymmetry or lateralized drop in power during
   the pump run.

Methods of Intervention:

1) Increasing cerebral perfusion pressure (MAP minus
   CVP) to 60 - 65 mmHg.
   a) Increase CPB pump flow.
   b) Increase MAP using phenylephrine.
2) Readjustment of the arterial cannula for a
   lateralized deficit.
3) Readjustment of the venous cannula.
4) Increase blood CO_2.

Single or multiple incremental interventions were used
until maximal CEEG power was restored. Pressure or flow
was maintained at or above the corrective level for a
period of 30 minutes to insure that reflow was well
established.

TABLE III.   Diagnostic Classifications

Diagnosis	Exam 1		Exam 2	
	Group A	Group B	Group A	Group B
Normal	36% (18)	76% (31)	64% (32)	80% (33)
Global Deficit	44% (22)	5% (2)	20% (10)	2% (1)
Focal Deficit	20% (10)	19% (8)	16% (8)	17% (7)*

* Two patients experienced postoperative strokes which resulted in focal deficits.

RESULTS - PART II

Following part two of the study, comparisons were made between control Group A and intervention Group B. The most dramatic finding was the reduction in global neurological deficits from 44% to 5% (Table III).   The effect was most significant (p<.001) for first post-operative examinations.

Additional statistically significant differences were found between Groups A and B (Table IV).   1) The mean PDI for Group A was found to be higher (p<.01) than for Group B.   2) The mean duration of CPB averaged an additional 19 minutes in Group B.   A positive correlation (r=.408, n=50, p<.01) was found between the averaged PDI and CPB duration in Group A.   No significant (r=-.107, n=41, p<.1) correlation was observed in Group B.   3) The average PDI was lower in Group B despite longer pump runs.   Comparable findings between the groups included mean age, history of prior neurological symptoms, types of surgical procedures and intraoperative cerebral perfusion pressures (Tables IV).   Hospital stay averaged 2.7 days less for the intervention group (Table IV).

CASE STUDY

RE is a 51 year old right handed male with no prior neurological complaints.   Preoperative neurologic exam revealed slight hyperreflexia of the right lower extremity without other abnormalities.   The patient underwent aortocoronary bypass involving 3 vessels.

Postoperatively on exam 1, the patient exhibited slowed mentation with mild memory dysfunction and reduced performance on calculation testing.   Deep tendon reflexes were diffusely brisk.   No focal findings were noted.   On exam 2, the patient continued to evidence signs of a mild encephalopathy without a focal deficit.

TABLE IV.   Comparison of Groups A and B

	Group A	Group B
Population	50	41
Mean PDI	143	73
Mean CPB (duration (min.)	97	116
Mean Age (Range)	61.6 (36-83)	61.8 (28-78)
Prior Neuro Findings	40%	41%
Mean Cerebral perfusion pressure	59.5	59.9
Mean Postop. lengh of stay (Range)	12.8 (7-49)	10.1 (6-13)
Coronary artery bypass	76%	63%
Valve replacement	18%	27%
Both	6%	10%

The power trend reveals a diffuse drop in EEG power with an averaged PDI of 243. The increase in power noted midway in the graph represents the increase in EEG power associated with rewarming.

DISCUSSION

Electroencephalographic monitoring during CPB has been advocated as a sensitive indicator of neuronal function since the early 1970s [11, 12]. Salerno et al. [6] using eight channel conventional EEG recorders detected diffuse EEG changes related to low perfusion pressures and superior vena cava obstruction from an unsuspected kink in the venous lines. Multichannel recordings also detected a focal area of dysfunction which resolved after repositioning the aortic arch cannula. Wright et al. [9] described patterns of EEG activity believed to be associated with the onset of CPB, venous hypertension, reduced perfusion pressure, embolism and hypoxia. These conventional EEG recordings are not characterized in a quantitative fashion; therefore, it is difficult to construct protocols for rapid intraoperative interventions. Global abnormalities are more difficult to discern on analog EEG. By applying digital computer techniques to the analysis of EEG, the sensitivity for the detection of ischemic changes has increased. Stockard et al. [7, 8], using six to fourteen channels of CEEG data analysis, found a correlation between intraoperative hypotension, postoperative neurologic complications and EEG dysfunction. Also demonstrated was an age-dependent cerebral vulnerability to hypotension. Neurologic complications were found to correlate with the duration of CPB.

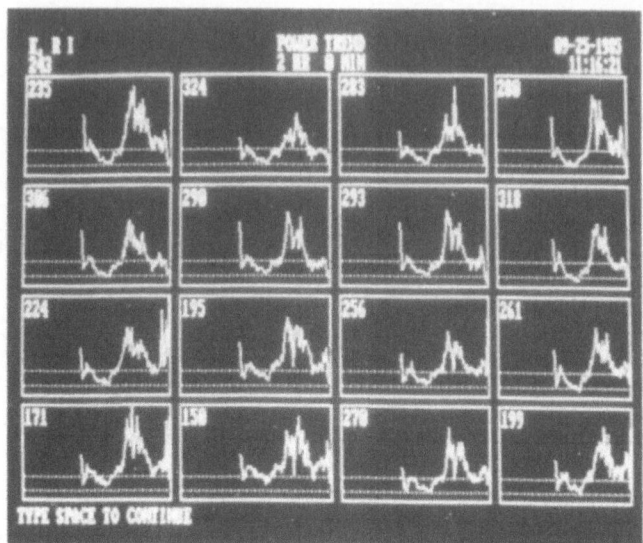

Figure 1.   Illustrates 16 EEG channels covering the whole
            head (Right is right; top is anterior). Each
            box represents 100% (top) to 0% (bottom) of
            the patient's own baseline. Dotted lines
            correspond with 25% and 10% power.

Åberg et al. [13], using adenylate kinase (AK)
measurements in the CSF, found that 50% to 60% of patients
undergoing CPB have evidence of ischemic brain lesions.
His results are comparable to the present findings in
Group A, exam one, and consistent with other studies
utilizing biochemical indicators of neurologic
damage [14].

Logas et al. also found the PDI to be predictive of
neurological outcome in patients receiving a narcotic
based anesthetic [15]. Isley and Kafer documented computer
processing of EEG to be a reliable and sensitive indicator
of neuronal function [16]. They also observed transitory
ischemic changes associated with head rotation or flexion
and hypotensive episodes. Pronk and Simons [17] have
conducted extensive research examining various aspects of
EEG monitoring during CPB. Their results add to and
support the other investigators. Studies in progress are
comparing pulsatile vs. nonpulsatile perfusion patterns
and the effect of intraoperative interventions on outcome.

This study corroborates prior investigations which
have indicated that no single cerebral perfusion pressure

will satisfy cerebral metabolic demands of all patients. Consequently, individualized treatment based upon measurements of organ perfusion would prove superior.

In our opinion, intraoperative interventions based on dynamic CEEG data offers an opportunity to significantly reduce the percentage of global neurological deficits following CPB. Further studies will continue to refine characteristics of adequate CPB/CPP and corrective interventions.

REFERENCES

1. T. Åberg, M. Kihlgren, L. Jonsson, Improved cerebral protection during open heart surgery. A psychometric investigation on 339 patients, in: "Psychopathological and Neurological Dysfunctions Following Open Heart Surgery," R. Becker, J. Katz, M. J. Polonius, H. Speidel, eds., Springer, Berlin, Heidelberg, New York (1982).
2. K. A. Sotaniemi, Brain damage and neurological outcome after open heart surgery. J. Neuro, Neurosurg, Psychiatry. 43:127-135 (1980).
3. L. Henriksen, Evidence suggestive of diffuse brain damage following cardiac operations, Lancet. 8381: 816-820 (1984).
4. P. J. Shaw, D. Bates, N. E. F. Cartlidge, J. M. French, D. Heaviside, G. J. Desmond, D. A. Shaw, Early neurological complications of coronary artery bypass surgery, Br. Med J. 291:1384-1387 (1985).
5. A. C. Breuer, A. C. Furlan, M. R. Hanson, R. J. Lederman, F. D. Loop, D. M. Cosgrove, R. L. Greenstreet, F. G. Estafanous, Central nervous system complications of coronary artery bypass graft surgery: Prospective analysis of 421 patients, Stroke. 14:682-687 (1983).
6. T. A. Salerno, D. P. Lince, D. N. White, E. J. P. Charrette, Monitoring of electroencephalogram during open-heart surgery. A prospective analysis of 118 cases, J Thorac Cardiovasc Surg. 76:97-100 (1978).
7. J. J. Stockard, R. G. Bickford, J. F. Schauble, Pressure-dependent cerebral ischemia during cardiopulmonary bypass, Neurology. 23:521-529 (1973).
8. J. J. Stockard, R. G. Bickford, R. R. Myers, M. H. Aung, R. B. Dilley, J.F. Schauble, Hypotension induced changes in cerebral function during cardiac surgery, Stroke. 5:730-746 (1974).

9. J. S. Wright, A. K. Lethlean, R. G. Hicks, T. A.
    Torda, R. Stacey, Electroencephalographic studies
    during open-heart surgery, J Thorac Cardiovasc
    Surg. 63:631-638 (1972).

10. K. V. Aron, P. M. Nicoloff, W. G. Lindsay, Should
    valve replacement and related procedures be
    performed in elderly patients? Ann Thorac Surg.
    38:466 (1984).

11. A. J. Furlan, A. C. Breuer, Central nervous system
    complications of open-heart surgery, Stroke.
    14:7-11 (1984).

12. M. M. Witoszka, H. Tamura, R. Indeglia, R. W. Hopkins,
    F. A. Simeone, Electroencephalographic changes and
    cerebral complications in open heart surgery, J
    Thorac Cardiovasc Surg. 66:855-863 (1973).

13. T. Aberg, G. Ronquist, H. Tyden, S. Brunnkvist,
    J. Huttman, K. Bergstrom, A. Lilja, Adverse effects
    on the brain in cardiac operations as assessed by
    biochemical, psychometric, and radiologic methods,
    J Thorac Cardiovasc Surg. 87:99-105 (1984).

14. T. Lunar, O. Stokke, Total creatine kinase activity in
    cerebrospinal fluid as an indicator of brain damage
    during open heart surgery. Scand J Thorac
    Cardiovasc Surg. 17:157-163 (1983).

15. W. G. Logas, B. Braverman, R. J. McCarthy, K. J. Tuman,
    B. D. Spiess, J. A. Hunter III, M. D. Goldin, M. O.
    Ivankovich, EEG power analysis is superior to
    frequency analysis for predicting adverse
    neurologic outcome after open heart surgery for
    narcotic anesthesia, Anesthesiology. 69:A315
    (1988).

16. M. R. Isley, E. R. Kater, Raw and computer processed
    EEG during cardiac surgery with cardiopulmonary
    bypass, Anesthesiology Review. 14(5):56 (1987).

17. R. A. F. Pronk, A. J. R. Simons, Automatic recognition
    of abnormal EEG activity during open heart and
    carotid surgery. Kyoto Symposia (EEG Suppl. No. 36)
    Elsevier Biomedical Press. (1982).

SUCCESS OF THE LOW FLOW - LOW PRESSURE PERFUSION IN

REDUCING POSTOPERATIVE PSYCHOLOGICAL DISTURBANCES

A. Tanzeem, C. Vahl, H. Schaefer, and
S. Hagl

Department of Cardiac Surgery
University of Heidelberg
Heidelberg, FRG

During the last 25 years, there has been a significant reduction in the mortality and morbidity of the
procedures necessitating the use of extracorporeal circulation. As most of the cardiac surgery procedures are
now performed with a very low mortality, attention is now
focussed on reducing complications and improving quality
of life after cardiac surgery. The incidence of psychological disturbances has been reported, in different
series, between 10 and 60%. The factors responsible for
such a high incidence of psychological changes after
extracorporeal circulation are still controversial. Most
cardiac surgeons believe the cause to be cerebral hypoperfusion and thereby react by increasing the flow during
ECC. On the other hand, neurophysiological experimental
data do not confirm this hypothesis. Astrup showed that
even at normothermia, cerebral blood flow has to be
reduced to less than 20% of the normal value (around 10
ml/100 mg/min.) before cell death related to perfusion
can be anticipated [1]. In practice, however, cerebral
blood flow during conventional perfusion never falls to
such low levels. It has been shown that particulate and
gaseous microemboli present prior to and generated during
the ECC may significantly influence the cerebral status
of postoperative cardiac surgery patients [2]. Willner
et al. [3] and other investigators have shown a reduction
in psychological disturbance in patients after the introduction of an arterial line filter. Allerdyce [4]
demonstrated the effects of microembolism on cerebral

Impact of Cardiac Surgery on the Quality of Life
Edited by A. E. Willner and G. Rodewald
Plenum Press, New York, 1990

function. Kessler and Patterson [5] provided evidence
that the oxygenator was an important source of microemboli.
Patterson reinforced this evidence by designing and
constructing a screen micropore filter, which when placed
in the arterial line reduced the number of gaseous
microemboli and very significantly improved the animals'
neurological status following CPB [6]. Pierce, in his
numerous studies on different oxygenators, demonstrated
that more gaseous microemboli were detected within the
arterial line when a bubble oxygenator was used, while
the membrane oxygenator produced no gaseous microemboli.
He also showed that gaseous microemboli may be present in
the priming fluid or may be produced by excessive
cardiotomy suction and during the rewarming period [7].

     A second possible cause of postoperative psycho-
logical disturbance may be the use of continuous flow.
The studies of Mavroudis [8] and the concepts of energy
equivalent pressure [9], capillary critical closing
pressure and microcirculatory patency [10] theoretically
support the use of pulsatile flow. Numerous studies of
Taylor et al. [11-14] show that the perfusion is better
at the cellular level with a pulsatile flow than with a
continuous flow. Taylor et al. [11, 12] have also demonstrated that the hypothalamic and pituitary stress
response patterns are significantly disordered during
the period of non-pulsatile flow. Restoration of normal
responses is seen soon after the return to pulsatile
perfusion. The studies of Wright and Sanderson [15] have
demonstrated that the diffuse brain cell damage associated with non-pulsatile flow may be prevented when
pulsatile flow is used. Studies of de Peepe et al. [15]
have demonstrated a significant reduction in arteriolar
and capillary diameter during non-pulsatile flow. The
above considerations convinced us to use membrane
oxygenators in our system routinely. In addition, we
started using an arterial line filter and a prebypass
filter to keep the level of particulate and gaseous
emboli at a minimum. Pulsatile flow was used in all
cases. In spite of these measures, the incidence of
postoperative cerebral dysfunction after cardiac surgery
remained unacceptable. A retrospective study of 100
patients operated on with ECC and cardioplegic arrest in
1987 showed that 21 patients had cerebral symptoms of
different degrees after cardiac surgery.

     Another cause of cerebral function disturbances may
be brain hyperperfusion during ECC as described by
Henricksen [17]. It is a common observation that the
patients are cooled to 28° C. rectal temperature without
a corresponding reduction in flow. Moreover, during this

period a high pressure is maintained, the hematocrit is usually kept low in order to save blood. The combination of these three factors may result in considerable tissue edema including brain celluar edema, with possible cerebral complications postoperatively, especially in long time perfusions.

Studies of Katogi [18] and of Yasuhiro Soma [19, 20] show that a flow of 40 ml/kg at moderate hypothermia (around 25° C) is within safe limits. Studies of Ellis et al. [21] show that a reduction of flowrate and arterial pressure do not result in cerebral dysfunction. This was further confirmed by impressive clinical results of Belcher and Lennox who reported that low-flow, low pressure perfusion resulted in better postoperative recovery of the patients, especially of respiratory, renal and cerebral function and needed less catecholamines postoperatively [22, 23]. In a study with prostacycline Aren et al. [24] could demonstrate that hypotension and low flow during perfusion do not increase postoperative cerebral damage. Wilson et al. [25] assessed online measurement of somatosensory evoked potentials during low flow - low pressure perfusion and reported that cerebral cortical function was preserved even after marked reduction in flow and pressure during CPB at 25° C.

These studies encouraged us to use low flow, low pressure perfusion without any further change in the perfusion system. After the commencement of CPB at around 2.0 1/min/m2, the bypass flow is gradually reduced to 2.0 1/min on reaching 26° C nasopharyngeal temperature. In patients with a body weight above 80 kg the flow is around 1.2 1/min/m2. The flow is gradually increased to the initial value during the rewarming phase. The rewarming is gradual. During the aortic crossclamping, the mean arterial pressure is maintained between 40-60 mm Hg. A clear prime is used to maintain hematocrit values between 20-25%. This lower hematocrit counteracts the increase in viscosity and vasoconstriction caused by hypothermia. At the same time the vasoconstriction due to hypothermia and also the reduced arterial pressure prevent building of tissue edema which may occur as a result of hemodilution. A pulsatile flow is used in all cases.

After changing the mode of perfusion, a drastic fall in the frequency of psychological disturbances after extracorporeal circulation was noticed. Subsequently a prospective study was designed to study the neurological and psychological complications accompanying this perfusion technique.

METHODS

    In our prospective study, all consecutive patients
were included who were admitted at least 12 hours before
operation. The patients were examined neurologically and
psychologically assessed at regular intervals. The
psychiatric evaluation included assessment of orientation,
social behavior, hostility, withdrawal, hallucinations
and delusions, and memory, both remote and recent. In
the event of neurological or psychological changes, a
neurologist and a psychiatrist were consulted. In all
cases an EEG and a cranial tomography were carried out.
In addition, 240 preoperative, operative and postoperative data were stored on computer for further analysis.
The patients were under neurologic and psychiatric care
until they were free of symptoms.

    The following criteria were used to exclude patients
from the study: Emergency operations, and patients who
were admitted from other hospitals on the day of operation. In these patients a preoperative psychological and
neurological assesssment was not possible. One patient
died on the operating table and was excluded from the
study. In the event of a neurological focal finding, the
patients were excluded from the study. This was the case
in 4 patients. This prospective study was designed for
350 patients.

RESULTS

    Figure 1 shows the diagnosis of patients operated
upon in our series. The most common procedure was an
aortocoronary bypass operation followed by single valve
replacement, double valve replacement and combined
procedures. In this study of 350 consecutive patients,
8 patients developed a psychosyndrome.

    Figure 2 shows the frequency of symptoms noted in
our patients. Eight patients were disorientated in time
and/or space. The same 8 patients showed disturbance of
memory. Five patients showed psychomotor disorders and
changes in social behavior - such as unfriendliness and
aggressiveness. Five patients showed paranoid fears and
3 of these patients had postoperative delerium.

    Figure 3 shows this group of 350 patients were
further analysed according to their age. Three of 127
patients who developed psychological disturbances were in
the 6th decade group, and 5 out of 46 patients were in

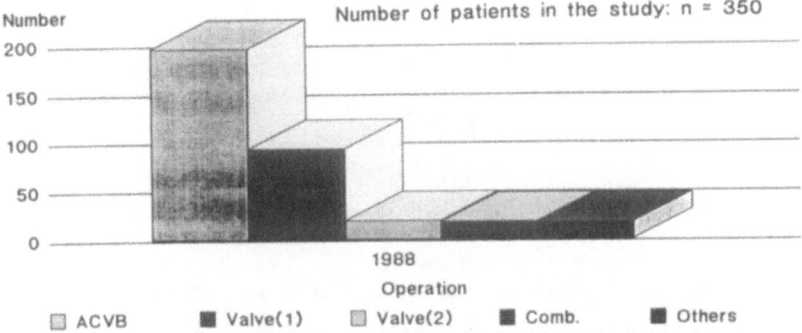

Fig. 1.   Frequency and nature of cardiac surgery,
          Heidelberg, FRG.

the 7th decade group.   Especially in this group one would
have expected a higher frequency of psychic disturbances.
Further analysis showed that 2 patients in the 6th decade
had a history of alcohol abuse and 2 patients in the 7th
decade who developed psychiatric disturbances had long
time sedative abuse preoperatively.

Figure 4 shows the duration of psychiatric disturbance in our 8 patients.   All the patients were free of
symptoms two weeks after the operation.   The relatives or
the general practitioner of the patients were contacted
two months after discharge from the hospital to report
any residual psychiatric symptoms or changes in personality of the patients.   All patients were free of symptoms.

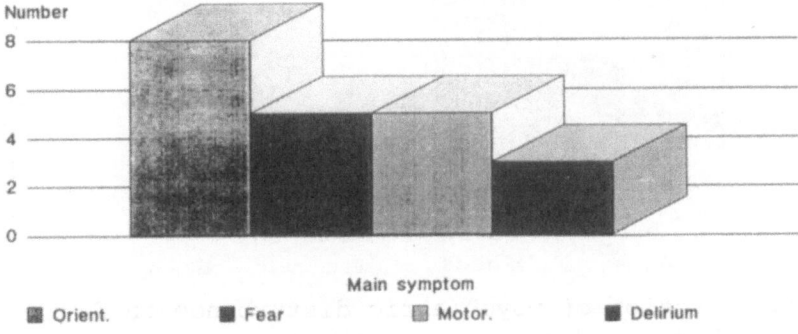

Fig. 2.   Frequency of major symptoms.

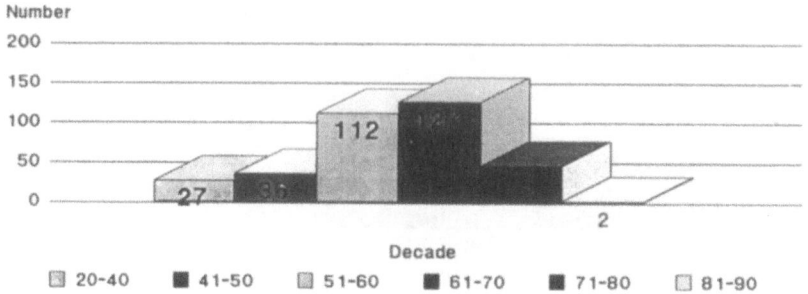

Fig. 3.   Distribution of patients according to age groups
          (n=350).

DISCUSSION

     The incidence of psychiatric disturbances in our
series is extremely low.   Much higher incidence is
reported by Javid and Tufo [26] (70%), Eggerton and Kay
[27] (31%), Blachly and Starr [28] (5-7%), Vahl et al.
[29] (15%).   The studies differ in the type of
investigation, the time the patients were examined
postoperatively and the follow-up period.   The method of
investigation varied from an impressionistic one to
elaborate psychometric tests. In some series the
determination of brain-specific markers in cerebrospinal
fluid has been used as an indicator of brain cell damage.

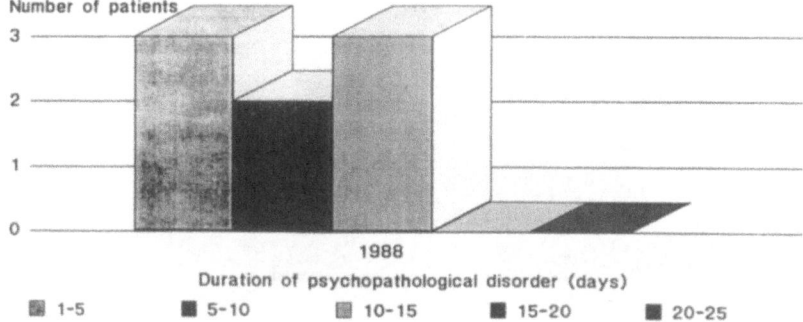

Fig. 4. Duration of psychiatric disturbance in days
        (n=8).

In our series we relied on full neurologic and psychiatric examinations at least 12 hours before the operation and at regular intervals after the operation, beginning from the day of extubation. Our studies are based on the classification of Rodewald et al. [30] for the recognition of postoperative psychological disturbances. The patients were examined independently by two surgeons following an examination protocol which was successfully used in a previous study at another heart center [29]. This gave us a unique opportunity to compare two different techniques using the same protocol and the experience of the same investigator.

This mode of perfusion technique raises the question of underperfusion of the brain and other organs. The experimental and clinical studies using somatosensory cortical evoked stimuli [25, 31], cerebral tissue gas analysis by mass spectrometer [18] and cerebral flow measurements [19, 20] prove that the cerebral tissue is adequately protected during low flow, low pressure perfusion. The studies of Kolka et al. [32] and Fedderson [33] with low flow moderate hypothermia and extreme hypotension (around 30 mm Hg) induced by prostacyclin infusion also report no higher incidence of postoperative cerebral damage.

An additional advantage of low flow, low pressure perfusion is a better conduction of cardioplegia. In recent years cardioplegia has gained widespread acceptance. Although no agreement has been reached on cardioplegic solution, there is a general agreement that one essential factor in the success of cardioplegic arrest is the lowering of myocardial temperature to around 15° C. Brazier et al. [34] reported noncoronary collateral flow. It is obvious that low flow, low pressure perfusion not only reduces this noncoronary flow but on account of the accompanying hypothermia, also facilitates the maintainance of lower myocardial temperature. This explains the better clinical results reported by Belcher and Lennox [22].

SUMMARY

By changing the mode of perfusion through reduction of bypass flow in accordance with the reduction of temperature, the incidence of psychiatric disturbances has been reduced in our series from 21 to less than 3%.

We believe that, in addition to the use of membrane oxygenator prebypass filter, arterial filter and pulsatile flow, a reduction of total bypass flow to the level necessary to guarantee adequate oxygenation may influence, in a positive way, the postoperative psychological recovery.

ACKNOWLEDGMENT

We are thankful to Miss Edtbauer for the typing of this manuscript.

REFERENCES

1. J. Astrup, L. Symon, M. N. Branston, et al. Cortical evoked potential and intracellular K+ and H+ at critical levels of brain ischemia, <u>Stroke</u>. 8:51-58 (1977).
2. T. Aberg, M. Kihlgren. Cerebral protection during open heart surgery, <u>Thorax</u>. 32:525-33 (1977).
3. A. E. Willner, L. Carmente, J. W. Garvey, et al. The relationship between arterial filtration during open heart surgery and mental abstraction ability. <u>Proceedings of the American Academy of Cardiovascular Perfusion</u>. Vol. 4, Jan. (1983).
4. D. B. Allardyce, S. A. Yoshida, P.O. Ashmore, et al. The importance of microembolism in the pathogenesis of organ dysfunction caused by prolonged use of pump oxygenator, <u>J Thorac Cardiovasc Surg</u>. 52:706-15 (1966).
5. J. Kessler, R. H. Patterson, The production of microemboli by various blood oxygenators. <u>Ann Thorac Surg</u>. 9:221-228 (1970).
6. R. H. Patterson, J. Kessler, P. M. Gergland. A filter to prevent cerebral damage during experimental cardiopulmonary bypass, <u>Surg. Gyn Obstet</u>. 132:71-4 (1971).
7. E. C. Pierce, Membrane oxygenation in cardiopulmonary bypass, <u>in</u>: "Cardiopulmonary Bypass. Principles and Management," K. M. Tayler, ed., Chapman and Hall, London (1986).
8. C. Mavroudis, To pulse or not to pulse, <u>Ann Thorac Surg</u>. 25:259-71 (1978).
9. R. B. Shepard, D. C. Simpson, J. Sharp, et al. Energy equivalent pressure, <u>Arch Surg</u>. 93:730 (1966).

10. R. J. Parsons, P. D. McMaster, The effect of the pulse upon the formation and flow of lymph, J Exp Med. 68:353 (1938).

11. K .M. Taylor, G. S. Wright, W. H. Bain, et al., Comparative studies of pulsatile and non-pulsatile flow during cardiopulmonary bypass, J. Thor Cardiovasc Surg. 75:579-584 (1978).

12. K. H. Taylor, G. S. Wright, W. H. Bain, et al. Comparative studies of pulsatile and non-pulsatile flow during cardiopulmonary bypass. III. Anterior pituitary response to thyrotrophin-releasing hormone, J Thor Cardiovasc Surg. 75:579 (1978).

13. K. H. Taylor, B. J. Devlin, S. M. Mittra, et al., Assessment of cerebral damage during open heart surgery. A new experimental model, Scand J Thor Cardiovasc Surg. 14:197-203 (1980).

14. K. M. Taylor, W. H. Brain, K. G. Davidson, et al., Comparative clinical study of pulsatile and non-pulsatile perfusion in 350 consecutive patients, Thorax. 37:342-30 (1982).

15. G. Wright, J. M. Sanderson. Brain damage and mortality in dogs following pulsatile and non-pulsatile blood flows in extracorporeal circulation, Thorax. 27:738 (1972).

16. J. de Paepe, P. M. A. Pomerantzeff, K. Nakiri, et al. Observations of the microcirculation of the cerebral cortex of dogs subjected to pulsatile and non-pulsatile flow during extracorporeal circulation, in: "A Propos du Debit Pulse," Cobe Laboratories, Inc., Belgium.

17. L. Henriksen, E. Ejelins, T. Lindeburgh, Brain hyperperfusion during cardiac operations. Cerebral blood flow measured in man by intra-arterial injection of Xenon 133: evidence suggestive of intraoperative microembolism, J Thorac Cardiovasc Surg. 867:202 (1983).

18. T. Katogi, Analysis of brain tissue gas tensions during hypothermic low flow perfusion, Nippon Kyobu Geka Gakkai Zasshi. 31:1505-12 (1983).

19. Y. Soma, T. Hirotani, R. Yozu, et al., A clinical study of cerebral circulation during extracorporeal circulation, J Thor Cardiovasc Surg. 97:187-93 (1989).

20. Y. Soma, T. Hirotani, R. Yozu, et al., A clinical study of cerebral circulation during extracorporeal circulation, J Thor Cardiovasc Surg. 97:187-93 (1989).

21. R. J. Ellis, A. Wisniewski, R. Potts, et al.
    Reduction of flow rate and arterial pressure at
    moderate hypothermia does not result in cerebral
    dysfunction, J Thorac Cardiovasc Surg. 79:173-180
    (1980).
22. P. Belcher, S. C. Lennox, The effects of low flow -
    low pressure pulsatile bypass, J Cardiovasc Surg.
    26:223-227 (1985).
23. S. C. Lennox, Brampton Hospital, London, Personal
    Communications (1986).
24. C. Aren, C. Glomstrand, Wikkelsoc, et al.
    Hypotension induced by prostacyclin treatment
    during cardiopulmonary bypass does not increase
    the risk of cerebral complications. J Thorac
    Cardiovasc Surg. 88:748-753 (1984).
25. G. J. Wilson, I. M. Rabeyka, J. G. Coles, et al.,
    Loss of the somatosensory evoked response as an
    indicator of reversible cerebral ischaemia during
    hypothermic low flow cardiopulmonary bypass, Ann
    Thorac Surg. 45:206-209 (1988).
26. H. Javid, H. M. Tufo, H. Majafi, et al. Neurological
    abnormalities following open-heart surgery,
    J Thorac Cardiovasc Surg. 58:502 (1969).
27. N. Egerton, J. H. Kay, Psychological disturbances
    associated with open heart surgery, Brit J
    Psychiatry. 110:433-439 (1964).
28. P. H. Blachly, A. Starr, Postcardiotomy delerium, Am
    J Psychiatry. 121:371-375 (1964).
29. C. E. Vahl, I. Carl, E. Struck. Psychiatric
    complications after extracorporeal circulation;
    computer-assisted prospective study on 2000
    patients, 17th Annual Meeting, Bad Nauheim, The
    Thoracic and Cardiovascular Surgeon, Vol. 36:86
    (1988).
30. G. Rodewald, H. J. Meffert, T. Emskotter, et al.,
    Head and heart - neurological and psychological
    reactions to open heart surgery, Thorac Cardiovasc
    Surgeon. 36:254-261 (1988).
31. T. M. Rabeyka, J. C. Coles, G. S. Wilson, et al. The
    effect of low flow cardiopulmonary bypass on
    cerebral function: An experimental and clinical
    study, Ann Thorac Surg. 43:391 (1987).
32. R. Kolkka, M. Hilberman, Neurological dysfunction
    following cardiac operations with low flow, low
    pressure cardiopulmonary bypass, J Thorac Cardio-
    vasc Surg. 79:432 91980).
33. K. Fedderson, C. Aren, N. J. Nilsson, et al. Cerebral
    blood flow and metabolism during cardiopulmonary

bypass with special reference to effects of hypotension induced by prostacyclin, <u>Ann Thorac Surg.</u>
41:395-400 (1986).
34. J. Brazier, C. Hottenrott, G. Buckberg. Noncoronary
collateral myocardial blood flow, <u>Ann Thorac Surg.</u>
19:426 (1974).

REVIEW: MEDICAL AND SURGICAL DATA

K. M. Taylor

Hammersmith Hospital
London

This session was set up to discuss the differences in drug therapy, surgical and anaesthetic protocols and the different components of the cardiopulmonary bypass circuit which might relate to neurological and psychological disturbance in the postoperative period.

Drs. Dahme and Pokar from the University of Hamburg, West Germany discussed the effect of anaesthetic regimes on psychometric test analysis. In particular, they focussed on the important question of the recovery of cognitive function after the deep levels of anaesthesia used during open heart surgery. The relationship between anaesthesia particularly for prolonged operative procedures and a subsequent period of deep sedation in the intensive care unit is known to affect cognitive function in patients undergoing major non-cardiac surgical procedures although there seems little doubt that defects in cognitive function are significantly greater in the cardiac surgical population.

The authors drew attention to the fact that some anaesthetic and sedative regimes often used in cardiac surgical practice may retain suppressed defects of cognitive recovery until at least the second or third post-operative day. This immediately raises the problem of the timing of postoperative tests. If the tests are carried out too early the results may be difficult to interpret in view of the anaesthetic and sedative effects. If the tests are carried out too late, the recovery process may have reduced the actual incidence of cognitive deficits.

Impact of Cardiac Surgery on the Quality of Life
Edited by A. E. Willner and G. Rodewald
Plenum Press, New York, 1990

The authors also drew attention to the choice of neurological and psychological tests used, preferring those tests which place little demands on cognitive and motor responses from the patients in the early post-operative period.

Their exclusion of studies carried out after the third postoperative day evoked some controversy. Some discussants felt that post operative testing at 7 or 8 days following surgery would give a much firmer indication of the actual incidence of cognitive deficits in the patient population. The use of Lindsley's method using an auditory stimulus and a simple motor response was thought to be a useful test. The authors also described the simple test battery proposed by Grabow et al. The preferred memory tests include the Benton-Recognition Test; the Bethune-Williams Test had been used with some success.

Inevitably there was some considerable discussion as to the relative merits of different types and times of testing. There was however a consensus that anaesthesia and sedative drugs will exert a profound and often variable effect on the recovery of cognitive function in the cardiac surgical population. Awareness of these effects must be an important consideration in the planning and interpretation of any research studies.

The use of EEG monitoring during cardiopulmonary bypass was reviewed by Drs. Strobl and Arom from the Minneapolis Clinic of Neurology, USA. Although conventional EEG monitoring has previously been shown to be difficult to interpret in cardiac surgical practice, a number of modified EEG systems have been developed, some of which are designed towards simplifying the standard EEG, and others designed as a more comprehensive and computerised system. The authors studied a new computerised 16 channel electroencephelograph (CEEG) to detect, quantify and where possible treat episodes of cerebral ischaemia during cardiopulmonary bypass. In their matched prospective controlled study, two groups of patients underwent comparable cardiopulmonary bypass procedures. In the control group, full CEEG monitoring was carried out together with pre- and postoperative neurological assessment. In the test group the same monitoring and neurological examinations were carried out but interventions made during surgery were on the basis of the changes in the power drop index (PDI) shown in the CEEG. The cardiopulmonary bypass regime utilised by the authors included a standard anaesthetic regime based on

Flurane, Fentanyl and Valium. Moderate hypothermia was used to 28 to 30 degrees Centigrade. Mean arterial pressures were maintained during perfusion at 50 to 60 mms of mercury.

In the first part of their study, neurological outcome was classified into 3 categories: 1) normal; 2) global deficit; and 3) focal deficit. No significant differences were found in the normal versus focal deficit group in relation to pump time, surgical procedure, diagnostic groups, previous arterial hypertension or previous neurological symptoms. Focal deficits could not be discerned by the drop in CEEG power, although this indicator did correlate with postoperative global neurological deficits. Where the CEEG information was used as a basis for therapeutic interventions during the operation, the incidence of global neurological deficits was reduced from 44% to 5% (p less than 0.001). These interesting results provoked considerable discussion. The authors indicated that they need to continue their studies to increase their interpretation skills with the CEEG device and also to develop appropriate therapeutic interventions.

The principal contribution to this section related to the preliminary results from the International Consortium Study. This data was presented by Professor Rodewald, University Hospital, Hamburg, West Germany and Dr. Willner, Hillside Hospital, Long Island Jewish Medical Center, USA. As a preliminary to the presentation of the data a description of the statistical methods used was given by Dr. Borenstein, a colleague of Dr. Willner. Following detailed discussion of the statistical methods, the potential medical and surgical variables chosen for inclusion in the study were reviewed. The authors discussed the apparent importance of mixed venous oxygen saturation in the context of adequate cerebral perfusion. Mixed venous saturation varies with the arterial oxygen saturation, tissue and vital organ oxygen consumption. It also relates to cardiac output (flow rate on bypass) and hematocrit. The health of tissue in general, or a vital organ in particular, relates directly to maintainance of energy supply/demand equality. Many of the techniques used in cardiac surgery, particularly those during the central period of cardipulmonary bypass, are designed specifically to reduce oxygen demand during the period of artificial perfusion and oxygenation. Of principal importance is the induction of moderate hypothermia, reducing body temperature to 28 degrees centigrade or lower. A brief discussion focussed on the current

attitudes towards blood gas control under conditions
of hypothermia. The differing approaches of alpha-stat
and pH-stat were reviewed. There is undoubtedly a growing
consensus that alpha-stat management of blood gases during
hypothermia maintains the relationship between cerebral
blood flow and cerebral metabolic rate. Accordingly,
pH-stat (in which the CO_2 content of the circulating blood
is artificially raised) may be associated with the so-
called "luxury perfusion" syndrome. From the preliminary
results presented in the first part of the consortium
presentation, the following tentative conclusions were
drawn.

1. Cognitive tests do seem to be a sensitive method for
   the detection of cerebral impairment following open
   heart surgery.

2. Cognitive defects do appear to correlate to methodological variables, in cardiopulmonary bypass. This
   is in contrast to the results from neurological
   investigations.

3. Changes in mixed venous oxygen saturation appear to
   show a highly significant correlation to cognitive
   outcome.

   In addition to focussing on mixed venous oxygen
saturation the effects of cardiopulmonary bypass equipment
variables were discussed. The principal components of the
cardiopulmonary bypass circuit include the oxygenator or
gas exchange device and the arterial line filter. The
duration of the cardiopulmonary bypass perfusion period,
the perfusion flow level and the nature of bypass flow
(pulsatile or non-pulsatile) should also be considered.

   A review of the bypass times from the 7 study centres
revealed that 47.8% of the patients had a bypass time from
60-120 minutes and 32.3% had a bypass time of 121-180
minutes. Considerable differences were seen in the bypass
times between the individual centres. Similar differences
in the selection of surgical equipment were evident. The
various study centres used a variety of oxygenator-types
and filter types. This variability in the protocols
between the centres inevitably makes statistical interpretation of the data extremely difficult. Submission of
the data to complicated multivariant analysis does allow
some tentative conclusions to be drawn.

1. Increasing bypass time does correlate with the probability of a fall in the test scores (CLAT and WAIS tests). In the assessment of bubble oxygenators used in combination with or without an arterial line filter, the finding of little difference in the drop in test scores between the filtered and non-filtered groups was challenged by discussants who had found significant changes in psychometric and neuropsychological test scores indicating that arterial line filtration did protect consistently. Similar controversy was raised over some results which appeared to indicate no significant difference between the flat sheet membrane and bubble oxygenator groups as far as fall in test score was concerned. This finding was also questioned by some discussants who produced data indicating that superior post-bypass neuropsychological performance results in patients perfused with a membrane oxygenator. The consortium team rightly drew attention to the fact that the statistical power of the consortium results would be improved by increasing the numbers of patients in each statistical cell.

Dr. Tanzeem from Heidelberg, West Germany reported his group's experience in reducing postoperative psychological disturbance by adopting a low flow, low pressure perfusion technique. In their uncontrolled prospective study of 350 consecutive cardiac surgery patients, their perfusion technique was changed according to the following protocols: 1) Perfusion flow was reduced from 1.8 litres per minute, per metre squared to 1.1 litre per minute per metre square, at 26 degrees C.; 2) Membrane oxygenation was used; 3) Pulsatile flow was used; 4) Hematocrit was reduced to between 18 and 22%; 5) Mean aterial pressure was maintained at 40-50 mm of mercury.

Using the above perfusion modifications they experienced a reduction in their postoperative psychological syndromes from their previous incidence of 10-15% down to 3%. The authors reviewed in great detail the various aspects of change in perfusion technique including their advocacy of pulsatile cardiopulmonary bypass which is known to provide superior capillary perfusion for any given level of mean arterial blood flow and pressure.

This paper evoked considerable discussion with a number of discussants suggesting that the use of historical controls was invalid. The Heidelberg group continue to study their improved perfusion technique and hoped to present further corroborative data in the future.

SUMMARY

This session proved both interesting and controversial. The large amount of consortium data offers a
rich source of potential variables which may be related to
neurological and psychological outcome following cardiac
surgery. In retrospect, the lack of tight control over
perfusion protocols and equipment used during the period
of cardiopulmonary bypass has undoubtedly diluted the
statistical power of the results. Despite this, a number
of interesting pointers came from the papers given in this
section and they will certainly provide a basis for
further studies in the future. There is no doubt that the
results of the consortium study thus far confirm the
results from other studies that the incidence of neurological and psychological disturbance following cardiac
surgery remains unacceptably high.

CORRELATIONS BETWEEN PSYCHIATRIC,
NEUROLOGICAL AND PSYCHOMETRIC VARIABLES

CORRELATIONS BETWEEN: PSYCHIATRIC, NEUROLOGICAL AND

PSYCHOMETRIC VARIABLES: PSYCHIATRIC AND PSYCHOMETRIC

ISSUES

Bellkiss Wilma Romano Lamosa

Instituto do Coracao
Sau Paolo, Brazil

One of our main tasks at this symposium is to discuss whether the psychopathology observed in cardiac surgery patients may be influenced by neuropsychological factors and whether these factors can be assessed by psychometric tests.

An overview of several relevant issues, the psychiatric, neurological, psychometric, and medical-surgical issues, has already been presented. We will see now to what extent two of those issues are related, to what extent variations in one go with variations in the other.

We studied the relationship between psychiatric and psychometric findings, both preoperatively and post-operatively. In order to facilitate comparison, the tables show preoperative and postoperative results for each psychometric test. In each table, the magnitude of the correlation is represented by the size of the bar, with significant correlations shown by dark bars.

Figure 1 shows correlations of the Conceptual Level Analogy Test (CLAT) with several psychiatric measures. Preoperatively, it shows significant correlation with the Hamilton Depression and Anxiety scales, although it is not significantly correlated to the composite measure of the Hamburg Rating Scale for Psychic Disturbance (HRPD). Some items of the HRPD however do have significant correlation with the CLAT, i.e.: disorientation, disturbed concentration and masked depression. In comparison, the results at discharge show a more restricted relationship.

Impact of Cardiac Surgery on the Quality of Life
Edited by A. E. Willner and G. Rodewald
Plenum Press, New York, 1990

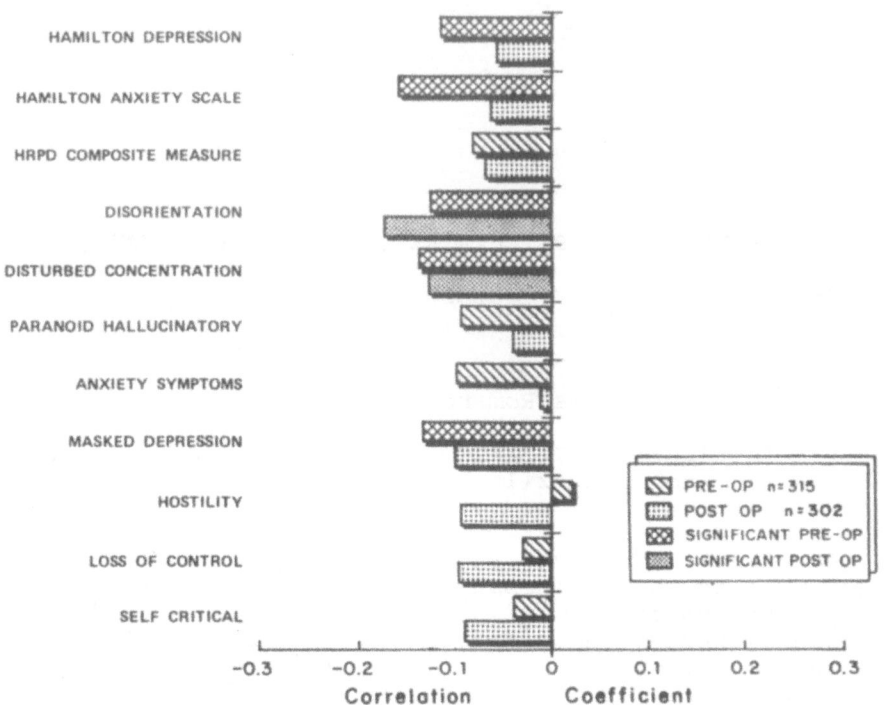

Fig. 1.   Correlations of CLAT scaled score preoperatively
          and at discharge.

Significant correlation persists only with disorientation
and disturbed concentration.

     In the CLAT Dichotomy (devastated versus non-
devastated scores) analysis (Figure 2), we can see that
preoperative results show a significant correlation with
the Hamilton Anxiety Scale but the Hamilton Depression
Scale correlation is no longer significant. The HRPD
factors that are significantly correlated are again:
disorientation, disturbed concentration and masked
depression. At discharge, disorientation and masked
depression remain significantly correlated.

     For the Weschler Adult Intelligence Scale (WAIS)
Digit Symbol subtest, significant correlation coefficients preoperatively are observed with the HRPD
factors: disorientation, disturbed concentration and
masked depression (Figure 3). Postoperatively significant correlations were found between digit symbol
scores and Hamilton Depression, HRPD composite and the

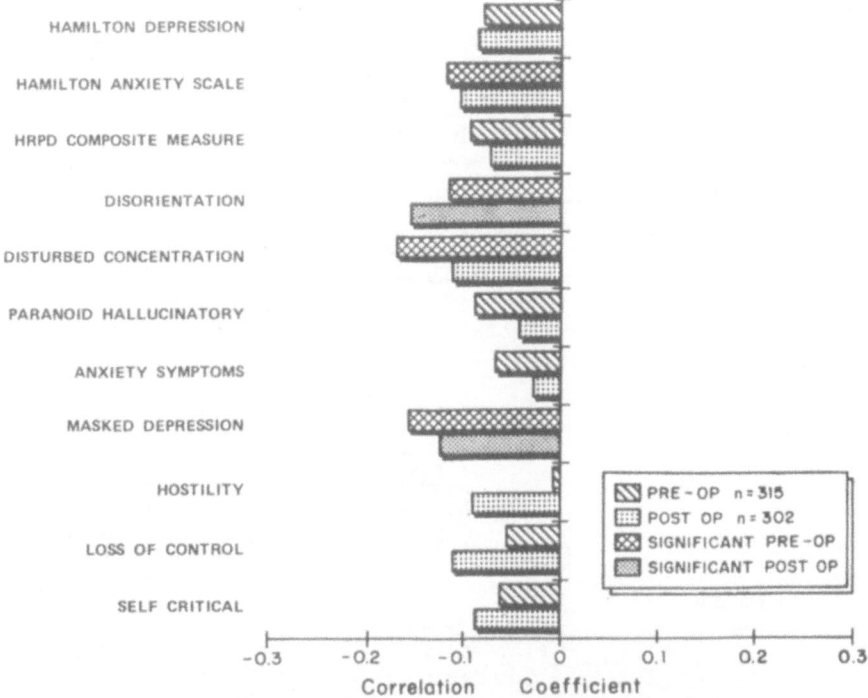

Fig. 2.   Correlations of CLAT Dichotomy Scores
          Preoperatively and at Discharge.

following HRPD factors: disorientation, disturbed
concentration, hostility and loss of control.

The WAIS Block Design results preoperatively showed
no correlation with the Hamilton scales, but a signficant
correlation with the HRPD composite measure, especially
with the factors: disturbed concentration, paranoid
hallucinatory, anxiety symptoms, masked depression and
self critical (Figure 4).   At discharge, all these correlations are non-significant, but the disorientation
factor becomes significantly correlated.

The Trail Making test (part B) has a signficant
correlation coefficient before the surgery with the
Hamilton Depression and Anxiety Scales, and also with the
following HRPD factors: disorientation, disturbed concentration and paranoid hallucinatory (Figure 5).   Postoperatively significant correlations persist only with
the Hamilton Depression Scale and the disorientation and
disturbed concentration factors.

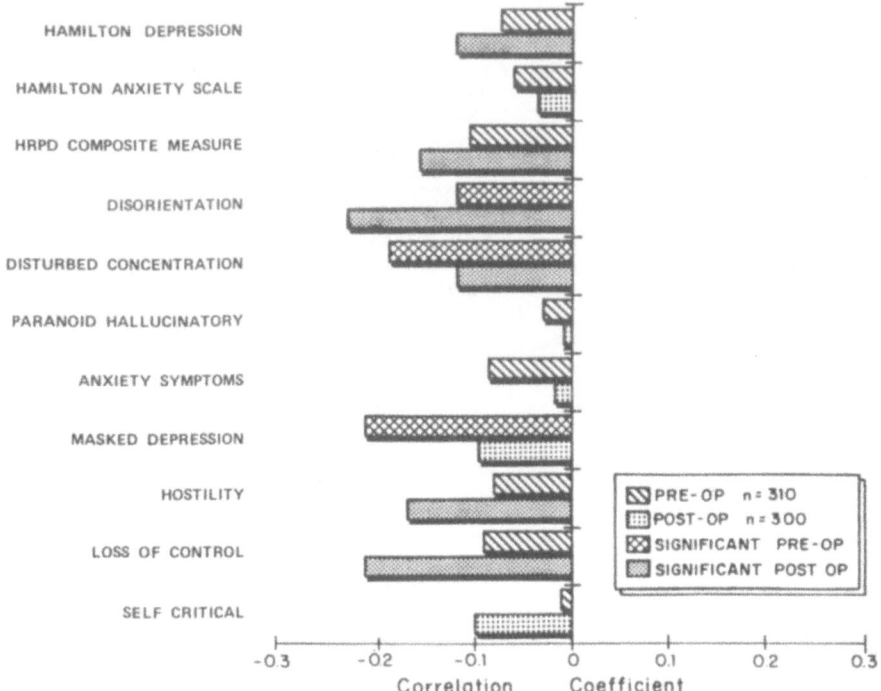

Fig. 3.   Correlations of WAIS Digit Symbol preoperatively
          and at discharge.

        Preoperatively, the Figure Rotation Test is not
signficantly correlated with the psychopathological
measures (Figure 6).   At discharge, correlations with the
following HRPD factors become significant: disorientation, disturbed concentration and self critical.

        The Bethune-Williams Visual Memory Test also has no
significant correlation with the psychiatric findings,
preoperatively (Figure 7).   At discharge, correlations
with the Hamilton Depression Scale and the disturbed
concentration and hostility factors become significant.

        In summary, we find that, preoperatively, four of
the six psychometric tests were significantly correlated
with the psychiatric measures.   Only two (the Figure
Rotation Test and Bethune-Williams Visual Memory Test)
were not significantly correlated with the psychopathology measures.

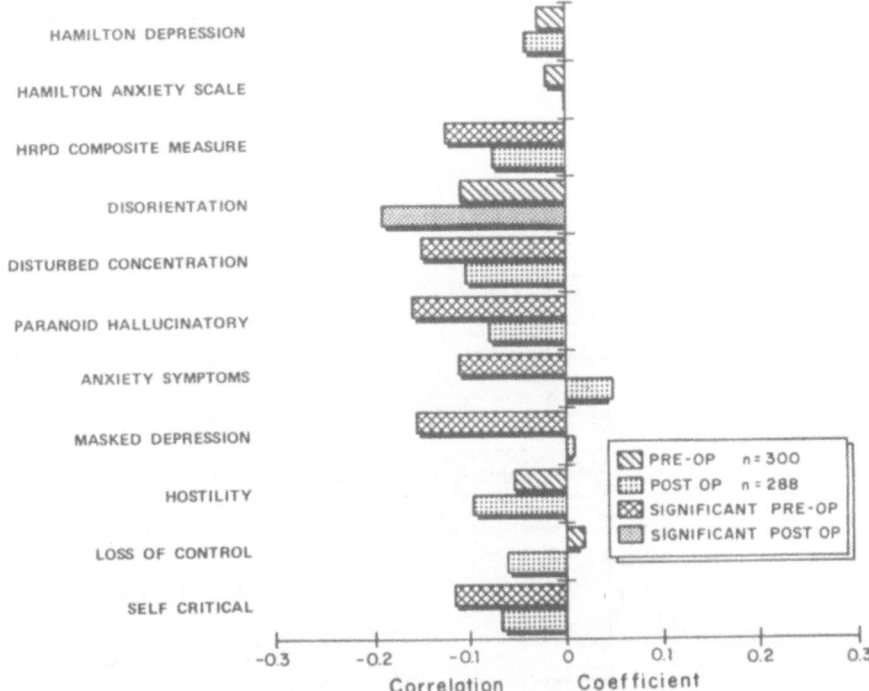

Fig. 4.   Correlations of WAIS Block Design preoperatively
and at discharge.

Postoperatively there was a change in the pattern of
correlation between the psychometric and psychiatric
measures. The two tests which were not correlated before
became correlated postoperatively with psychopathology.
The other tests tended to become less correlated with the
psychiatric measures.

In general, the correlations between psychometric
and psychiatric measures, while significant, were rather
weak. Presumably several identifiable but weak neuropsychological factors influence the patient's psychopathology.

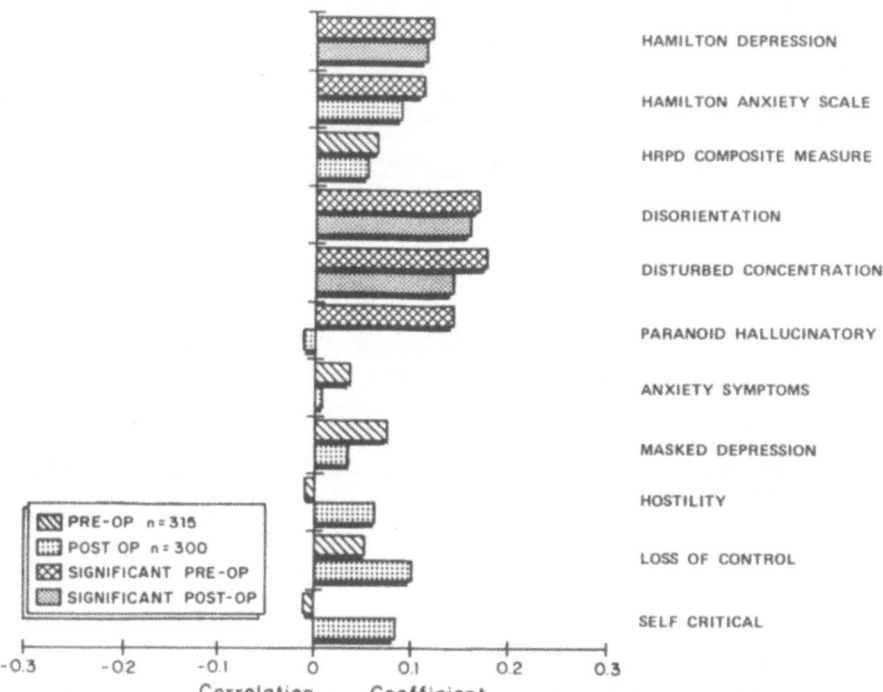

Fig. 5. Correlations of the Trail Making Test, Part B,
          preoperatively and at discharge.

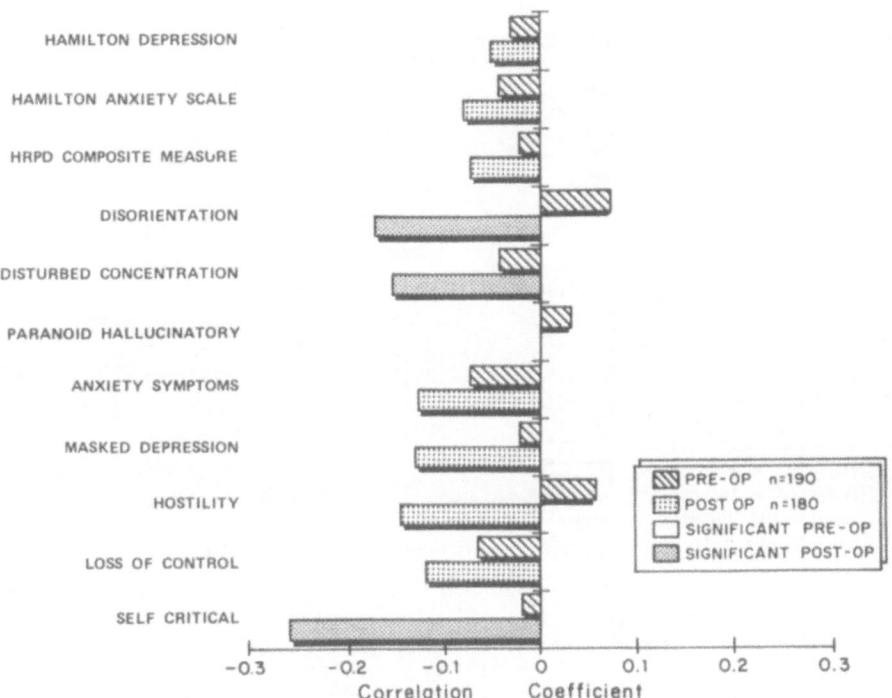

Fig. 6. Correlations of Figure Rotation, preoperatively and at discharge.

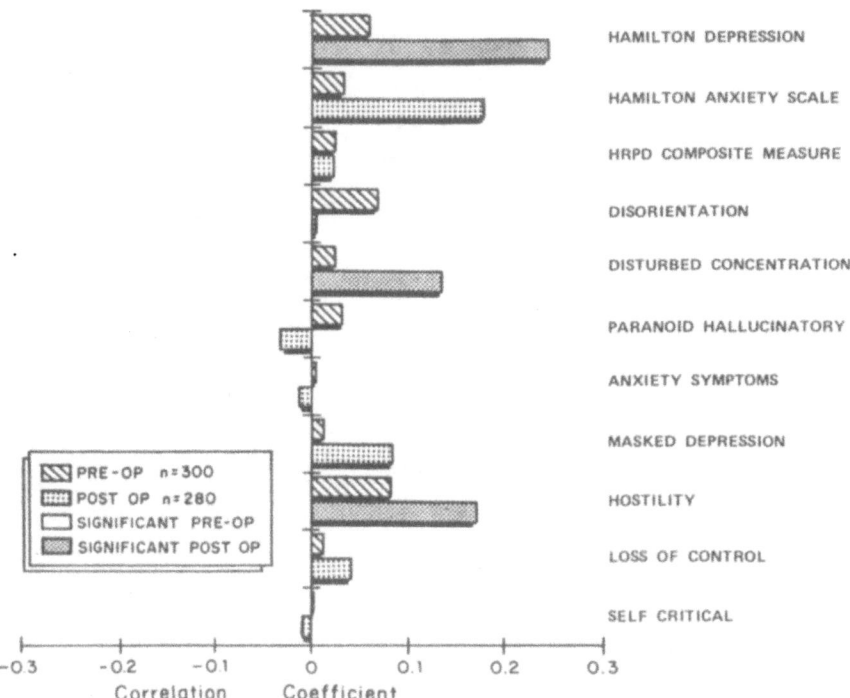

Fig. 7.   Correlations of the Bethune-Williams Visual
Memory Test, preoperatively and at discharge.

CORRELATIONS BETWEEN PSYCHIATRIC AND NEUROLOGICAL FINDINGS

Pekka Tiénari

Department of Psychiatry
University of Oulu
SF-90210 Oulu, Finland

We would expect many correlations between psychiatric and neurological findings. The psychopathological syndromes we see clinically are usually either organic mental syndromes or adjustment disorders [1, 2].

In the DSM-III-R, organic mental syndromes are grouped thus: 1) delirium and dementia in which cognitive impairment is relatively global; 2) amnestic syndrome and organic hallucinosis in which relatively select areas of cognition are impaired; 3) organic delusional syndrome, organic mood syndrome and organic anxiety syndrome, which have features resembling schizophrenia, mood and anxiety disorders; 4) organic personality syndrome in which the personality is affected [3].

Among DSM-III-R categories of organic mental syndromes, delirium is the most common. The cardinal feature of delirium is day to day, hour to hour and even minute to minute fluctuation in brain dysfunction. These fluctuations, especially in the level of arousal, orientation, attention, perception, and affect may be caused by alterations in the underlying systemic etiology. These fluctuations may also be influenced by external events, such as changes in the environment or increased or decreased stimuli. A reduced level of consciousness makes the patient misunderstand the surroundings.

Disturbed brain functioning has much impact on

Impact of Cardiac Surgery on the Quality of Life
Edited by A. E. Willner and G. Rodewald
Plenum Press, New York, 1990

behavior because of disturbed integration of perceived
stimuli, difficulties in the understanding of environment,
proneness to anxiety, disrupted communication, etc. All
this increases odd behaviors. On the other hand, anxiety
is a physiological stress and can have an impact on brain
functioning.

Organic mental disorders are a heterogeneous group;
therefore no single description characterizes them all.
The difference in clinical presentation reflects differences in localization, mode of onset, progression, duration, and the nature of underlying pathophysiological
process.

Behavior can hardly be divorced from its anatomical
substrate in the brain. On the other hand, psychopathology normally cannot be treated as a pure neurological
phenomenon without reference to psychological development,
psychodynamics, learning, illness behavior and the treatment environment. Different pathological processes do not
necessarily affect the nervous system in precisely the
same way. It is important to recognize that the diagnosis
of organic syndrome does not preclude the diagnosis of a
functional disorder as well.

Although every person has the potential for developing
delirium if the provocation is severe, there appears to be
wide variation in individual susceptibility. It is
probably more accurate to consider surgery as a factor
predisposing a person to delirium. In a sense, therefore,
delirium may be conceptualized as a threshold phenomenon.
Each individual probably has a certain threshold for
delirium. Pre-existing brain damage and certain medical
disorders possibly bring the patient close to this
threshold, even if they do not exceed it, so that relatively small metabolic changes may then push the patient
beyond threshold into delirium.

Intense psychological reactions, especially anxiety
and fear, have been reported in general to predispose
patients to delirium, and it would not seem unreasonable
for these intense affects to be accompanied by metabolic
changes of the sort that might increase the brain's
susceptibility to delirium. There is some evidence to
suggest that patients who are most fearful of medical and
surgical procedures are the ones most likely to become
delirious [4, 5].

Psychopathology most likely results from an interaction of multiple factors, with the relative importance

of any one varying from patient to patient. Preoperative
and operative factors probably contribute to subclinical
cerebral dysfunction which makes the patient vulnerable to
the subsequent stresses of the open heart recovery room.

RESULTS

        The following results report the first 330 of a total
sample of 1,000 cardiac surgery patients collected in a
multicenter study at 9 medical centers. The details of
the study are described in other chapters in this book.

        Since there may be a neurological component in the
psychopathology seen in cardiac surgery patients, we
examined the relationship between neurological abnormality
and several measures of psychopathology: The Hamburg
Rating Scale for Psychic Disturbance (HRPD), the Hamilton
Depression Scale and the Hamilton Anxiety Scale.

        Significant correlations were found between neuro-
logical abnormality and Hamilton Depression scores:
preoperatively (p < .01), postoperatively (p < .01), and
at hospital discharge (p < .01) (Figure 1).

        Similarly, significant correlations were found
between neurological abnormality and Hamilton Anxiety
Scale score: preoperatively (p > .01), postoperatively
(p < .05), and at discharge (p > .05) (Figure 2).

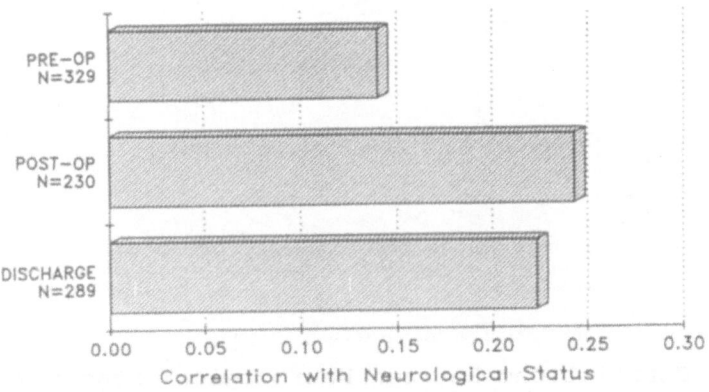

Fig. 1.   Correlations Between Neurological Status and
          Hamilton Depression Scores.

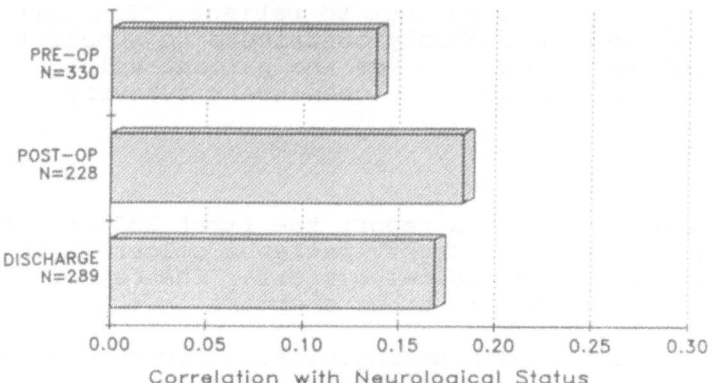

Fig. 2.   Correlations Between Neurological Status and
          Hamilton Anxiety Scores.

     On the Hamburg Rating Scale for Psychic Disturbance
significant correlations were found for the following
factors: disturbed concentration and thinking preoperatively (p > .01), postoperatively (p > .001), and at
discharge (p > .001) (Figure 3).

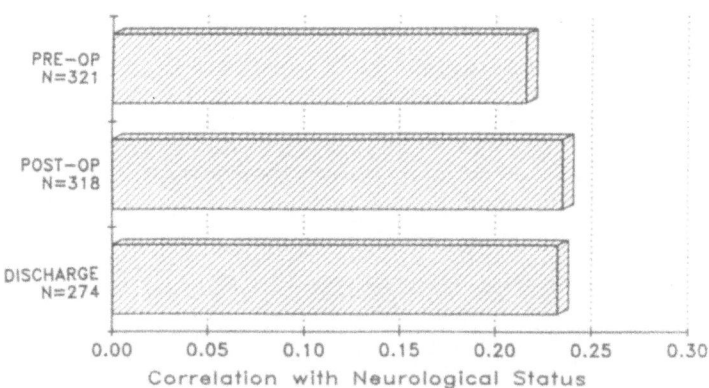

Fig. 3.   Correlations Between Neurological Status and
          HRPD, Disturbed Concentration/Thinking.

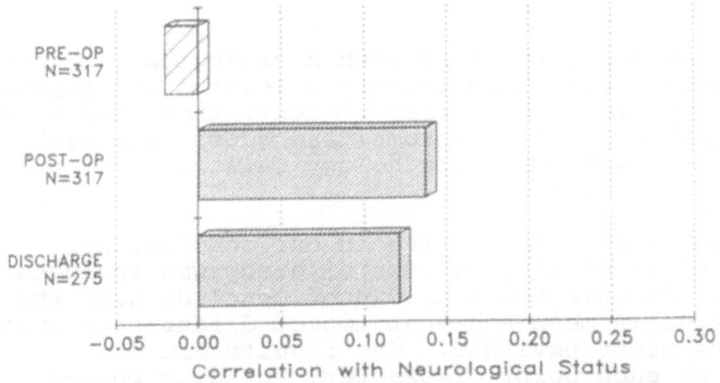

Fig. 4. Correlations Between Neurological Status and HRPD, Masked Depression Symptoms.

Significant correlations were also found for masked depression postoperatively and at discharge (p > .02) (see Figure 4), and for hostility postoperatively (p > .01) (see Figure 5). In addition, significant correlations were also found for paranoid hallucinatory symptoms pre-operatively (p > .05) and at discharge (p > .05). Overall, the number of patients in whom HRPD critical values were exceeded on 3 items (or more), meaning an abnormal HRPD, was significantly increased postoperatively. The same was true for the HRPD number of critical items (the number of items in the abnormal range).

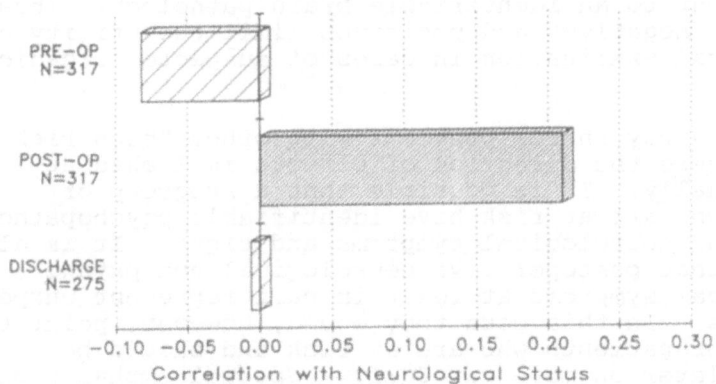

Fig. 5. Correlations Between Neurological Status and HRPD, Hostility.

DISCUSSION

The symptoms correlated with neurological abnormality, i.e., anxiety, depression and signs related to "psycho-organic" conditions (disturbed concentration, thinking and paranoic hallucinatory symptoms) are consistent with previous reports of psychopathology related to organic mental syndromes [1].

We should be conservative in our conclusions, however. First of all, no control group was included in the study. In this phase we cannot conclude what the results actually mean and what impact differences among the centers might have had. The results are cross-sectional at each point. Moreover, in later phases of the study longitudinal results can be brought in, which allows us to consider causality and also direction of effects.

In evaluation of the psychiatric syndrome itself, the neurological examination is probably the least helpful of the elements. The simple truth is that in most patients with organic psychiatric syndromes the neurological examination is normal and remains so until the disease is far advanced. For some time hope was maintained that so-called soft neurological signs might prove reliable indicators of organic disease. Although some of these neurological features have been found with greater frequency in patients with established brain disorders, none has proven to be pathognomonic of organic disease. In addition, it is well established that even focal abnormalities in the neurological examination do not always point to an identifiable brain pathology. Thus, both false negatives and positives limit the utility of neurological examination in cases of suspected organic disease.

This study shares problems with other "high risk" studies where the direction of effects is looked at longitudinally. It is possible that a subgroup of patients who are at risk have identifiable psychopatho-logical and neurological symptoms and signs. It is also possible that postoperative neurological and psycho-pathological symptoms at least in part represent unspecific indicators. In this case they would, however, point to a subgroup of patients who are at risk and should be observed later on more carefully. Special emphasis on them would undoubtedly improve their treatment and rehabilitation. Clinical methods may help to identify preoperatively "at risk" patients, on whom more attention should be focused to improve the outcome of operation [2, 6].

REFERENCES

1. S. Heller, and D. Kornfeld, Psychiatric aspects of
    cardiac surgery, <u>Adv. Psychosom. Med.</u>, 15:124-139
    (1986).
2. P. Tienari, Adjustment disorder in cardiac surgery,
    <u>in</u>: "Cerebral Damage Before and After Cardiac
    Surgery," A. Willner, ed., MTP Press Ltd.,
    Lancaster (in preparation).
3. "Diagnostic and Statistical Manual of Mental
    Disorders." Third Edition, Revised. Washington,
    D.C., American Psychiatric Association (1987).
4. M. Johnston, Pre-operative emotional state and
    post-operative recovery, <u>Adv. Psychosom. Med.</u>,
    15:1-22 (1986).
5. P. Tienari, J. Outakoski, R. Hirvenoja, A. Juolasmaa,
    and J. Takkunen, Postoperative psychosis in open
    heart surgery. A longitudinal study on valve
    replacement patients, <u>Psychiatria Fennica</u>, 63-70
    (1984).
6. P. Tienari, J. Outakoski, A. Juolasmaa, R. Hirvenoja,
    Open heart surgery: The psychiatric point of view,
    <u>in</u>: "Psychosomatic Medicine," A. J. Krakowski, and
    C. P. Kimball, eds., Plenum Publishing Corporation,
    New York (1983).

THE CORRELATION BETWEEN NEUROLOGICAL AND

NEUROPSYCHOLOGICAL VARIABLES

Reijo Hirvenoja

Department of Psychiatry
University of Oulu
Finland

Patients undergoing coronary artery bypass surgery may be influenced by short-term neurological and neuro- psychological deficits. In order to assess these deficits, we have assessed the neurological and neuropsychological sequelae of patients undergoing coronary artery bypass surgery at several points in time. This paper presents preliminary findings on the correlations between neuro- logical and preoperative neuropsychological variables observed in the first 340 coronary bypass surgery patients in this multicenter study.

METHODS

Neuropsychological examination was carried out to assess several areas of cognitive functioning. A battery of psychometric tests was administered 3 to 5 days pre- operatively; and 7 to 10 days and one year postoperatively. The battery includes the Conceptual Level Analogy Test (CLAT), Trail Making Test, WAIS Block Design, WAIS Digit Symbol, Aberg-Kihlgren Figure Rotation Test and Bethune Williams Delayed Memory Test. To assess patients' fatigue and anxiety the Feeling Tone Checklist and Spielberger State-Trait Anxiety Scale were included in the study.

Prior to surgery a neurological history was taken and a standard neurological examination performed. To assess changes in neurological status, the examination was repeated three times: in the intensive care unit, one week postoperatively, and at follow-up one year later.

Impact of Cardiac Surgery on the Quality of Life
Edited by A. E. Willner and G. Rodewald
Plenum Press, New York, 1990

389

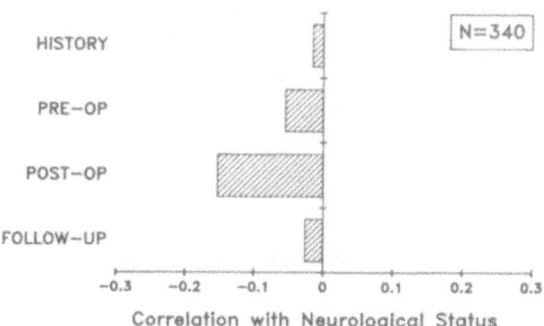

Fig. 1.   Correlation Between Pre-Op CLAT Score and
          Neurologicl Status.

RESULTS

     Figure 1 represents the correlation between the
preoperative CLAT-scores and neurological status at
several points in time.   Each bar represents the size of
the correlation.   There is a significant (p < 0.01)
correlation between the preoperative CLAT score and the
postoperative neurological status.

     Figure 2 also indicates a significant correlation
between the preoperative CLAT Dichotomy and postoperative
neurological status.   Patients with low scores had many
postoperative neurological symptoms.

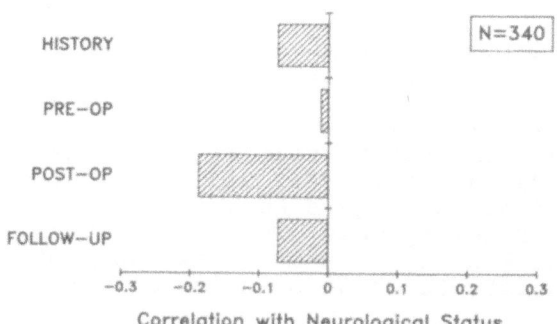

Fig. 2.   Correlation Between Pre-Op CLAT Dichotomy and
          Neurological Status.

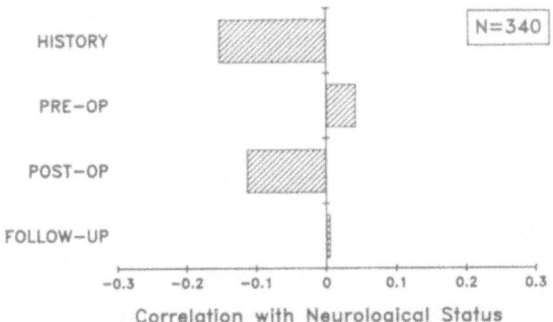

Fig. 3.   Correlation Between Pre-Op WAIS Digit Symbol and
           Neurological Status.

        Figure 3 shows significant correlation between the
WAIS Digit Symbol test score, the neurological history
(p < 0.01), and postoperative neurological status
(p < 0.04).   It seems that patients who are identified
as having symptoms in the neurological history are
vulnerable to postoperative cerebral dysfunctions.

        Figure 4 shows that we have a significant correla-
tion between the preoperative WAIS Block Design test
score and the neurological history (p < 0.02).

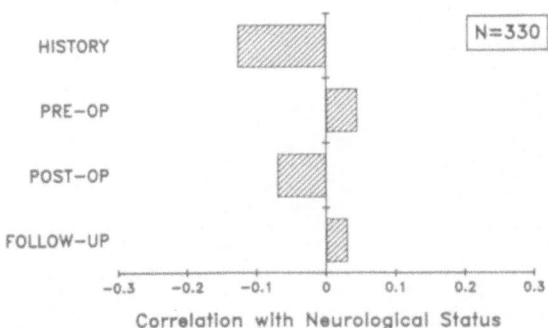

Fig. 4.   Correlation Between Pre-Op WAIS Block Design and
           Neurological Status.

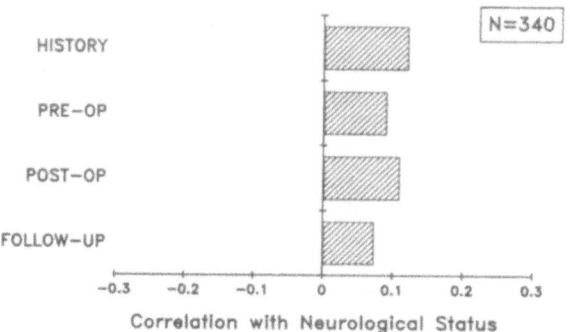

Fig. 5.   Correlation Between Pre-Op Trails B and
           Neurological Status.

        Figure 5 shows a significant correlation between the
preoperative Trail Making test score and the neurological
history (p < 0.02) and postoperative neurological status
(p < 0.04).

        Figure 6 shows no significant relationship between
the Figure Rotation test score and neurological status at
any point in time.

        Figure 7 represents no significant correlation
between the preoperative Bethune Williams memory test
score and neurological status at any point in time.

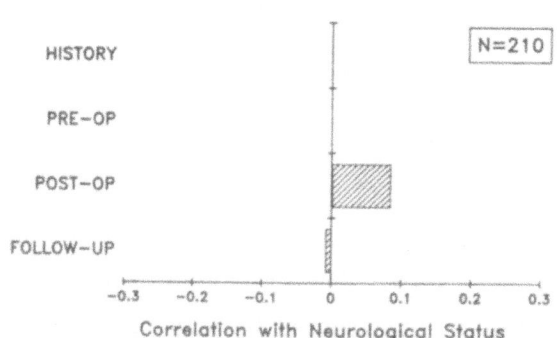

Fig. 6.   Correlation Between Pre-Op Figure Rotation and
           Neurological Status.

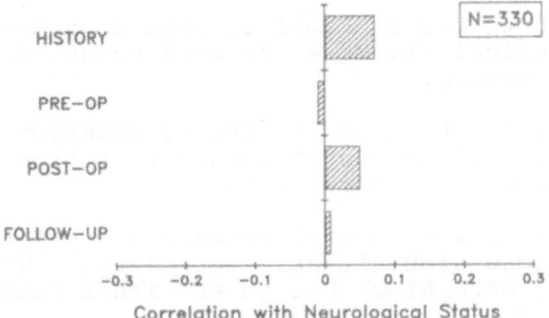

Fig. 7. Correlation Between Pre-Op Bethune-Williams and Neurological Status.

TABLE 1. Probability Levels of Correlations Between Neurological Status and Cognitive Test Scores N = 340

	Psychometric Tests						
	CLAT	CLAT Dichotomy	WAIS Digit Symbol	WAIS Block Design	Trail-making B	Figure Rotation	Bethune Williams
History	.760	.159	.004***	.019**	.022**	.986	.196
Preoperative	.293	.825	.430	.215	.088	.987	.850
Postoperative	.004***	.009***	.037*	.201	.040*	.220	.364
Discharge	.631	.187	.919	.608	.189	.905	.887

*** p < .01

** p < .02

* p < .04

Table 1 shows the probability levels of correlations between neurological status at several points in time and cognitive test scores.

Results of the P value for the correlation analysis between neurological and psychometric test findings show that preoperative test scores were:

1. correlated with neurological history data (3 of 6 tests were significantly correlated: WAIS Digit Symbol, WAIS Block Design and Trail Making B)

2. poorly correlated with preoperative neurological examination data (only one of the tests significantly correlated: Trail Making B)

3. correlated with postoperative neurological examination data (4 of 6 tests were significantly correlated: CLAT-scores, CLAT-dichotomy, WAIS Digit Symbol and Trail Making B)

4. poorly correlated with neurological examination data at hospital discharge (0 of 6 tests were significantly correlated).

CONCLUSIONS

The results support the notion that neurological abnormality is most striking while the patient is in the ICU, before the immediate symptoms have had a chance to subside. Furthermore, a neurological history identifies many symptoms that have occurred at some earlier point in a patient's life, even if they are not present now. On the other hand, the preoperative and discharge neurological examinations note abnormalities present at those times, i.e. that occur either before or after the most acute symptomatology. Apparently the correlation of neuropsychological and neurological findings is higher under conditions in which the salience of the neurological symptoms is greatest.

Psychometric tests have usually failed to predict the postoperative course but some recent results have been encouraging. Willner, et al [1] have shown that the CLAT test has some ability to predict immediate as well as late postoperative outcome. Also in this study, the CLAT correlated to postoperative neurological outcome. It might be possible to predict postoperative neurological outcome with the CLAT and WAIS Digit Symbol tests.   Interesting for prognostic results is also the Trail Making test, which measures attention, concentration, arousal and mental flexibility.   These functions are easily affected by any kind of cerebral dysfunction. In that sense, the results of this study give support to the earier findings that pre-existing, even slight cerebral dysfunction makes the brains of these patients especially vulnerable to the strains of surgery.

Both the present and earlier results suggest that it might be possible to construct a test battery to identify patients with high risk of cerebral complications. Further research is needed to get information about reliability of various predictive signs, as well as to reach a practically significant level of prediction.

REFERENCES

1. A. E. Willner, C. J. Rabiner, Psychopathology and cognitive dysfunction five years after open heart surgery, Comprehensive Psychiatry, 20: 409-418 (1979).

PREDICTION AND POSTOPERATIVE OUTCOME

CAN ONE PREDICT THE PATIENT'S POSTOPERATIVE PSYCHIATRIC

AND NEUROLOGICAL CONDITION?

Allen E. Willner

Hillside Hospital
Glen Oaks, NY

During the last 30 years, many studies have found a
significant relationship between the preoperative
psychological state of cardiac surgery patients and their
postoperative psychiatric outcome [1-10]. Psychometric
test scores have also been found to be significantly
related to postoperative psychiatric outcome [11-13].

This paper investigates the degree to which one can
predict postoperative quality of life from preoperative
examination. Specifically, to what degree can one predict
the neurological and psychiatric outcome of cardiac
surgery from a set of psychometric, psychiatric and neurological measures administered preoperatively.

There were three classes of predictors:

Psychometric tests. The six tests used were the
CLAT, WAIS Block Design, WAIS Digit Symbol, Trail Making
Test B, Aberg Figure Rotation and Bethune-Williams Visual
Memory Test, described in the chapters by Feys-Dunne and
Willner. The tests were administered preoperatively and
about a week postoperatively.

Personality measures. The five personality measures
used are described more fully in the chapters by Gotze and
Dahme, et al., and by Strauss and Paulsen. They were the
Hamburg Rating Scale for Psychic Disturbance (HRPD), the
Hamilton Anxiety Scale, the Hamilton Depression scale, the
Spielberger Anxiety State, and Spielberger Anxiety Trait

Impact of Cardiac Surgery on the Quality of Life
Edited by A. E. Willner and G. Rodewald
Plenum Press, New York, 1990

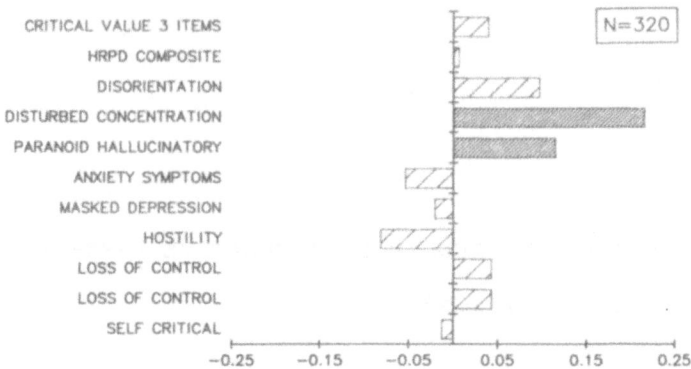

Fig. 1.   Pre-op Status as Predictor of Pre-Op Neurological
          Status.

scales.   They were administered preoperatively, 2 to 3
days postoperatively and about a week postoperatively.

     Neurological examination.   A standard neurological
examination was administered.

RESULTS

     The figures below depict the relationship between
several preoperative variables and postoperative measures
of neurological and psychiatric status.

Predicting Neurological Status

     Figure 1 shows the relationship between preoperative
HRPD factor ratings and preoperative neurological status.
The magnitude of the correlation between the variables is
indicated by the length of the respective bars; significant correlations are indicated by filled-in bars.
Positive correlations extend to the right and negative
correlations to the left.   Only two significant correlations are depicted here, e.g. preoperative Disturbed
Concentration and Paranoid Hallucinatory states are
positively related to Neurological Status before the
surgery.

     Figure 2 depicts the relationship between pre-
operative HRPD factors and postoperative neurological
status.   There are no significant correlations here.

     The relationship between neurological status at
hospital discharge and preoperative HRPD factors is

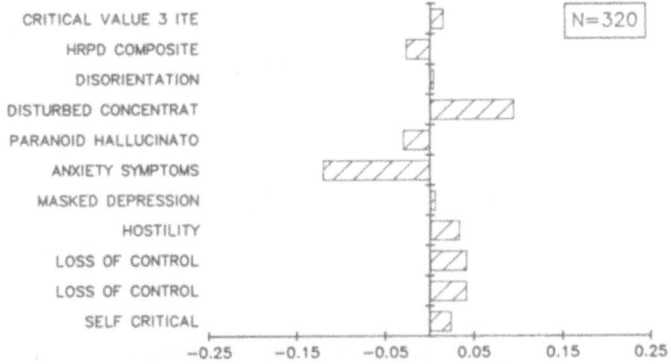

Fig. 2.   Pre-Op Status as Predictor of Post-Op
          Neurological Status.

indicated in Figure 3.   A significant positive correlation
with disturbed concentration and a significant negative
correlation with anxiety symptoms was found.

The next two figures show the relationship of
preoperative measures of anxiety and depression with
postoperative neurological status.   Figure 4 shows no
relationship for preoperative ratings of anxiety and
depression with early postoperative neurological status.
The negative findings for anxiety apply both to interviewer ratings (Hamilton) and patient ratings
(Spielberger) of anxiety.   Figure 5 shows that similar
findings apply to predicting neurological status at
discharge.

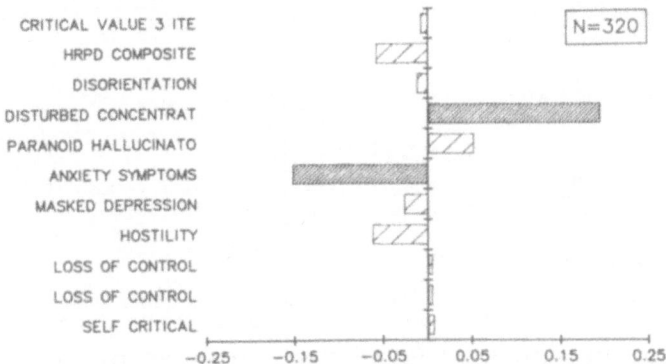

Fig. 3.   Pre-Op Status as Predictor of Discharge
          Neurological Status.

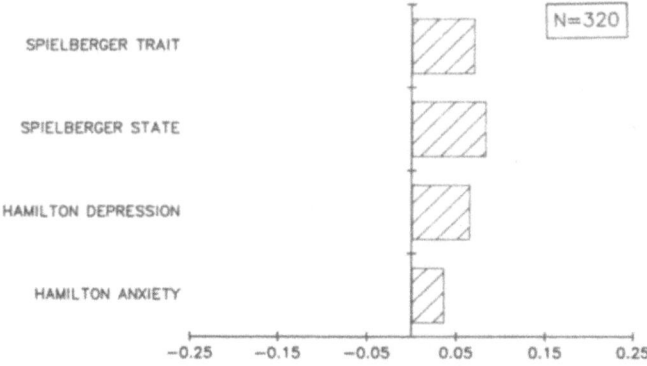

Fig. 4.   Pre-Op Status as Predictor of Post-Op
          Neurological Status.

The ability of preoperative psychometric, psychiatric
and neurological measures to predict postoperative neurological status is shown in the next two figures. Figure 6
shows that preoperative psychometric and psychiatric
measures are not related to early postoperative neurological status whereas preoperative neurological status is
significantly related to postoperative status. The
findings for prediction of discharge neurological status
are quite similar, as shown in Figure 7.

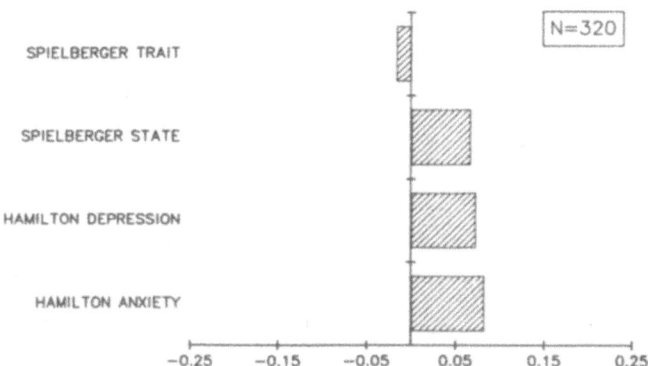

Fig. 5.   Pre-Op Status as Predictor of Discharge
          Neurological Status.

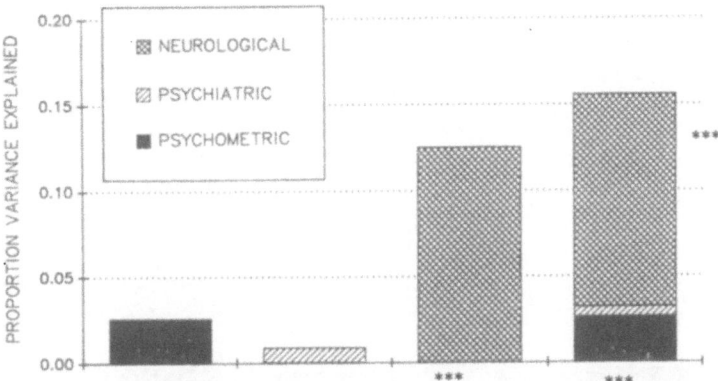

Fig. 6.   Pre-Op Status as Predictor of Post-Op
Neurological Status.

Predicting Postoperative Psychiatric Status

The remaining analyses assess the ability of preoperative psychometric, psychiatric and neurological
measures to predict early postoperative and discharge
psychopathology. Figure 8 shows postoperative ratings on
the Hamilton Anxiety Scale were significantly predicted by
preoperative psychopathology ($p < .001$) and neurological
status ($p < .01$) measures but not by psychometric measures.

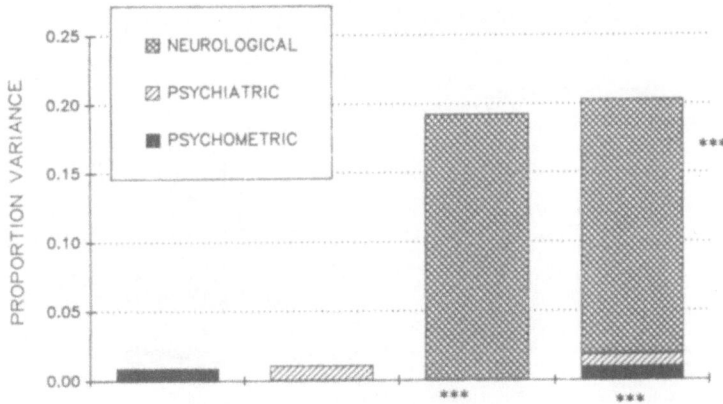

Fig. 7.   Pre-Op Status as Predictor of Post-Op
Neurological Status.

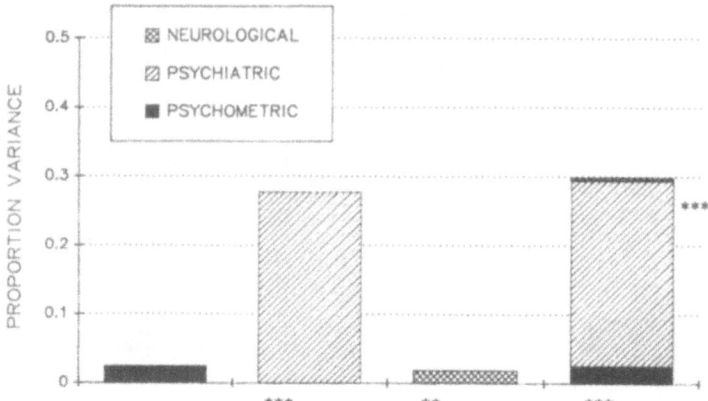

Fig. 8.   Pre-Op Status as Predictor of Post-Op Hamilton
          Anxiety.

The overall measure on the extreme right indicates that
the neurological status measure did not make a significant
contribution to the overall prediction beyond that of the
psychopathology measures.   Figure 9 indicates much the
same picture when discharge ratings on the Hamilton
Anxiety Scale were predicted.

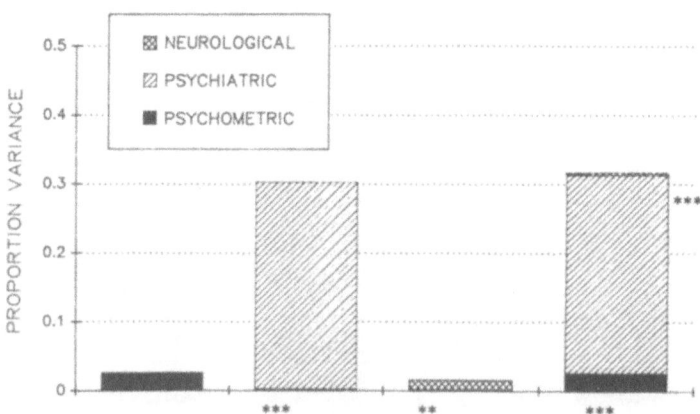

Fig. 9.   Pre-Op Status as Predictor of Discharge Hamilton
          Anxiety.

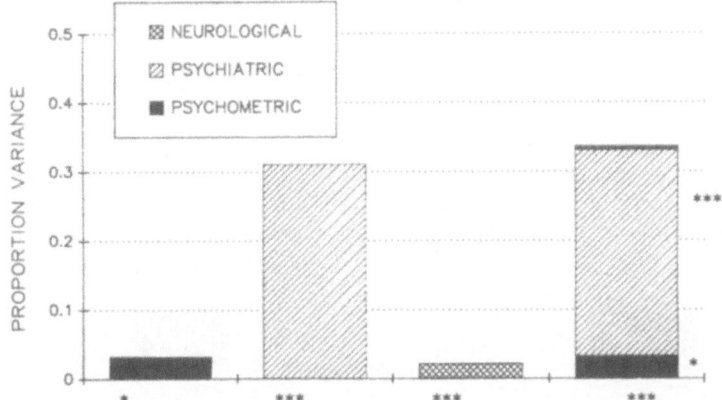

Fig. 10. Pre-Op Status as Predictor of Post-Op Hamilton Depression.

Figures 10 and 11 evaluate the effectiveness of the same 3 sets of measures (predictors) in predicting postoperative and discharge Hamilton Depression ratings. Figure 10 shows significant relationships for all 3 predictors (psychopathology measures p < .001, neurological status p < .001, psychometric measure p < .05) with early postoperative Hamilton Depression Ratings.

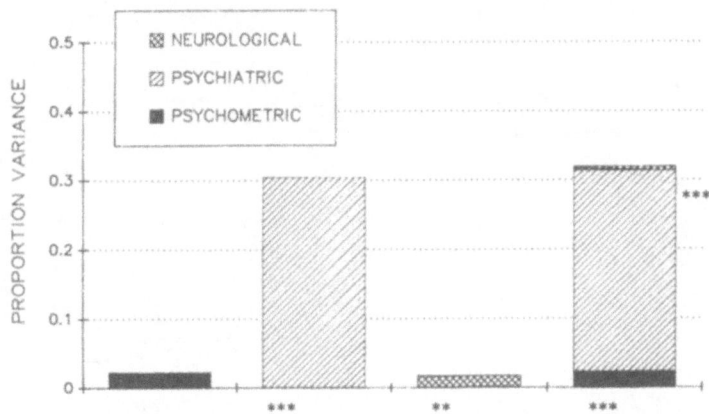

Fig. 11. Pre-Op Status as Predictor of Discharge Hamilton Depression.

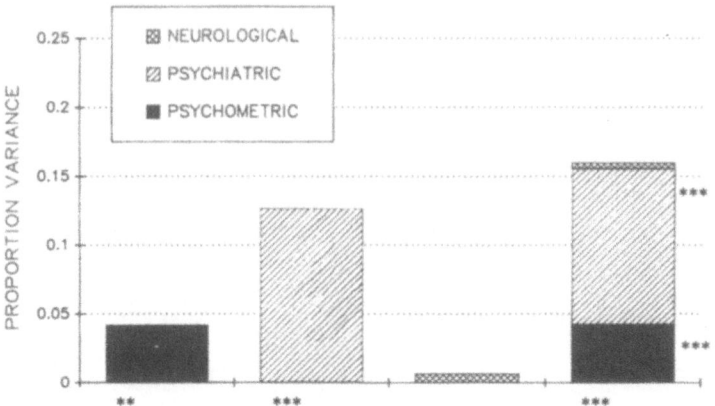

Fig. 12.   Pre-Op Status as Predictor of Discharge
           Speilberger State.

However, the overall measure on the right shows signficant
independent prediction only for psychopathology (p < .001)
and psychometric measures (p < .C5).   When discharge
Hamilton Depression ratings were the criterion, only
psychopathological (p < .001) and neurological (p < .01)
ratings were significantly related.   In the overall comparison, only the psychopathological (p < .001) ratings
remained significant.

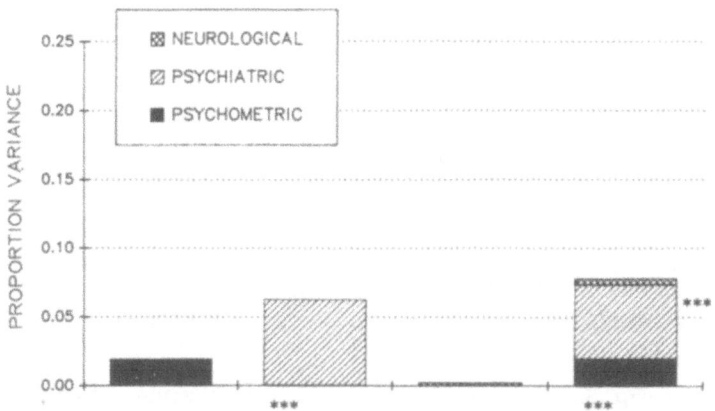

Fig. 13.   Pre-Op Status as Predictor of Discharge
           Speilberger Trait.

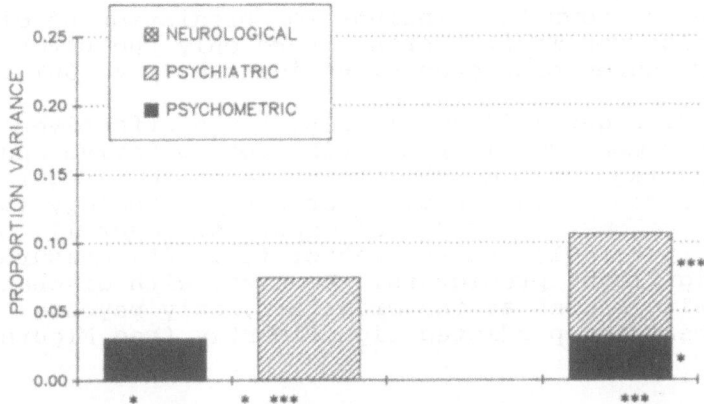

Fig. 14.   Pre-Op Status as Predictor of Post-Op HRPD
            Composite.

Figures 12 and 13 assess whether the same 3 sets of
preoperative measures can predict postoperative and discharge Spielberger State Anxiety measures. Significant
prediction of postoperative Spielberger State Anxiety
scores was found for psychopathological (p < .001) and
psychometric (p < .01) variables. In the overall comparison both psychiatric (p < .001) and psychometric (p <
.001) measures remained significant (Figure 12).

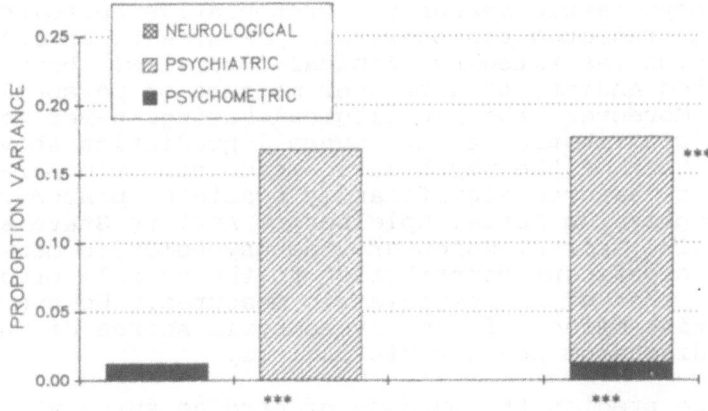

Fig. 15.   Pre-Op Status as Predictor of Discharge HRPD
            Composite.

Figure 13 shows the findings for prediction of discharge Spielberger Trait scores. Here only the psychopathology measures predicted significantly (p < .001).

Finally, Figures 14 and 15 depict the effectiveness of the same 3 measures in predicting postoperative and discharge ratings on the HRPD composite score. Figure 14 shows significant relationships for psychopathology (p < .001) and psychometric (p < .05) measures. Overall, both the former (p < .001) and the latter (p < .05) measures remained signficant predictors. However, with discharge HRPD composite scores as the criterion, only psychopathology measures predicted significantly (see Figure 15).

DISCUSSION

We studied the degree to which psychometric, neurological and psychiatric predictors could predict neurological and psychiatric outcome after cardiac surgery. In general we found that:

Neurological outcome was best predicted by preoperative neurological status, and much more weakly predicted by preoperative cognitive functioning. Preoperative anxiety and depression measures did not predict neurological outcome, except for the anxiety scale of the HRPD which was negatively correlated with neurological outcome (as if preoperative denial of anxiety might be weakly related with outcome).

Psychiatric outcome was best predicted by preoperative psychiatric measures. Preoperative neurological examination predicted postoperative measures of anxiety and depression (as rated by clinical interview), but not patient-rated anxiety or a broader measure of personality, the HRPD. Moreover, the neurological ratings never made a signficant contribution to the overall prediction above and beyond that of the psychiatric measures. Preoperative psychometric measures significantly predicted postoperative Hamilton Depression Scale, Spielberger Anxiety State and HRPD composite scores. Moreover, the psychometric measures did make a signficant contribution to the overall prediction beyond that of the psychiatric measures. However, the predictive effect of the psychometric scores did not extend to discharge psychiatric ratings.

Can one predict the outcome of cardiac surgery? We found that the combination of three predictors significantly predicted the outcome of the surgery. The proportion of true variance accounted for, however, varied between 8 and 34 percent. This represents a significant relationship, but one not strong enough to permit accurate prediction in individual cases. It also was clear that prediction of immediate postoperative functioning was more accurate than prediction of functioning just before hospital discharge. Presumably, there was more observable pathology on the ICU rather than later, and this increased the accuracy of some predictors.

Will we ever be able to develop techniques powerful enough so that we can predict the outcome for individual patients? On the one hand, that would require the development of much more powerful tests and assessment devices, as well as more powerful techniques of statistical analysis. On the other hand, the increasingly patient-friendly aspects of the surgery may render this a moot question, as the incidence of psychological and neuro-logical morbidity becomes very small. Just as one no longer tries to predict mortality rates after cardiac surgery, because the rates are very low, so one may in the future have too little psychological and neurological morbidity to serve as a useful criterion.

REFERENCES

1. S. J. Denker, A. Sandahl, Mental disease after operations for mitral stenosis, Lancet II. 1230 (1961).
2. N. Egerton, J. H. Kay, Psychological disturbances associated with open-heart surgery, Br. J. Psychiatry. 110:433 (1964).
3. P. H. Blachy, A. Starr, Postcardiotomy delirium, Am. J. Psychiat. 121:371 (1964).
4. H. S. Abram, Adaptation to open-heart surgery: A psychiatric study of response to the threat of death. Annual Meeting of Am. Psychiatric Assoc. 121, New York (1965).
5. C. P. Kimball, Psychological responses to the experience of open-heart surgery, Am. J. Psychiatry. 126:348 (1969).
6. S. S. Heller, K.A. Frank. J.R. Malm, F.A. Bowmann, Jr., P. D. Harris. M. H. Charlton, D.S. Kornfeld, Psychiatric complications of open-heart surgery: A reexamination, N. Engl. J. Med. 283:1015 (1970).
7. O. L. Layne, Jr., and S. C. Yudofsky, Post-operative psychosis in cardiotomy patients. The role of organic and psychiatric factors, N. Engl. J. Med. 284:518 (1971).

8. T. J. Henrichs, J. W. MacKenzie, C. H. Almond,
    Psychological adjustment and psychiatric
    complications following open-heart surgery,
    J. Ner. Ment. Dis. 152:332 (1971).
9. B. Flemming. H. -J. Meffert, The role of personality
    traits for psychic disturbances after open-heart
    surgery, in: "Psychic and Neurological Dysfunctions
    After Open Heart Surgery," H. Speidel and G.
    Rodewald, Eds., Georg Thieme Verlag, Stuttgart, New
    York (1980).
10. H. -J. Meffert, B. Flemming, Psychic and Psychosocial
    stress before open-heart operations and their
    relationships with postoperative psychic
    disturbances, in: "Psychic and Neurological
    Dysfunctions After Open-Heart Surgery," H. Speidel
    and G. Rodewald, Eds., Georg Thieme Verlag,
    Stuttgart, New York (1980).
11. A. E. Willner, C. J. Rabiner, B. G. Wisoff, J.
    Fishman, B. Rosen, M. Hartstein, and D. F. Klein,
    Analogy tests and psychopathology at follow-up
    after open heart surgery, Biological Psychiatry.
    11:698-705 (1976).
12. A. E. Willner and C. J. Rabiner, Psychopathology and
    cognitive dysfunctions five years after open heart
    surgery, Comprehensive Psychiatry. 20:409-418
    (1979).
13. A. E. Willner and C. J. Rabiner, Psychiatric
    complications following coronary bypass surgery,
    in: "Return to Work After Coronary Artery Bypass
    Surgery," P. J. Walter, ed., Springer-Verlag,
    Berlin, Heidelburg (1985).

PSYCHODYNAMIC PREDICTION OF POSTOPERATIVE MENTAL

VULNERABILITY

U. Lamparter, P. Götze, H.-J. Meffert

Universitäts-Krankenhaus Eppendorf
Hamburg, Federal Republic of Germany

INTRODUCTION

Considering the frequent occurrence of psychopathological disturbances after open heart surgery, the
question of preoperative detection of at-risk patients
arises. Ideally, those patients should be pointed out
preoperatively to the cardiac surgeon who are more
vulnerable to postoperative psychopathological disturbances because of certain individual characteristics,
certain attitudes or their way of coping. This identification should be possible under routine clinical conditions. The most practical opportunity for identifying
at-risk patients, in our opinion, arises in the first
preoperative interview between the psychological investigator and the patient. Our question is: Does the
systematized clinical psychodynamic impression we have
obtained from this first interview, enable us really to
make a valid prediction, even in the complex field of
cardiac surgery? This question was the starting point of
an investigation within the framework of the International Study in Hamburg. In this paper we want to
present our preliminary results.

Materials and Method

Our sample consists of 66 coronary patients, 52 men
and 14 women. They took part in an open psychodynamic
interview of about half an hour. The patients were asked

to talk about their present condition, their anxieties
and their expectations concerning the operation, but also
about their life-history. All information received from
this interview served as a basis for the assessment we
will describe now.

The instrument we used for the assessment was the
Index of Vulnerability, which includes 10 items with 5
levels each.

The first category, spontaneous impression, means
how does the patient seem in the first contact; anxiety,
depression, self-esteem, body-image, defense, quality of
infantile and actual object relationships are evaluated,
and finally a global impression is arrived at. That is,
the overall feeling of the interviewer about the patient
is noted. Every item was assessed in relation to the
question: How vulnerable does the patient appear to be
in respect to this psychic dimension? How easily can the
patient's integration be disturbed by the imminent operation? The score for each item can be summed up to get a
total score. After the interview, and before the items
were rated, the investigator was supervised by a psycho-
analyst.

Table 1

Index of Vulnerability

Spontaneous Impression	1	2	3	4	5
Anxiety	1	2	3	4	5
Depression	1	2	3	4	5
Body Self	1	2	3	4	5
Self Image	1	2	3	4	5
Defense	1	2	3	4	5
Quality of Infantile Relationship	1	2	3	4	5
Quality of Actual Relationship	1	2	3	4	5
Global Impression	1	2	3	4	5

Presumably, this method may seem strange to surgeons, anesthetists and neurologists. The psychologists, but especially the psychoanalysts, will know that this method can help obtain important information about the patient. In a psychoanalytic supervision setting the investigator tells the supervisor about the interview and his impressions. In the supervision, psychodynamically relevant phenomena arise, helping us to understand unconscious processes within the patient. As psychoanalysts, we speak of the unconscious and the conscious, about defense and resistance, transference and countertransference. Subsequent to the supervision session, the investigator and the supervisor separately rated the items of the Index of Vulnerability. In this way, psychodynamically relevant considerations could be included.

Results

First, we will give a general view of the rating differences between investigator and supervisor on all patients. There was no difference in the rating of the Total Score of Vulnerability. However, the results concerning single items showed significant differences. Compared with the investigator, the supervisor rated higher vulnerability in the items "body-image," "defense" and "general impression." The investigator rated a comparatively higher vulnerability in the item "quality of infantile object relationships." These differences can be interpreted from a psychodynamic point of view.

The investigator, knowing the patients personally, is more identified with them. Just like the patient, he denies the danger to the integrity of the body-self by the operation. Therefore on a conscious level, he considers the patient to be less vulnerable than the supervisor does. The supervisor, in his more distant position, does not deny the threatening danger of the operation to the same extent. According to his opinion, the patient is more vulnerable in regard to his body image and weaker concerning his defense mechanisms.

On the other hand, the investigator feels more affected by the directly given information of the patient's life-story, especially with regard to early trauma and losses. These circumstances make the investigator expect the patient to be more vulnerable.

Let us now consider the relationship between the above mentioned assessment and the postoperative psycho-

logical disturbances. The postoperative HRPD-data served
as criteria variables. Following the cluster analyses by
Götze and Dahme, we distinguished two groups of patients
differing in their postoperative condition: the psycho-
pathologically disturbed patients and the psychopatho-
logically normal group. Twenty-seven patients showed
psychopathological disturbances in the course of the
second through seventh day. Thirty-nine patients showed
no disturbances.

Table 2

INDEX OF VULNERABILTY

Direction of the differences between psychopathological
"normal" and "disturbed" postoperative patients.

	Investigator		Supervisor	
Spontaneous Impression	+		+	*
Anxiety	+		+	**
Depression	+		+	
Body Self	+		+	
Self Image	+		+	*
Defense	+	**	+	**
Quality of Infantile Relationship	+		+	
Quality of Actual Relationship	+		+	
Global Impression	+	**	+	
Total Score	+	**	+	

Significance: U-Test (Mann-Whitney)   *   p<0.1
                                       **   p<0.05
                                       ***   p<0.01

The table shows direction and significance of the observed mean differences between these two groups in each item of the Index of Vulnerability. The postoperatively disturbed patients achieved higher scores in all vulnerability items, both in investigator's ratings as well as in supervisor's. Some assessments even show significant differences between the two groups. Concerning the investigator's assessments, the largest differences were achieved in the items "defense," "global impression" and "total score." Regarding the supervisor's assessments, the items "defense" and "anxiety" discriminated most, "spontaneous impression" and "self image" showed tentative significant results.

Discussion

Obviously a psychoanalytically oriented clinical impression makes it possible to give a valid prognosis of postoperative psychopathological disturbances. Prognostic impressions on "anxiety" and "defense" proved to be of the best predictive value. At this point our results correspond with those of Lazarus and Hagen [2], Kimball [3] and Flemming and Meffert [4] who identified the dynamic interaction of anxiety, defense and ego-strength as a relevant predictor.

Our reflections on patients' ability to cope with depression proved to be comparatively less valuable as a predictor. Also our attempt to introduce "vulnerability of narcissistic regulation" as a predictor as assessed by the items "self-esteem" and "body-image," yielded unsatisfactory results. Presumably, narcissistic regulation is too complex to be recorded adequately by our rating method. More precise formulations of different aspects narcissistic regulation might help achieve better results.

The relatively low predictive value of "quality of object relationships" surprised us. The following reflection may provide an explanation. During preoperative pressure the patient has a strong tendency to idealize his object relationships. So, each object becomes a good object, and negative object experiences are split off.

Preoperatively the interviewer is not allowed to weaken this very important defense mechanism by confron-

tation or a deeply given interpretation. Thus, the
investigator may not get a correct picture of the
patient's inner world of objects.

Overall, we believe this paper demonstrates that
systematic psychodynamic considerations can make a
helpful contribution toward evaluating prognosis.

REFERENCES

1. P. Götze, B. Dahme, M. Wessel, Die Hamburger
    Schätzkala fur psychische Storungen nach
    Herzoperationen (HRPD)., Eur. Arch. Psychiatr.
    Neuro. Sci., 234: 308-318 (1985).
2. H. R. Lazarus, J. H. Hagen, Prevention of psychosis
    following open heart surgery, Am. J. Psychiatry
    124: 1190-1195 (1968).
3. C. P. Kimball, The experience of cardiac surgery and
    cardiac transplant, in: Modern perspectives in the
    psychiatric aspects of surgery, J. G. Howelles,
    ed., Brunner and Mazel, New York (1976).
4. B. Flemming, H. J. Meffert, The role of personality
    traits for psychic disturbances after open heart
    surgery. in: Psychic and neurological
    dysfunctions after open heart surgery, H. Speidel,
    G. Rodewald, eds., Thieme, Stuttgart, New York,
    169-180 (1980).

THE RELEVANCE OF HEALTH RELATED COGNITIONS AND ATTITUDES

FOR THE PREDICTION OF SURGICAL OUTCOME

B. Strauss, M. Amirmansouri, K. Oltmann,
G. Paulsen, D. Regensburger, H. Speidel,
S. Schmolling, H. Strenge, S. Tiemann, and
M. Tobias

Departments of Psychosomatics and Psychotherapy,
Psychiatry, Neurology and Cardiac Surgery
Kiel University
Kiel, Federal Republic of Germany

The relevance of specific attributions, coping strategies, and health-related cognitions for the development of chronic diseases and adaptation to their treatment is currently undisputed. Recent psychological reports concerning adaptation to cardiac surgery have emphasized that cognitive factors may be important for the process of coping with surgery and for rehabilitation. But there are still some authors who object that the isolated situation of the surgical procedure has been over-emphasized as the factor responsible for the kind and the intensity of stress experienced by patients. They suggest that the individual strategies of patients for coping with stress have been neglected just as the integration of coping processes into the patients' general psychological conditions was neglected [1]. Meanwhile there is much evidence for specific coping strategies which determine how patients experience the period prior to and following surgery; these sometimes correlate with the incidence of psychopathological impairment. Accordingly, it has been suggested that "psychological interventions preparing a patient for surgery have to be different for different patient groups, depending on their coping styles, cognitions, and attributions" [2].

Since suggestions like these indicate that cognitive and attributional factors are potentially important for

Impact of Cardiac Surgery on the Quality of Life
Edited by A. E. Willner and G. Rodewald
Plenum Press, New York, 1990

the outcome of surgery, we tried to assess these aspects by asking the patients we investigated during the International Study at Kiel to complete several questionnaires on health related coping styles, attitudes, and cognitions prior to surgery. The sample presently comprises 86 patients in our center. Fifty-four of these completed the questionnaire prior to coronary bypass surgery. The mean age of this subsample was 59 years; 83% of the patients were males. The main part of the questionnaire consisted of the Hamburg Health Questionnaire [3] which is based on a complex theory of hypochondriasis and attitudes towards a person's physical health. The subscales are entitled a) somatization/anxiety, b) self-devaluation/depression, c) phobic-aversive hypersensitivity, d) paranoid-hallucinatory hypersensitivity, e) medical locus of control, and f) ecological locus of control.

        This comprehensive health questionnaire was presented to the patients along with several shorter instruments: the first was a German version of a locus of control questionnaire derived from Rotter's attributional theory. It has three scales measuring orientation toward internal control, powerful others external control, and chance control [4]. We further used a Coping Questionnaire with subscales concerning 1. active vs. passive coping with illness; 2. competence vs. helplessness (as part of an emotional-cognitive self image); 3. a subscale covering high vs. low social support; 4. an Attribution-Coping Scale consisting of three scales differentiating between a. organic vs. psychosomatic attribution of illness; b. certainty about being in active control of the recovery process vs. powerlessness; and c. high vs. low social desirability [5].

Comparisons with other groups

        The Coping Questionnaire and the Attribution-Coping Scale were administered in a study of patients undergoing renal dialysis and another group suffering from cancer [5]. In comparison with those two groups (Fig. 1), patients undergoing coronary bypass surgery described themselves as more active in coping with their illness (which means that they use their initiative to arrange their lives better), they seem more competent than the cancer patients, and report more social support. They further differed from the other two groups in preferring psychosomatic rather than somatic attribution of their physical impairment and in showing less belief that they could take over active control of necessary medical procedures.

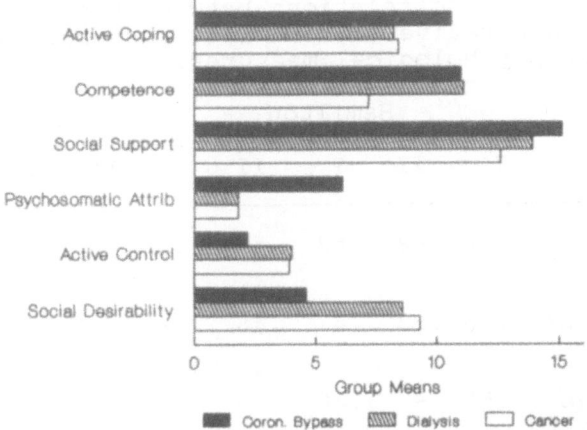

Fig. 1.   Comparison of 54 patients undergoing coronary
          bypass surgery with a group of patients undergong
          renal dialysis (n=35) and a group suffering from
          cancer (n=25):   Coping and Attribution
          Questionnaire;   data from Ziegler and Schuele
          [5].

Health related attributes and psychopathological impairment

        Significant correlations (Table 1) indicate a marked
positive correlation between the questionnaire scales and
psychiatric and neuropsychological measurements.   The
former include anxiety and somatization, selfdevaluation
and depression, phobic-aversive hypersensitivity (which
could be described as hypochondriasis in its narrow sense)
as well as ecological locus of control (i.e., an attitude
made up of a belief in a natural cure, a tendency to
reflect on one's state of health, and a preference for
psychosomatic explanations for physical complaints and
changes).   The latter include the preoperative and late
postoperative amount of anxiety and depression as
assessed by the Hamilton Scales.   Furthermore, three of
the four scales correlated significantly negatively with
the patients' postoperative scores in one neuropsychological test, the Block Design subtest of the Wechsler
Intelligence Scale.

Table 1. Significant correlations between health related attitudes and preoperative (I) and late postoperative (II) psychiatric/neuropsychological measures.

| | Hamilton | | | | | | WAIS | |
| | Anxiety | | Depression | | HRPD* | | Block Design | |
	I	II	I	II	I	II	I	II
Somatization/ Anxiety	.56	.42	.52	.34	.48	-	-	-.42
Selfdevaluation/ Depression	.50	.53	.47	.46	-	.44	-	-.44
Phobic-aversive hypersensitivity	.51	-	.46	-	.42	-	-	-.48
Ecological locus of control	-	.33	-	-	-	-	-	-

(p<.01); * composite.

The scores on these scales did not reveal any correlation with the psychiatric condition <u>immediately</u> after the operation. We only found a correlation between the amount of psychopathology at this time and a medical locus of control (Fig. 2). A comparison between extreme groups (one showing a decrease of symptoms in the HRPD from the preoperative to the early postoperative measure, and one showing a marked increase of symptoms) indicates that patients who describe themselves as "compliant" and endeavouring to take care of their physical health are obviously better adjusted immediately following surgery.

Coping/attributions and psychopathological impairment

As far as the remaining variables are concerned, we first found no relationship between general attributional styles (internal vs. external control) as measured with the Rotter Scale and any of the pre- and postoperative measures. Further, there was a negative correlation between the patients' subjective impression of competence and the degree of anxiety and depression, and psycho-pathological symptoms (HRPD composite) observed pre-operatively (r=-.36, r=-.43, r=-.35, p< .05). This

attitude, expressing self confidence in coping with new
situations and a more optimistic view of the future
therefore seems favorable for the emotional status of a
cardiac patient.

In contrast to subjective competence, a positive
correlation was found between patients' scores in the
subscale called "active control" and pre- and late postoperative levels of depression and anxiety ($r \geq .36$, $p < .05$).
This might seem surprising, but if one considers the
special situation of the approaching surgery it seems
understandable that patients who usually keep control over
their behavior and actions, experience more anxiety and
depression at a moment when this control is restricted.

A third important variable was the extent of social
support experienced by the patients. This aspect was the
only one out of the different scales of the coping instruments which was significantly related to the early postoperative psychiatric condition, in a sense that a high
level of social support was combined with a low degree of
anxiety, depression, and psychopathological symptoms.
This could be confirmed by comparing the extreme groups of
patients mentioned earlier, based on the change scores in
the HRPD (Fig. 3).

Conclusion

Taken as a whole these preliminary results indicate
that patients with a high level of preoperative anxiety
and depression tend to have an anxious and pessimistic
attitude towards their physical health and describe themselves as hypochondriacal and worried about their physical
state. Such health related attitudes and cognitions are
further accompanied by higher levels of late-postoperative
anxiety and depression. Results like these - especially
the relationship between depression and hypochondriasis -
are in line with those of other studies [6].

The early postoperative psychopathological condition
turned out to be related to a medical locus of control.
In other words: Patients who trust in their physician
prior to surgery and who are willing to follow medical
advice seem to be less affected by psychopathological
symptoms than patients who care less about their physical
state and have a sceptical attitude towards medical action
and advice.

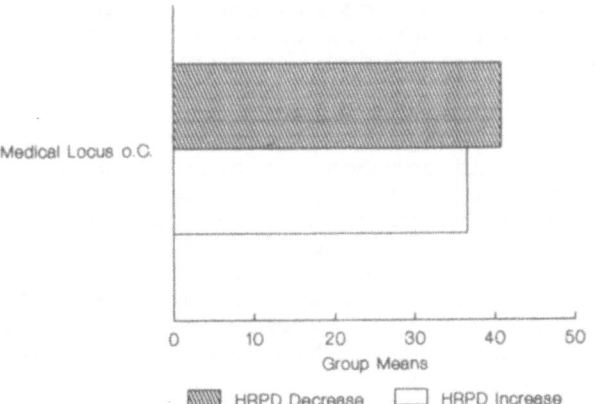

Fig. 2.   Comparison of subgroups with a decrease in HRPD
          symptoms and an increase in HRPD symptoms from
          preoperative to early postoperative
          investigation: Medical locus of control
          (t(29)-2.37; p<.05)

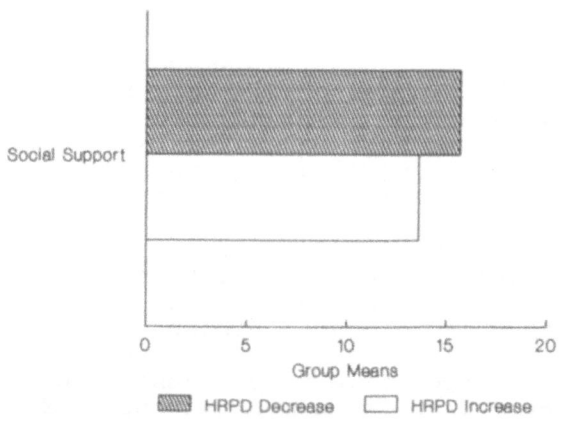

Fig. 3.   Comparison of subgroups with a decrease in HRPD
          symptoms and an increase in HRPD symptoms from
          preoperative to early postoperative
          investigation: Social support (t(28)=2.14;
          p<.05)

Furthermore, according to our results, the patient's early postoperative condition seems better in those who at least think they have a satisfying social support system that backs them up. We therefore have a slight indication that social support might be equally as important a factor for patients undergoing coronary bypass surgery as for many other chronic diseases and medical operations, such as heart transplantation, for instance.

If we are interested in providing psychological help for patients prior to surgery, several aspects stressed in our study seem promising in helping develop concepts for psychological intervention. Psychological variables such as attitudes and cognitions about the patients' health and their potential to actively influence their state can of course be influenced by psychotherapeutic means. One possible conclusion on the basis of our results is that it may be useful to foster a patient's competence, while also promoting a realistic expectation of his own ability to affect developments prior to and following cardiac surgery.

REFERENCES

1. A. Salm, Psychische Adaptationsprozesse bei Operationspatienten: Untersuchungsansatze und Modellvorstellungen, in: "Psychosoziale Kardiologie," B. F. Klapp, B. Dahme, eds., Springer, Heidelberg (1988).
2. K. Moehlen, S. Davies-Osterkamp, Psychische und korperliche Reaktionen bei Patienten der offenen Herzchirurgie in Abhangigkeit von Praoperativen psychischen Befunden. Zeitschr. Psychosom. Med. Psychoanal. 25: 128 (1979).
3. B. Andresen, "Der Hamburger Gesundheitsfragebogen." Unpubl. Manual, Hamburg (1988).
4. G. Krampe, "IPC Fragebogen," Hogrefe, Gottingen (1982).
5. G. Ziegler, I. Schuele, Psychische Reaktionen und Krankheitsverarbeitung bei Dialysepatienten. Psychother. med. Psychol. 35: 62 (1985).
6. A. Boll, Psycholigische Adaptation 3-5 Jahre nach der Herzoperation. Dissertation, Hamburg (1986).

THE RELATIONSHIP OF PREOPERATIVE ANXIETY AND

POSTOPERATIVE COMPLICATIONS IN PATIENTS HAVING

OPEN HEART SURGERY

Barbara C. Carlson

Director of Psychological Services
Las Encinas Hospital
Pasadena, California

INTRODUCTION

The purpose of this study was to determine if a relationship existed between preoperative anxiety, coping styles and postoperative complications in patients having open heart surgery. The study questions tested were:

I. Is there a relationship between preoperative anxiety level among cardiac patients:

a. Immediately after being scheduled for surgery
b. 48 hours preoperatively
c. 24 hours preoperatively

and postoperative complications as indicated by:

d. premature ventricular contractions
e. chest tube output
f. pain medications
g. delirium
h. discharge date
i. cardiac arrest with fatal outcome

It cannot be concluded that anxiety is necessarily responsible for the specified complications. If it is possible to describe a significant relationship, however,

Impact of Cardiac Surgery on the Quality of Life
Edited by A. E. Willner and G. Rodewald
Plenum Press, New York, 1990

the nurse practitioner should be aware of such a relationship in order to institute the most effective and
appropriate nursing interventions.

Two variables which are commonly cited as influencing
responses to a negative stimulus are the individual's
chronic level of anxiety and the characteristic defense
mechanisms he uses to reduce that anxiety, as shown by De
Long [1]. Three basic types of coping styles have been
identified. Subjects using avoidant types of defenses
have been labeled "avoiders," those using vigilant
defenses are referred to as "copers," and those who use
both types of defenses apparently without preference, are
called "non-specific defenders (NSD)" [1]. The hospitalized patient experiences anxiety from three basic
sources: (1) separation from home and family, (2) being
forced to conform to the sick role with anticipation of
pain, and (3) the threat to life itself.

HYPOTHESIS

There is a positive correlation between preoperative
anxiety level, coping styles, and postoperative complications in patients having open heart surgery.

METHOD

Study Variables

Independent variables: Preoperative anxiety
                          Preoperative coping styles

Dependent variables: Premature ventricular contraction
                          Chest tube fluid output
                          Postoperative delirium
                          Number of pain medications
                              administered
                          Cardiac arrest with fatal outcome
                          Number of postoperative hospital
                              days

Assumptions

A certain amount of stress and anxiety unavoidably
accompany the patient into his new hospital role.

Sample

A convenience sample of 75 adult subjects, both male and female, was selected. Changes in surgical scheduling, however, reduced the actual study population to 37. Each subject was given a standard explanation of the study and asked to sign a form stating his willingness to participate. None refused participation. All subjects were first seen by the researcher in the surgeon's office. All had a long history of cardiac symptoms, had recently completed a series of cardiac catheterization studies and had no previous heart surgery.

Instrumentation

The instrument used to measure preoperative anxiety levels was the State-Trait Anxiety Inventory (STAI). The instrument consists of two scales: The State Anxiety Inventory and the Trait Anxiety Inventory. Speilberger, Gorsuch and Lushens [2], who developed this brief paper and pencil test, report validity correlations of .75, .80, .52 with the Institute for Personality and Ability Testing Anxiety Scale (IPAT), the Taylor Manifest Anxiety Scale and the Affect Adjective Check List respectively [2].

Observation of Variables

The independent variable of anxiety was measured by the researchers using the STAI first in the surgeon's office immediately after it was confirmed that the subject was a candidate for surgery, second in the hospital for 48 hours preoperatively and third in hospital 24 hours preoperatively.

Postoperative observations on the six dependent variables were collected by the investigators from the subject's medical chart.

Analysis of the Data

The data were computer analyzed using Chi-square. All findings showing a significance of $p < .05$ were accepted.

The possible raw scores ranged from 20 to 80 on both the State and Trait Anxiety scales. Groups were formed by dividing the scores into thirds for each testing time.

Coping patterns were determined by subtracting the raw scores on the State and Trait Anxiety Scales to obtain a plus or minus number. Groups labeled avoiders, copers, and NSD were then formed by dividing the scores into thirds for each testing time.

Limitations of Design

1. The physical environment of the Intensive Care Unit as well as the doctor-nurse, nurse-nurse, and nurse-patient relationships in this area could produce postoperative anxiety (and thus possibly complications) that would not be measured in a preoperative anxiety scale.

2. The preoperative physical condition of the patient could lead to postoperative complications strictly on a physiological basis and without intervening anxiety.

3. The small sample and method of sample selection does not permit generalizations to be made to other populations.

4. The effects of various anesthetic agents, e.g., Succinylcholine and electrolyte imbalance, e.g., low serum sodium and potassium, can produce transient postoperative delirium, as shown by Meyer and Blacker [3].

5. No attempt was made to ascertain a single subject's anxiety level or coping style through the three testing times, since the statistic used is limited to the analysis of groups.

Results

The data were analyzed and all findings showing a significance at the 0.05 or greater level of confidence when compared with the independent variables of anxiety and coping styles were accepted. The dependent variable which met this criterion was survival. The other dependent variables of premature ventricular contractions, chest tube output, amount of pain medication administered, delirium and postoperative hospital days, failed to reach the acceptable level of significance when compared with either independent variable of anxiety or coping style and were therefore rejected.

The score on the State Anxiety Scale forty-eight hours preoperatively was significant with the dependent variable of survival (X^2 = 10.14; 4 df; p = 0.038). Eight percent of those classed as having low anxiety survived surgery but expired later during hospitalization. Two percent of those with medium anxiety expired in the operating room, as did five percent of those with high anxiety (see Table 1).

When coupled with the fact that only 19 percent of those scoring low on the same scale at the same time survived and only 29.7 percent of those scoring high survived (those scoring high had the highest incidence, 5.4 percent of death in the operating room), apparently supports the studies done by Janis [4].

TABLE 1

STATE OF ANXIETY FORTY-EIGHT HOURS
PREOPERATIVELY AND SURVIVAL

Level of Anxiety		Expired in Operating Room	Expired Later in Hospital	Survived	Row Total
Low	f	0	3	7	10
	%	0	8.1	19.0	27.1
Medium	f	1	0	13	14
	%	2.7	0	35.1	37.8
High	f	2	0	11	13
	%	5.4	0	29.7	35.1
Column Total	f	3	3	31	37
	%	8.1	8.1	83.8	100.0

Source: STAI and subject hospital record.

$$x^2 = 10.141; \quad 4df; \quad p = 0.038$$

Discussion

According to Janis [4], either extremely low or extremely high levels of preoperative anxiety interfere with postoperative recovery. A moderate level of anxiety is most likely to be reflective and stimulate what he calls the "work of worry" prior to surgery, thus leading to a smoother recovery.

Extremely low preoperative anxiety leads to denial in which warnings are ignored and this predisposes the individual to stress when it occurs. Extremely high levels of fear preoperatively are more likely to be neurotic in nature. The neurotic component does not stimulate the "work of worry" [4] and thus the subject does not adequately prepare himself for the stress of surgery. De Long's [1] interpretation of the way in which Janis' [4] "work of worry" reduces anxiety is as follows: (1) through rehearsal of the event, (2) reduction of ambiguity, and (3) allowing the subject to develop self-delivered reassurances that he can cope with the situation, as shown by De Long [1].

In this study those with low anxiety were least capable of dealing with postoperative stress in the Invensive Care Unit because none in this category expired in the operating room. All deaths occurred during their stay in that unit. All of those subjects with high anxiety who died did so in the operating room.

Apparently the medium level subjects did stimulate the "work of worry" because only one death occurred in this category (in the operating room), thus giving this group the highest survival rate.

Implications for Further Research and Nursing Practice

The data indicated that 48 hours preoperatively was a critical anxiety period. This needs to be validated by further study. Nursing interventions which could reduce this anxiety level should be explored. The STAI has proven to be a simple, easily administered tool that could continue to be the first step in the medical and nursing assessment of patient anxiety.

Since the researchers are unsure of the effects that preoperative teaching or counseling had on these subjects, both structured and informal sessions could be organized and anxiety measured at various intervals in the pre-operative period to see what effect these sessions have on anxiety.

REFERENCES

1. R. D. De Long, "Individual Differences in Patterns of Anxiety Arousal Stress-Relevant Information and Recovery from Surgery," unpublished Doctor's dissertation, University of California at Los Angeles (1970).
2. R. Gorsuch, R. Lushens, "STAI Manual," Consulting Psychologists Press, Palo Alto, CA (1970, 1984).
3. B. Meyer, R. Blacker, A traumatic reaction induced by suscinylcholine chloride," New York State Journal of Medicine, 44:1255-1261 (1961).
4. I. Janis, "Psychological Stress," John Wiley and Sons, New York (1958, 1973).

QUALITY OF LIFE

QUALITY OF LIFE OF FINNISH HEART SURGERY PATIENTS RELATED

TO RESULTS FROM PREOPERATIVE AND FOLLOW-UP EXAMINATIONS

Hannu Rahikkala

Department of Psychiatry
University of Oulu
Finland

This article is based upon the clinical experiences
and preliminary results of studying one hundred Finnish
coronary bypass surgery and combined valve and bypass
surgery patients. The study was done at Oulu University
Central Hospital, Finland, as part of the international
study organized by the International Consortium for the
Study of Neurological and Psychological Reactions to
Cardiac Surgery. The author did the psychiatric interviews of all patients.

INTRODUCTION

Finland is traditionally a country with an exceptionally high incidence of coronary heart disease. In
1985 approximately 23,500 citizens were permanently
retired because of this disease. Annually 20,000-25,000
people go through a myocardial infarction; as an example,
20,430 persons died of a heart attack in 1984. The death
rate for ischemic heart diseases was 332.4 deaths per
100,000 mean population between 1981 and 1984 according
to Finnish official statistics.

The significance of coronary heart disease to the
health of the population and therefore to the whole
society has thus been extremely high. Several research
projects have been carried out in Finland, with the goal
of reducing the health risks of this disease. As an
example, I would like to mention the so called Northern

Impact of Cardiac Surgery on the Quality of Life
Edited by A. E. Willner and G. Rodewald
Plenum Press, New York, 1990

Carelia Project, in which the objective has been to reduce smoking and use of animal fat and to treat hypertension adequately in a restricted area in eastern Finland where the morbidity and mortality of coronary disease have been exceptionally high. In recent years, the crucial issue of national health education has been reduction of the use of animal fat. On the whole, public discussion about healthy nourishment and ways of life has been lively.

The first coronary bypass operation in Finland was performed in 1970 in Helsinki. Nowadays bypass patients are operated on in all five university central hospitals and also in two private hospitals in Helsinki. Some Finnish patients have, in addition, been operated on abroad, in Sweden, England and Spain. Compared with the high incidence of coronary disease, the number of bypass operations has been remarkably low in Finland. In 1984, 113 operations per one million people were done (compared with 800 in the USA, 240 in Sweden). In 1985 the number was 147 per one million people, but still at the end of that year approximately one thousand patients (equivalent to 50,000 patients in the USA) were lining up for the operation, many of them for 2 or 3 years. During the beginning of our study in Oulu there was a very intensive public discussion about the state of coronary surgery in Finland.

CARRYING OUT THE STUDY IN OULU

The preparatory phase of this study lasted several years, until autumn 1985. On the surgical ward we settled how the patients arrive at the ward and where and when we best can examine them. In the ICU we planned how the psychiatrist can interview and the neurologist examine the patients without disturbing the intensive treatment. We had several meetings with the cardiologists, anaesthetists, surgeons and neurologists to standardize the collection of data. The practice of pre- and post-operative CT scanning was arranged with the radiological department, etc. Finally we gave an information booklet about the study project to every person participating in the study and to all units where the examinations would be performed. This information contained also a detailed time schedule for the various clinical examinations and tests. Our plan was to have the same persons working in the research until the end of the project, but we did not succeed in that. The psychiatrist and neuropsychologist

were the persons who in reality examined the patients
from the beginning to the end.   All other researchers
changed.

        After a pilot study with a couple of patients in May
1985, we started the actual study in November 1985.   All
the operative phase examinations were done between
November 20th, 1985 and June 16th, 1987.   Follow-up examinations were performed between December 4th, 1986 and
June 6th, 1988.

        The sample consisted of all electively operated
bypass or combined bypass and valve patients who were
operated on certain weekdays and who had no congenital
heart disease.   We examined preoperatively 103 patients,
three of whom were left out of the final sample.   Two
patients died during the follow-up period.   The other 98
patients went through the follow-up examinations.

        During our study the patients arrived at the
surgical ward from three to five days before the operation and were discharged approximately on the twelfth
postoperative day.   Most patients came to the hospital
from their homes and were discharged home.   In some cases
complications required further treatment in another
hospital.

        In addition to the standard research protocol of the
international consortium, the psychiatrist obtained information about the general life history of the patient and
he also gave the Rorschach test preoperatively to the
patient.   The preoperative interviews were tape-recorded,
and likewise a summary of the postoperative interviews.

        Pre- and postoperative CT scanning was performed on
almost all patients.   In the beginning neurophysiological
tests (SSEP,. etc) were also given to approximately ten
patients with obviously minor findings, so we did not
continue with them.

        The psychiatrist had plenty of time for interviewing
the patients, and the doctor/researcher - patient relationship became very intense and confidential.   The
psychiatrist and the psychologist were two of the very
first persons whom the patient met after arriving at the
surgical ward.   In the beginning some patients were a
little embarrassed with our study but not after we
decided to mail an informative letter by the psychiatrist
and chief surgeon to the patients preoperatively.   During

the first interview the psychiatrist told the patient
that he would also meet him in ICU and before discharge
from the hospital. He also told about the follow-up
examinations one year after the operation and said that
the patient would be contacted by letter and telephone
some months before those examinations.

In the beginning of the follow-up examinations the
patient usually had a physical examination on the following day in our hospital. Patients who did not live very
far away from the hospital visited us on an out- patient
basis. Other patients could stay overnight at a patient
hotel of another hospital in Oulu. The psychiatrist
personally contacted all the patients or their families
about the arrangements. So the contact between the
psychiatrist and the patients was also very personal in
the follow-up examinations. This perhaps had some disadvantages, which I will discuss later. In follow-up the
psychiatrist interviewed the patient first, followed by
the neuropsychological tests and neurological examination.

RESULTS

Ninety-two of the one hundred patients were men, and
86 of them had bypass surgery. The mean age of these men
was 52.6 years, ranging from 33.9 to 65.2 years. A combined bypass and valve operation was performed on 6 men,
whose mean age was 57.7 years, ranging from 51.7 to 63.4
years. Twenty-eight point three percent of all the male
patients were between 55 and 59 years and 26.1% between
50 and 54 years. The third largest group were the
patients between 45 and 49 years with a percentage of
16.3.

The number of female patients was eight, five of whom
had a bypass and three a combined valve and bypass operation. The mean age for female bypass patients was 52.4
years (range 45.7-61.4 years) and for female combined
surgery patients 63.0 years (range 59.9-64.5 years).

Preoperatively, 50 patients already had a documented
myocardial infarction. Fourteen of them had been infarcted
twice and two patients as many as three times. Both
deaths during the follow-up period were observed in this
group. One of the preoperatively infarcted patients had
to be operated again approximately six weeks after the
first operation.

TABLE 1

PREOPERATIVE NYHA-CLASSIFICATION OF SOMATIC STATE

1.	ALL PATIENTS	2.	BP & V - PATIENTS
1.1	ANGINA CLASS	2.1	ANGINA CLASS

1.1 ANGINA CLASS		2.1 ANGINA CLASS	
I :	4%	I :	22%
II :	21%	II :	45%
III :	61%	III :	33%
IV :	14%	~IV :	0%

1.2 FUNCTIONAL CLASS		2.2 FUNCTIONAL CLASS	
I :	16%	I :	11%
II :	67%	II :	33%
III :	17%	III :	56%
IV :	0%	IV :	0%

You can see the preoperative somatic status according to NYHA classification in Table 1. Angina pectoris was in most cases rated at class three and most patients were in functional class two. The classification of function was performed preoperatively in 75 cases. Angina pectoris in patients who had combined bypass and valve surgery was classified as milder than in pure bypass patients but their functional status was worse.

TABLE 2

WORK STATUS (ALL PATIENTS)

PREOPERATIVE	AT TWELVE MONTH'S FOLLOW-UP
1. FULLTIME......... 10%	1. FULLTIME........... 26%
good 5 pat.	good 20 pat.
fair 12 "	fair 4 "

Table 2 (cont'd)

poor   2 "   poor   1 "

2. PART-TIME........ 5%   2. PART-TIME........... 6%

   good   0 pat.   good   2 pat.

   fair   3 "   fair   3 "

   poor   2 "   poor   1 "

3. SICK-LEAVE....... 31%   3. SICK-LEAVE........ 4%

4. RETIRED/HEART.... 34%   4. RETIRED/HEART...... 51%

5. RETIRED/AGE, OTH.   5. RETIRED/AGE, OTH.
   MED. CAUSES...... 11%   MED. CAUSES...... 10%

                                 6. UNEMPLOYED......... 1%

                                 7. DEAD.............. 2%

        The background data for the patient sample showed
that 42% of the patients had heavy physical work, 28%
lighter or partly physical work and 7% extremely stressful
mental work. Table 2 shows the work status preoperatively
and after the twelve month follow-up period. We see that
the proportion of working patients increased by seven per
cent and most of the working patients subjectively experienced their ability to work as very good. Many patients
who preoperatively were on a sick-leave had been pensioned.
Separate examination of work status of preoperatively
non-infarcted and infarcted patients revealed that the
proportion of working patients both preoperatively and in
follow-up was markedly higher in the former group of
patients. The proportion of working patients in the
not-infarcted group was 28% preoperatively and 40% at
twelve-month follow-up. In the infarcted group the
corresponding numbers were 16% and 24%. The same applies
also to the proportion of retired patients before the
operation but not at follow-up.

        The study also investigated the patients' subjective
evaluation of the coping of their important persons

TABLE 3

PATIENT'S ESTIMATION OF IMPORTANT PERSONS' COPING

PREOPERATIVE COPING

1. Spouse's/Other Imp. Person's

    Very Well................ 34%

    O.K. 53%

    Poor.................... 11%

    No Such a Person........ 2%

2. Children's

    Very Well................ 49%

    O.K. 32%

    Poor.................... 0%

    No Children............. 19%

COPING AT TWELVE MONTH'S FOLLOW-UP

1. Spouse's/Other Imp. Person's

    Very Well................ 51%

    O.K. 41%

    Poor.................... 5%

    No Such a Person........ 3%

2. Children's

    Very Well................ 62%

    O.K. 18.5%

    Poor.................... 1%

    No Children............. 18.5%

(Table 3). I think this is also an expression of the
patient's projection of his own feelings onto his
important object. As you might expect, the patients
assessed the coping of nearest persons as better in the
follow-up than in the preoperative phase. Incidentally,
I would like to mention the high proportion of childless
patients (almost every fifth patient) in our sample.

The quality of sexual life, subjectively estimated by
the patients, is shown in Tables 4 and 5. The preoperative
assessment included the period since developing heart
disease and the follow-up assessment the period since the
surgery. There seem to be some differences between non-
infarcted and infarcted groups. In follow-up 10% of the
non-infarcted and 20% of the infarcted patients regarded
their sexual activity as decreased since the surgery, and
almost half of the patients regarded it unchanged since
the surgery. However, 44% of the non-infarcted and 38%
of the infarcted patients felt that satisfaction of
sexual life had increased after the operation. Sixteen
percent and 18% of the patients respectively thought that
their satisfaction had decreased.

TABLE 4

QUALITY OF SEXUAL LIFE. NOT-INFARCTED PATIENTS (N=50)

PREOPERATIVE (N=50)   AT 12 MONTH'S FOLLOW-UP (N=50)

1. FREQUENCE OF SEXUAL   1. FREQUENCE OF SEXUAL
   ACTIVITY   ACTIVITY

   Increased......... 2%   Increased.......... 38%

   Unchanged......... 30%   Unchanged.......... 48%

   Decreased......... 64%   Decreased.......... 10%

   No information.... 4%   No information..... 4%

2. SATISFACTION   2. SATISFACTION

   Increased.......... 2%   Increased.......... 44%

   Unchanged......... 58%   Unchanged.......... 38%

   Decreased......... 36%   Decreased.......... 16%

   No information..... 4%   No information...... 2%

TABLE 5

QUALITY OF SEXUAL LIFE. INFARCTED PATIENTS

PREOPERATIVE (N=50)

AT TWELVE MONTH'S FOLLOW-UP (N=48)

1. FREQUENCE OF SEXUAL ACTIVITY

Increased.......... 0%

Unchanged.......... 16%

Decreased.......... 82%

No information..... 2%

1. FREQUENCE OF SEXUAL ACTIVITY

Increased.......... 40%

Unchanged.......... 37%

Decreased.......... 21%

No information...... 2%

2. SATISFACTION

Increased.......... 0%

Unchanged.......... 52%

Decreased.......... 46%

No information..... 2%

2. SATISFACTION

Increased.......... 39%

Unchanged.......... 42%

Decreased.......... 19%

No information...... 0%

In additon to the foregoing description of these rough and not very sophisticated results, I would like to report briefly the following results from the data analysis of four factors of the Hamburg Rating of Psychic Disturbances. The analysis revealed that the anxiety of the patient is high preoperatively and again just before discharge from the hospital. In the ICU, anxiety is lowest, perhaps because of the patient's experience of surviving the surgery and because of the sedation by the anaesthetics and analgesics. There are statistically significant differences in the levels of anxiety in different phases of the hospital treatment. Moreover, masked depression, symptoms of hostility, and signs of losing control show also a tendency to be highest during the discharge phase and to decline significantly during the follow-up period. The data analysis showed further that the follow-up neurological findings were significantly related to follow-up psychiatric ratings for both the Hamilton Depression and Anxiety Scales (p = 0.01). In addition, the entire HRPD scale and four of its eight

factors (paranoid-hallucinatory symptoms, anxiety, masked
depression and loss of control) were significantly
related to follow-up neurological symptoms. As a whole
the level of neurological abnormalities at follow-up was
significantly larger than the level in the preoperative
phase (p = 0.01).

DISCUSSION

    When I think about our results in Oulu it is impor-
tant to pay attention to the arrangements of our study.
We must also remember that special publicity was given to
coronary surgery in Finland during our research.

    It seems to me that the fact that the same psychia-
trist saw the patients several times during the hospital
treatment when the patient was treated in different
hospital units, meant a lot to many patients. The continuity of the relationship with the psychiatrist seemed
to be important. The psychiatrist and the psychologist
were among the first persons who contacted the patient
after his arrival at the surgical ward. During the
follow-up patients did not have extensive medical examinations, only the neurological examination was done.
Therefore, many patients wanted to ask advice from the
psychiatrist about various medical, mental or social
problems. The patient-doctor/researcher relationship
became very intense and confidential. So perhaps we in
Oulu had an exceptionally good chance to observe psychic
symptoms in our patient sample.

    Only in a few cases did the psychic disturbance seem
severe and apparently influence the convalescence, rehabilitation and further quality of life of our patients.
In these cases there seemed often to be some manifest
clinical neurological abnormality postoperatively, for
instance mild hemiplegia or TIA. These clinical findings
support the statistical relationship between psychopathology and neurological pathology. Our clinical
experience of this patient sample is that organic neurological pathology and psychopathology manifest themselves
often in the older, valve surgery and female patients.
This is true especially with patients who had preoperative signs of psychopathology. I also observed
clinically how stressful the discharge phase was to the
heart surgery patients. This is understandable, because
most patients were discharged home less than two weeks

after their major operations. They were anxious and worried about coping without the nursing and medical care of the hospital.

On the other hand, only severe psychopathology seemed to be important to Finnish patients. The long waiting lists for the operation perhaps influenced our findings of psychopathology in the Finnish heart surgery patients. Candidates for heart surgery perhaps form a selected group of patients. Many of them may persistently try to get the operation and try to stay alive. The most hopeless, pessimistic or anxious patients have possibly died or given up. They, for instance, do not phone their doctor to use preoperative angiography or heart surgery itself in spite of worsening symptoms.

Most Finnish bypass surgery patients are relatively young and still very able to adapt. During the long waiting time they might have adapted to possible psychic disturbances as well as to somatic problems. They also are often physically rather healthy in spite of their heart disease. So the significance of psychopathology, e.g. to the quality of life in general may often be not as vital as it would be to older patients who may have more difficulties in adaptation.

Finally, I believe that the research project constituted an important supportive intervention which presumably helped the patients to anticipate the possible physical and psychic problems. Anticipation perhaps helped the patients to cope with the disturbances better. It is also possible that the study as a psychological intervention influenced the incidence of psychopathology and/or its significance to the patients. Many patients perhaps, consciously or unconsciously, left out of the conversation some topics that were unpleasant or negative because the interaction with the researchers was in most cases a close, positively charged and supportive one. With a more neutral and distant interaction one might have obtained other kinds of information.

The persons who carried out the study were identified as a part of the hospital staff, and most patients seemed to have deep feelings of gratitude towards the hospital and its staff. Many patients also felt that they were privileged because they were operated on despite the prevailing scarcity of coronary surgery in Finland. Our research group believes that these issues may have influenced the content of the information given by the patients.

So, with this background it may be easy to understand why in the one year follow-up after the operation so many patients were quite satisfied with their surgery, even though the quality of life, regarding ability to work, closest object relationships or sexual life had not improved much.

List of references is available from the Author.

BECK DEPRESSION INVENTORY SCORES OF CORONARY BYPASS

PATIENTS WITH OR WITHOUT PSYCHOLOGICAL INTERVENTION

June B. Pimm
James R. Jude

Department of Psychiatry
University of Miami
Miami, Florida

My paper will deal with ongoing research conducted in Miami, Florida, on the effectiveness of several intervention strategies on post surgical Beck Depression scores in coronary bypass patients.

The initial findings are from a 1985 study conducted at the Miami Heart Institute and South Miami Hospitals where counselors provided psychological counseling in the form of "crisis intervention" to half a sample of 104 male coronary bypass patients. The other half of the patients received the support provided routinely by their cardiologists and the nursing faculty of the hospital. Crisis intervention followed the model of Caplan of the Harvard Community Medical Health Center. It consisted of a preoperative session of "anticipatory guidance" and weekly sessions of supportive counseling for 8 weeks following discharge. These sessions were held initially in the hospital and later in the patient's home after hospital discharge. They included the wives and family of the patient. The intention of crisis intervention counseling was to help the patient recover his usual coping strategies in order to make it possible for him to re-establish his former level of psychological functioning.

Impact of Cardiac Surgery on the Quality of Life
Edited by A. E. Willner and G. Rodewald
Plenum Press, New York, 1990

All patients were assessed the day prior to surgery on a battery of psychological tests which included the following:

1) Beck Depression Inventory;
2) SCL-90-R;
3) Jenkins Activity Survey;
4) Conceptual Level Analogy Test;
5) Locus of Control Scale;
6) Recent Life Changes Questionnaire;
7) Minnesota Multiphasic Personality Inventory-Depression Scale;
8) Millon Behavioral Health Inventory.

At the end of the 12 weeks, all patients were reassessed on the same battery of tests and their wives were asked to rate the amount of depression they saw in their husbands. Three years after surgery, 34 of the original 104 patients were again interviewed in their homes and again participated in a battery of psychological tests.

A full report of all of these data is available elsewhere but the Beck was found to be the most robust dependent measure of depression. Therefore, we will discuss only these scores here.

At the time of our study there was no one generally accepted cutoff for clinical depression on the Beck Depression Inventory, but 14 had often been used in other research studies; therefore it was selected for our data. Table 1 displays the numbers of patients who were clinically depressed and not clinically depressed by treatment and control. Treatment and control patients had equivalent probabilities of clinical depression presurgery. Three months after surgery, however, control patients were significantly more likely to suffer from clinical depression. At the three year mark the trend was clearly in the same direction but no longer significant, possibly because of the small sample size. Thus it appeared that crisis intervention counseling reduced the occurrence of clinical depression at three months after surgery, and this effect could still be noted three years later.

Multiple regression analysis of presurgical variables on post surgical depression showed several significant interactions. Table 2 shows the very significant multiple regression for the Beck Depression Inventory at 3 years. The significant variables and their directions were as follows:

(1) Group by RLCNE: being in the control group
and having many life changes tended to increase later
depression;
(2) Triple Coronary Disease: having this disease
tended to increase later depression (the coding of this
and other dichotomous medical items lead to a negative
coefficient if the items' presence tends to increase
with depression);
(3) GSI: increases in the SCL-90 Global Severity
Index tended to relate to increased postsurgical
depression;
(4) New York Heart Association Functional Class:
higher levels on this scale tended to lead to higher
levels of later depression; and
(5) Age: older patients tended to have higher
levels of later depression. Together these variables
accounted for more than 90% of the variance in this
sample for Beck Depression Inventory scores at 3 years
after surgery.

TABLE 1. Frequency Distribution of Clinical Pathology
          Using Beck Depression Scores

A. Patients before Surgery

	Not clinically depressed	Clinically depressed	Total	
Treatment	31	5	36	
Control	24	7	31	$x^2(1)=0.86$
Total	55	12	67	$p > .10$

B. Patients 3 months after surgery

	Not clinically depressed	Clinically depressed	Total	
Treatment	47	4	51	
Control	35	10	45	$x^2(1)=3.97$
Total	82	14	96	$p = .05$

C. Patients 3 years after surgery

	Not clinically depressed	Clinically depressed	Total	
Treatment	14	1	15	
Control	13	5	18	$x^2(1)=2.45$
Total	27	6	33	$p > .19$

TABLE 2.   Regression Analysis of Beck Depression
            Inventory at 3 Years.

Variable	Standardized regression coefficient	Standard error of standard regression coefficient	F	P
Group by Recent Life Changes Number Endorsed	.79	.11	55.14	.0001
Triple Coronary Disease	-.34	.09	14.71	.0024
SCL-90 Global Severity Index before surgery	.24	10	5.79	.0331
New York Heart Association Functional Class prior to surgery	.28	10	7.62	.0172
Age	.30	.11	8.00	.0152

(Beck Depression Inventory at 3 years is dependent
variable) R = .95, R^2 = .91, R^2Adj. = .87, F(5,12) =
23.37, p = .001

The equation for the Beck Depression Inventory at
3 months presented in Table 3 was also highly significant.   Four independent variables were selected for
inclusion in this equation, all with very significant
regression coefficients.   The direction of these four
variables was as follows:
(1)   Beck Depression Inventory: high presurgical
Beck Depression Inventory scores tended to be associated
with high Beck Depression Inventory Scores at 3 months
after surgery;
(2) Group by Number of Bypasses: having a greater
number of bypasses and being in the control group tended
to result in higher levels of later depression;
(3)   Group by Recent Life Changes: the greater the
number of recent life changes and being in the control
group tended to lead to greater postsurgical depression;
(4) Group by Left Main Coronary Disease: being in
the control group and having left main coronary disease
tended to reduce postsurgical depression.   Together
these four variables account for 80% of the variance in
this sample in depression at 3 months after surgery as
measured by the Beck Depression Inventory.

TABLE 3. Regression Analysis of Beck Depression
Inventory at 3 Months.

Variable	Standardized regression coefficient	Standard error of standard regression coefficient	F	P
Beck Depression Inventory before surgery	.51	.12	17.42	.0004
Group by Number of Bypasses	.37	.10	13.22	.0014
Group by Recent Life Change Number Endorsed before surgery	.33	.12	7.31	.0127
Group by Left Main Coronary Disease	-.26	.10	6.50	.0180

(Beck Depression Inventory at 3 months is dependent
variable) $R = .90$, $R^2 = .80$, R^2Adj. $= .77$, $F(4.23) =$
23.70, $p = .0001$

It appears as if the Beck Depression Inventory is
an instrument sensitive enough to participate in prediction of coronary bypass patients "at risk" for postsurgical depression and is also capable of reflecting
the effect of intervention programs with this group of
individuals.

We are currently comparing the effectiveness of a
patient handbook to that of crisis intervention in lowering Beck Depression Scores in heart surgery patients
who have had the book available. Because of the cost of
providing individual counseling according to the Caplan
model to all hospital patients, we worked with a pro-
fessional health writer to translate the principles of
crisis intervention into a comprehensive handbook for
the use of the patient and his family. At the moment we
are providing all heart surgery patients, both male and
female, with this book and we are following them after
surgery in order to evaluate the book's effectiveness.

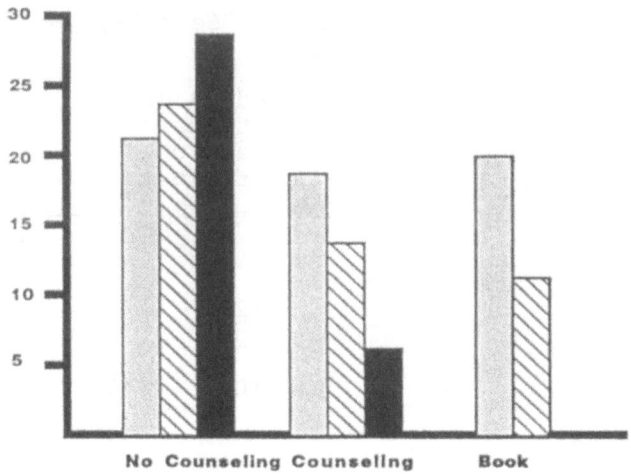

Fig. 1. Percentage of Clinically Depressed Patients

Because the frequency of post-surgical depression
appears to be now well documented, we have not included
a specific control, or "no intervention" group but are
comparing our results to our previous findings. Our
initial findings are based on a small initial sample of
20 patients but we now have over 50 patients enrolled.
Our preliminary results suggest that the book may compare well to counseling if you look at the Beck Depression scores of the three groups. You can see that the
pattern of scores is similar to those found in our
crisis intervention group (Figure 1).

Very recently we have begun a cooperative study
with Presbyterian Hospital in Albuquerque, New Mexico,
where they routinely give a relaxation and information
tape to patients prior to surgery. We are administering
the Recent Life Events Scale and the Beck Depression
Inventory prior to surgery and will follow up with the
patients 3 months after surgery to obtain Beck Depression scores.

We feel that the Beck is singularly applicable to
our type of intervention research as Beck's cognitive

theory suggests that individuals are depressed because
they view the world in a negative fashion. In order to
help a patient overcome his depression, according to
Beck, it is necessary to change his negative cognitions
and enable him to see events more "realistically." The
crisis intervention approach to patients would fit this
model in that it is short term, cognitive, and intended
to assist the individual to view events more positively.

We found the Beck items helpful in understanding
the patients' cognitive view of themselves. We noted
that heart surgery patients express their depression
through somatic complaints as they see themselves as
sick and not depressed. Over half of the items in the
Beck Depression Inventory relate to a view of self and
events which could be termed morbid and full of despair.
Examples include items such as "I feel the future is
hopeless and that things cannot improve." The remaining
items on the other hand, are more typical of feelings
which relate to physical illness. An example would be
"I get tired more easily than I used to." Thus the
total Beck scores could be divided into two groups
termed affective and somatic. We found that heart
patients endorsed more of the latter. In looking at the
pattern of scores in our two groups of patients in our
1984 study we found that patients were more likely to
endorse "somatic" items than "affective ones" before
surgery. Only from 7% to 11% of the total possible
score of affective items were endorsed by our patients
whereas 20 to 26% of the somatic items were endorsed.
It seems that the cognitive structure of a heart surgery
patient encourages him to express depression through
medical complaints.

Interestingly, when we compare the compositon of
Beck scores in our current studies with those obtained
in 1984 we continue to see a similar pattern of scores.
In our current group of Miami patients from Northridge
General Hospital we find that 7% of items out of the
"affective items" are endorsed whereas 20% of the
somatic items are included. In the Albuquerque group
11% of the items endorsed fall in the affective category
compared to 26% in the somatic group.

If counseling succeeded in changing patients' cognitive view of themselves, this would be reflected in a
drop in somatic items post surgery. This proved to be
the case. In our 3 year follow-up data of 1984 we found
that overall Beck Depression scores dropped in the
treatment or counseling group. This drop was in the

somatic items.   The percentage of affective items
endorsed remained the same whereas the percentage of
somatic items dropped by 30%.

This finding is important to cardiologists who
supervise the post-operative care of coronary bypass
patients.   If patients do not <u>appear</u> significantly depressed, they are unlikely to be recognized.   Moreover
if patients do not recognize depression and still per-
ceive themselves to be vaguely unwell and present
somatic complaints, they will continue to be a source of
concern to their physicians.   This could result in
multiple medical visits, repeated diagnostic tests and
increased health care costs.

QUALITY OF LIFE AFTER OPEN-HEART SURGERY

P. J. Walter, B. J. Amsel

University Hospital Antwerp
Antwerp, Belgium

Until recently the physical results of open-heart
surgery have been of major interest to physicians and
surgeons. The actual quality of life as experienced by
the patients has, however, been neglected. Now doctors
have begun to realize the importance of these aspects for
the integral success of heart operations.

Because quality of life is a relatively new concept,
a precise definition has not yet been fixed in the
literature. This discussion of the recent literature
will follow the subdivision by S. Levine and S. Croog [1]
of the aspects of quality of life: physiological state
of the individual; intellectual functioning; emotional
state of the individual; general satisfaction or feeling
of well-being.

Physiological State of the Individual

Coronary bypass surgery has yielded good improvement
of symptoms and event-free survival (no death, angina,
repeat bypass surgery, myocardial infarction, and less
than 5 days of hospitalization) of 40 to 50% depending on
patient age [2].

Medication use is halved postoperatively. Survival
and symptoms are improved after valvular replacement with
freedom from thromboembolism in 76 to 99% of patients at
10 years depending on the type of valve, and with 71 to
88% freedom from reoperation. In desperately ill
patients requiring heart transplantation (HTX), survival
is greatly improved, approaching 70% at two years in most
centers, and with preserved left ventricular function.

Impact of Cardiac Surgery on the Quality of Life
Edited by A. E. Willner and G. Rodewald
Plenum Press, New York, 1990

Intellectual Functioning

Intellectual functioning, comprising memory, conceptual reasoning, mental flexibility, attention, concentration, fine motor dexterity, and affect, while deteriorated
10 days after coronary bypass surgery is improved 6
months later [3] (Figure 1). The prevalence of cognitive
disorders correlated with reduced social and sexual
activity up to five years after open-heart surgery [4].

Emotional State of the Individual

Although 30% felt much less nervous 3-5 years after
coronary bypass surgery, 47% actually had no improvement
or even some aggravation [5]. In another study, however,
both anxiety and depression were improved 6 months after

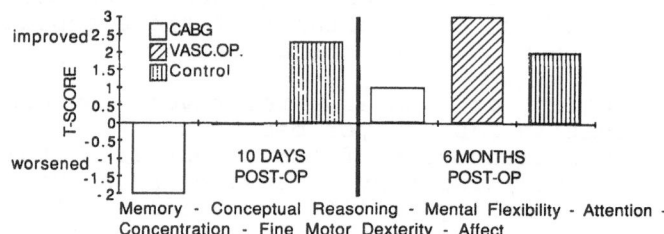

Fig. 1 Intellectual functioning - emotional state after
        cardiac operation. From Ref. 3.

valvular surgery [6, 7]. To some extent, working status
determined the emotional changes, the latter being best
in those working, worst in those forced to retire, and
intermediate in those not working, but by choice [8]
(Figure 2). After heart transplantation worry, not only
about somatic factors such as biopsy results and weight
gain, but also about finances and burden upon the family,
weighed upon the patient. However, from discharge to 12
months, posttransplantation depression was significantly
less than before heart transplantation [9].

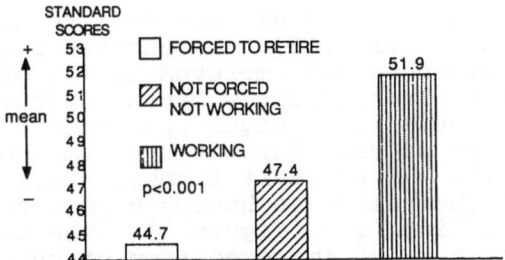

* ANXIETY, NERVOUSNESS, RESTLESSNESS, SADNESS,HAPPINESS, CONTENTMENT

Fig. 2   Emotional changes* after major heart surgery
affected by working status.   From Ref. 8.

Performance of Social Roles

Social adjustment, that is the relationship with
spouse, children, and coworkers is related to medical
aspects of recovery. Patients hospitalized for cardiac
complaints were more poorly socially adjusted than those
hospitalized for other reasons [8].

Coronary bypass surgery had a positive effect on
family relations, the latter having improved in 70%
3-5 years postoperatively [5]. Relationship with friends
was good in 80% both before and 1 year after open heart
surgery [10]. Psychosocial problems after coronary
bypass surgery seem to have a negative effect on sexual
activity. While 62% of patients engaged in sexual
activity at least once a week preoperatively, only 38%
did so 9 months after the operation [5]. The rate of
return to work after bypass surgery varies from 58 to 91%
depending on the country studied. Further factors
determining this rate are physical recovery, age, gender,
duration of preoperative work interruption, social class,
and, to a great extent, physicians' advice. Housewives
return to home duties up to 98% of the time; about 2/3
of them full time [11]. Return to work after heart valve
replacement is somewhat less, 38% at a mean of 1.7 years
and 33% at a mean of 4.7 years in our own study [12]
(Figure 3). Even after heart transplantation, return to
work is possible, varying from 18% to 66% in various
studies.

General Satisfaction or Feeling of Well Being

Pleasure in life was most negatively affected in
males by forced or voluntary retirement. However, in

women those voluntarily retired did not seem to have this
reduction in quality of life [13].   In another study,
overall feeling of pleasure was improved in 77% of
patients, 3 1/2 years after coronary bypass surgery,
while only 11% felt worse [5].   Vigor was increased 6 and
12 months after bypass or valvular surgery compared to
preoperatively [6, 7].   After heart transplantation most
patients considered themselves as having a good to
excellent quality of life [14] (Figure 4).   The Campbell
Well-Being score seems to be improved from discharge to
at least 12 months postoperatively, compared to the
pretransplant score [9].

Quality of Life in the Elderly

        In the future, the concept of quality of life will
become as important for the elderly as for younger people,
because of a sheer increase in the population of the
elderly.   According to a 1984 United States Census Bureau
report, the estimated population above 80 years of age in
the USA would be 2.7 million in 1985, 7.4 million in 1990,
and 12 million in 2010. According to a study from the CASS
registry, hospital survivors of coronary bypass surgery 65
years or older had significantly greater freedom from angina
recurrence than those younger than 65 years old from 1 to 5
years postoperatively [2].   Roughly 1/5 of elderly patients
were working up to 10 years past retirement age after bypass
surgery [15]. When questioned at a mean of 31 months after
coronary bypass surgery, more than 3/4 of men and women
above 70 years of age indicated they had a good to excellent
quality of life [16] (Figure 5).

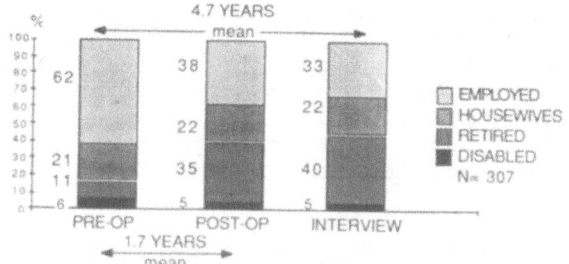

Fig. 3   Return to work after heart valve replacement.
          From Ref. 12.

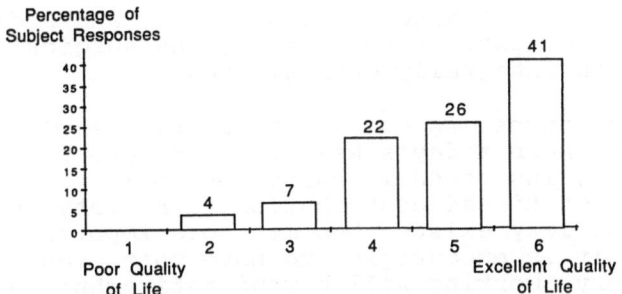

Fig. 4 Current quality of life after heart
         transplantation.   From Ref. 14.

Discussion

The technical results of open-heart surgery have
improved over the last 20 years resulting in greater
longevity and reduction of cardiac symptoms.   However,
little note has been taken of patients' emotional,
psychosocial, and subjective condition, which are greatly
related to the quality of life.   It appears now that
there is no perfect correlation between somatic improvement and this life quality.   Not only is this frequently
unknown to physicians, but also the physicians may
unknowingly negatively affect quality of life.   In the
future it will be necessary to better inform the treating
physician, the general practitioner, and the cardiac
surgeon of the importance of positively influencing the
psychosocial problems of these patients in order to
improve the success of the operation.   This process
should be begun in as early a stage as possible and

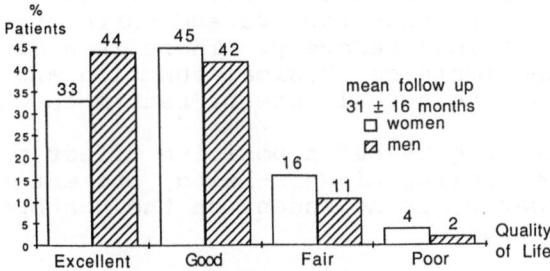

Fig. 5   Quality of life after coronary artery bypass
         surgery in patients older than 70 years.*
         From Ref. 16.

patients' families, trained psychologists, and social
workers should be part of the medical and surgical team
to arrive at an integrally optimal result.

With the increasing number of elderly people in the
population which in today's welfare structure would prove
to be an increasing economic burden on society, the
importance of continued contribution to society as long
as physical ability exists, becomes more important. In
this regard, it is encouraging to note that even after
cardiac surgery, working well beyond retirement age is
often possible, in spite of negative attitudes of doctors
today. By working, even these elderly patients enjoy an
improved quality of life.

Summary

1.   Physical condition after open-heart surgery improves
     with a relatively low incidence of cardiac events
     and a reduction in drug requirements. In other
     words, cardiac surgery is able to achieve its
     somatic goals in most patients.

2.   In the early postoperative phase cognitive disorders
     and intellectual dysfunction occur and are related
     to reduced social and sexual activity. These
     improve later after surgery, but do not reach normal
     levels.

3.   Psychological state is better after successful heart
     surgery than before and depends on the heart condi-
     tion and the functional state of the patient.

4.   A small positive change in family relations and
     contact with friends appears and correlates with the
     extent of medical recovery. There is a discrepancy
     between the improved physical function and ability
     to work and the actual rate of return to work.

5.   Open-heart surgery has a positive effect on the
     subjective feeling of well-being, the extent of
     which, however, is dependent on the postoperative
     working status.

6.   The improvement in functional class and quality of
     life also holds true for elderly patients.

REFERENCES

1. S. Levine and S. H. Croog: What constitutes Quality
    of Life? A conceptualization of the dimensions of
    life quality in Health Population and patients
    with cardiovascular disease, in: "Assessment of
    quality of life in clinical trials of cardio-
    vascular therapies," N. K. Wenger, M. E. Mattson,
    C. D. Furberg, J. Elinson, eds., Le Jacq
    Publishing Inc., New York (1984)
2. B. Gersch, R. Kroumal, H. Schaff, R. Frye, Th. Ryan,
    W. Myers, W. Athearn, B. Athur, J. Gosselin, G.
    Kaiser and Th. Killip, Long-term (5 year) results
    of coronary bypass surgery in patients 65 years
    old or older: a report from the coronary artery
    surgery study, Circulation, 68, II:190 (1983).
3. Th. A. Hammeke and J. E. Hastings, Neuropsychologic
    alterations after cardiac operations, J. Thorac.
    Cardiovasc. Surg. 96:326 (1988).
4. C. J. Rabiner, A. E. Willner and K. Detmer, Effects
    of Environmental stress upon the long-term outcome
    of open-heart surgery: a five year follow-up
    study, in: "Psychopathological and Neurological
    dysfunction following open-heart surgery," R.
    Becker, J. Katz. N. J. Polonius and H. Speidel,
    eds., Springer Publishing Co., Berlin, Heidelberg,
    New York (1982).
5. D. S. Kornfeld, S. S. Heller, K. A. Frank, S. N.
    Wilson and J. R. Malm, Psychological and behavioral
    responses, in: "Return to work after coronary
    artery bypass surgery," P. Walter, ed., Springer
    Publishing Co., Berlin, Heidelberg, New York,
    Tokyo (1985).
6. C. D. Jenkins, B. A. Stanton, S. A. Savageau, D. S.
    Ockene, Ph. Denlinger and M. D. Klein, Physical,
    psychologic, social and economic outcome after
    cardiac valve surgery, Arch Intern Med. 143:2107
    (1983).
7. C. D. Jenkins, B. A. Stanton, R. L. Bergh, R. L.
    Goldstein and R. A. Aucoin, Quality of life 12
    months after coronary artery bypass surgery,
    Quality of life and cardiovascular care, 4:29
    (1987, 1988).
8. St. J. Zyzanski, B. A. Stanton, J. D. Jenkins, M.
    Klein, Medical and psychosocial outcomes in
    survivors of major heart surgery, J. Psychosom.
    Res., 25:213 (1981).
9. B. M. Jones, V. P. Chang, D. Esmore, Ph. Spratt,
    M. X. Shanahan, A. E. Farnsworth, A. Keogh and

K. Downs, Psychological adjustment after cardiac transplantation, Med. J. Aust., 149:119 (1988).

10. B. Bunzel and F. Eckersberger, Changes in life quality after aortocoronary bypass and valve replacement: a subjective criteria for assessing operative results, Thorac Cardiovasc Surgeon, 35:242 (1987).

11. G. J. Maddern, D. R. Craddock, P. I. Leppard, I. K. Ross, J. Stubberfield and J. L. Waddy, The costs of coronary artery surgery to the community, J. Cardiovasc. Surg., 27:469 (1986).

12. P. J. Walter, B. Ibe and M. Gottwik, Return to work after heart valve replacement, in: "Return to work after coronary artery bypass surgery," P. J. Walter, ed., Springer Publishing Co., Berlin, Heidelberg, New York, Tokyo (1985).

13. S. T. Zyzanski, R. Ronse, B. Stanton and C. Jenkins, Employment changes among patients following coronary bypass surgery: social, medical and psychological correlates, Public Health Reports, 97:558 (1982).

14. M. Lough, A. Lindsey, J. Shinn and N. Stotts, Life satisfaction following Heart Transplantation, Heart Transplantation, IV:446 (1985).

15. H. V. Liddle, P. Jones, B. Gould and P. Clayton, The rehabilitation of patients following coronary revascularization surgery: social and economic aspects in: "Return to work after coronary artery bypass surgery - psychosocial and economic aspects," P. J. Walter, ed., Springer Publication, Berlin, Heidelberg, New York Tokyo (1985).

16. D. Jeffery, R. R. Vijayanagar, D.A. Bognolo, and P. F. Eckstein, Results of Coronary Bypass Surgery in elderly women, Ann Thorac Surgery, 42:550 (1986).

QUALITY OF LIFE AFTER CARDIAC SURGERY:

SOCIAL AND ENVIRONMENTAL ASPECTS

H. -J. Meffert, W. Roediger

Department of Cardiovascular Surgery and
Experimental Cardiology
University Hospital
Hamburg-Eppendorf, FRG

A. Boll, W. Huhmann

Rehabilitation Center
Bad Segeberg, FRG

ABSTRACT

This article gives an overview of some results of
the follow-up investigation of the first 45 International Study patients operated on because of coronary
heart disease at the University Hospital, Hamburg, FRG.
The sample contains 41 men and 4 women, with an average
age of 57 years. For organizational reasons this is a
two-year follow-up rather than the intended one-year
follow-up. That is no problem, because the rationale for
the follow-up investigation was to get an impression of
the patients' situation after they had dealt with postoperative vocational, social and personal issues.

The following topics will be discussed: The
patients' actual cardiac situation, their pre- and
postoperative work-status, their financial adjustment,
their social environment and personal relationships,
including sexuality, family and friends. The patient's
psychic situation, although not the focus of this
article, has to do with discrepancies between objective

Impact of Cardiac Surgery on the Quality of Life
Edited by A. E. Willner and G. Rodewald
Plenum Press, New York, 1990

and subjective rehabilitation leading to the final issues of the patients' general attitudes toward the surgical outcome.

1. Cardiac Situation

The patients' cardiac situation (Table 1) two years after the surgery is quite good. According to the NYHA-angina-class, 78% of the patients don't show any signs of angina, 16% experience angina under heavy physical stress, and only 6% under mild physical stress. According to the NYHA-functional-class (Table 2), the patients present an even better picture: the physicians classified 87% as not being restricted in their everyday routine because of angina or dyspnea. Eleven percent were assessed as mildly restricted and only one patient of the total of 45 was unable to manage his everyday life without cardiac problems except at rest.

TABLE 1

CARDIAC SITUATION

NYHA_ANGINA CLASS

I	35	78%
II	7	16%
III	3	6%
IV	-	-

TABLE 2

CARDIAC SITUATION

NYHA FUNCTIONAL CLASS

I	39	87%
II	5	11%
III	1	2%
IV	-	-

2. Vocational Situation

The vocational situation (Table 3) at first glance doesn't fit with the patients' good overall physical rehabilitation.

Before surgery 5% were unemployed, 20% were already retired and 67% were working, whereas after the operation only half the patients went back to work but the other half got old age pensions. The 52% who went on working, either continued their work as it was before surgery or arranged specific changes. In order to understand the impressive number (29%) of the patients who retired postoperatively, one has to look at the average age of both groups. This was 52 years for those who continued working and 60 years for those who retired. In this context one must know that today in Germany every disabled person 60 years or older (and heart surgery patients are disabled persons by official rules) can retire in good financial circumstances. In addition, with an average unemployment rate of about 10% for the Hamburg region, it is very difficult for those who are unemployed for an extended time, older than 45 years, or disabled persons, to find a new job. Considering the alternatives, it is understandable that only 3 of the 13 patients who retired were not content with their new situation.

TABLE 3

WORK STATUS

	PREOPERATIVE		POSTOPERATIVE	
Unemployed	2	4%	−	− .
Retired	9	20%	22	49%
Working	34	76%	23	51%

3. Financial Situation

Financial questions might be interesting in comparison with other countries, but according to the Hamburg figures they don't seem to play an important role in connection with heart surgery. For all patients, the

cost of the surgery itself, the hospital stay and the
rehabilitative facilities were approximately 100% covered
by their insurance. Furthermore, practically no financial
problems resulted from surgery or its consequences, e.g.
early retirement.

4. Personal Situation

        Besides health and financial resources, the personal
situation, meaning the family and social life, is an
important area in the quality of life. Given their good
health and the acceptable financial situation of nearly
all patients, this area was expectd to be satisfying,
too. The figures (Table 4) show that surgery didn't
change much in their social lives, including leisure
time. If something changed, it usually changed for the
better rather than for the worse. While the patients
themselves obviously coped well with the surgery, in
their eyes a third of their partners and families coped
poorly with the surgery. One explanation might be that,
again in the patients' eyes, about a quarter of their
partners and families were not adequately prepared for
adjustments after surgery. This might be a hint for
physicians and psychologists in the surgery departments
and rehabilitation centers to pay more attention to the
patients' relatives and family problems and to prepare
them better for the time after discharge.

TABLE 4

SOCIAL LIFE

POSTOPERATIVE CHANGE
IN SOCIAL LIFE?

Positive	9	20%
No	33	73%
Negative	3	7%

        Sexuality is known to be a special problem after
heart surgery. Sexual activity decreases for most
patients in frequency and in satisfaction as well. This
is not so obvious with our sample. Besides explanations
in terms of anxiety and pain, the average age of 59 years

at the time of the follow-up investigation should be
taken into consideration. Sexuality was a topic of
discussion in all interviews, preoperatively, at time of
discharge after surgery, and at follow-up. There were a
number of sexual problems within this group of patients
which persisted over the years, but the surgery itself
initiated few new problems.

5. Psychic Situation

        Objective ratings by physicians and psychologists
concerning the patients' state of health and the
patients' subjective point of view often differed,
indicating an unsatisfying psychic situation. This
discrepancy is striking, for example with respect to
cardiac complaints (Table 5). While the physicians rate
87% of the patients as unrestricted in everyday routine
by their cardiac situation, only 49% of the patients
declare themselves as unrestricted. Eleven percent of
the patients were objectively rated as mildly restricted,
whereas 42%, that is four times as many, claimed this
restriction for themselves. Nevertheless, things seem to
have changed over the last ten years (Table 6).

        Whereas today only 2% are objectively diagnosed to
have major symptoms under mild or no physical stress, in
a comparable investigation with cardiac surgery patients
in Hamburg ten years ago [1], it was 16%. While today
only 9% of the patients themselves complain of major
symptoms, then it was 53%. Cardiac problems in general,
either mild or severe, this year were diagnosed in 13%

TABLE 5

OBJECTIVE-SUBJECTIVE-DISCREPANCIES

NYHA FUNCTIONAL CLASS	OBJECTIVE PHYSICIANS CLASSIFICATION		SUBJECTIVE PATIENTS' CLASSIFICATION	
I	39	87%	22	49%
II	5	11%	19	42%
III	1	2%	3	7%
IV	-	-	1	2%

TABLE 6

OBJECTIVE-SUBJECTIVE-DISCREPANCIES

	FOLLOW UP INTERNAT'L STUDY 1989		FOLLOW UP HAMBURG STUDY 1979	
	Objective	Subjective	Objective	Subjective
Heavy symptoms under mild or no physical stress (NYHA functional Class III+IV)	2%	9%	16%	53%
Cardiac problems (NYHA functional Class II-IV)	13%	51%	32%	74%

and subjectively complained about in 51%, but ten years ago were diagnosed in 32% and subjectively complained about in 74%. There are various reasons for these discrepancies. One is, no doubt, that a number of patients pretend to be more ill than they are in reality, hoping to have a better chance for an early retirement. Another reason might be a persisting psychic lability, either due to the basic personality structure, or from fears and depressive moods since the time of surgery.

Nevertheless, these discrepancies at first glance do not seem to affect the patients' general attitude about the surgical outcome. Only two patients, 4%, complain of a poor general outcome while most look at it positively and 45% even rate it an excellent success (Table 7).

However, positive or negative results or answers obviously are consequences of the direction of the questions, today as well as ten years ago. When patients were asked to compare their postoperative cardiac situation with their preoperative symptoms ten years ago, 79% described a definite success which corresponded to objective physical improvement as measured by surgeons and cardiologists. But when asked to compare their immediate cardiac situation with their expectations, about 70% complained of unexpected problems! Of course in the International Study the patients were asked again whether their expectations had been fulfilled (Table 8).

TABLE 7

GENERAL ATTITUDE TOWARD OUTCOME

Poor	2	4%
Good	21	47%
Excellent	20	45%
Can't tell	2	4%

Instead of the 70% who said "no" ten years ago, today about 70% say "yes," another 25% "in part" and only 4% "no." The most probable explanation is that the Hamburg team has learned a lot over the years and today does not let patients go home after surgery with unrealistic expectations.

Quality of life means joy of life, too (Table 9). Seventy-eight percent of the patients experience more joy of life after surgery than before, for 11% it has not changed and for the last 11% joy of life has decreased. The International Study provides another chance to learn more about the cardiac surgery patients' situation and to improve it objectively and subjectively.

TABLE 8

GENERAL ATTITUDE TOWARD OUTCOME

EXPECTATIONS FULFILLED?

Yes	32	71%
In part	11	25%
No	2	4%

TABLE 9

GENERAL ATTITUDE TOWARD OUTCOME

JOY OF LIFE COMPARED TO PREOP.

More	35	78%
Equal	5	11%
Less	5	11%

REFERENCES

1. M. J. Meffert, A. Boll, G. Huse-Kleinstoll, F. Lempp,
    G. Rodewald, H. Speidel, Benefits and psycho-
    logical problems of aortocoronary bypass and valve
    replacement surgery, in: "Return to Work After
    Coronary Artery Bypass Surgery," P. J. Walter,
    ed., Springer, Berlin, Heidelberg, New York, Tokyo
    (1985).

QUALITY OF LIFE AND COPING IN HEART TRANSPLANT RECIPIENTS

Beth E. Meyerowitz, Jennifer Vasterling,
Jan Muirhead and William Frist

Vanderbilt University
Nashville, TN   37240

As the frequency of successful heart transplantations increases, there is a growing need for information about how recipients and their families can adjust successfully to the many ongoing medical and psychological demands that follow transplantation. Patients are asked to engage in a wide range of adherence behaviors, to remain vigilant daily to the possibilities of infection or rejection, and to change longstanding life styles and habits. Patients attempt to meet these challenges at the same time that they and their families strive to resume "normal" lives. It is likely that these competing demands can tax the coping resources of even the most well-adjusted patients.

Previous research has documented that recipients experience both physical symptomatology and psychological distress. Transplant coordinators have identified a wide range of psychosocial problems that they believe patients encounter during initial hospitalization and after discharge [1]. Similarly, patients have reported experiencing many physical symptoms, some of which they find to be upsetting and disruptive [2]. Nonetheless, during the first one or two postoperative years, psychiatric morbidity appears to abate for most survivors of transplantation [3] and recipients' quality of life ratings are high [4]. These findings suggest that some, but not all, areas of quality of life are negatively impacted. Moreover, it appears that many patients may find ways to cope with

Impact of Cardiac Surgery on the Quality of Life
Edited by A. E. Willner and G. Rodewald
Plenum Press, New York, 1990

distress and disruptions during the first two years
following transplantation and, thus, avoid serious
psychiatric difficulties.

The purpose of the present study is to provide a comprehensive assessment of aspects of quality of life that
are and are not disrupted during these important first two
post-operative years and to identify the coping strategies
that appear to be most common and helpful to patients in
facing the variety of problems that may arise during this
period. These data could help recipients, their families,
and their caregivers to prepare for the likely impacts of
transplantation and ongoing treatment. Physicians and
nurses can reassure patients when their reactions fall
within normal limits or can provide early referrals for
mental health intervention when reactions are extreme.
Knowledge of common and successful coping strategies can
be useful both to individual patients and to transplantation centers in developing patient programs.

MATERIALS AND METHODS

Subjects

All adult heart transplant recipients at Vanderbilt
University were approached for participation in this study
if they: (1) were at least one-month post-transplantation
(2) were not hospitalized at the time of the study, and
(3) had received their surgery within the preceding two
years. One patient was excluded who was unable to complete
questionnaires due to serious visual and memory deficits.
Of the 20 eligible patients, 18 participated (response
rate = 90%). Table 1 provides descriptive data on this
sample. Fourteen of the 18 participating patients had
partners or spouses, all of whom agreed to participate.

Table 1. Characteristics of Patient Sample

Gender	
Male	78%
Female	22%
Age	
21-30	11%
31-40	11%
41-50	33%
51-60	39%
> 60	6%

Education
<pre>
    < 12 years of school   17%
    High school graduate   56%
    College graduate   22%
    Postgraduate education   6%

Months Since Transplant
         < 7   39%
        7-12   22%
       13-18   17%
       19-24   22%
</pre>

Procedures

The transplant clinical nurse specialist (JM) approached each patient and his or her partner or spouse at the time of a scheduled medical visit. She described the study and, if they consented, provided the patient and spouse or partner with a questionnaire packet. The questionnaire packets were identified by code number and were returned to a separate data collection office in a stamped envelope that accompanied the questionnaires. The physicians and nurses involved in patient care never saw individual patient responses. The transplant nurse completed a questionnaire packet on each recipient as well.

Instruments

We developed the questionnaire packets to provide a multi-faceted assessment of quality of life and coping. Key variables relevant to the present report are listed on Table 2. Both patients and spouses/partners completed the Profile of Mood States [5] (POMS), a 65-item adjective checklist that provides ratings of the levels of six moods experienced over the preceding week, and the Dyadic Adjustment Scale [6] (DAS), a two-page questionnaire that assesses the quality of an intimate relationship. Scores of over 100 on the DAS are indicative of a stable and satisfying relationship. We measured additional aspects of patients' quality of life through two questionnaires designed for this study. A symptom/feeling checklist was fashioned after a scale designed by Lough and her colleagues [2]. On 5-point Likert-type scales patients rated both the frequency with which they experienced and the extent to which they became upset by each of 50 symptoms or fears/concerns. A quality of life scale contained 42 questions that tapped functional status, sexual functioning and satisfaction, social support, overall level of and

satisfaction with quality of life, and adherence to
medical recommendations on 7-point Likert-type scales.
Patients also completed Derogatis' Symptom Checklist-90
[7] (SCL-90), which assesses level of psychopathology, and
Folkman and Lazarus' Ways of Coping Checklist [8]. On the
Ways of Coping Checklist, respondents indicate on 4-point
scales the extent to which they had used each of 66
specific coping strategies in the past month to deal with
any problems caused by their physical condition and
medical treatments. Respondents also indicate whether
they found the strategies that they used to be helpful.

The nurse completed three questionnaires: (1) a
demographic and medical data form; (2) a nurse rating
form that assessed each patient's level of physical
symptomatology, functional ability, social support,
quality of life, and adherence to medical recommendations;
and (3) the Global Adjustment to Illness Scale [9] (GAIS).
On the GAIS, an observer rates a patient's overall level
of psychosocial adjustment to illness on a scale ranging
from 1=severely impaired adjustment to 100=excellent
adjustment. The scale contains clear operational
definitions for each decile.

Table 2. Key Constructs Assessed

Demographic and Medical Data+

Quality of Life

        Mood state*
        Physical symptomatology+
        Functional abilities+
        Fear/concerns
        Marital satisfaction*
        Sexual functioning and satisfaction
        Social support+
        Other sources of difficulty
        Overall rating of quality of life and level of
            satisfaction+

Psychopathology

Coping+

Adherence to Medical Recommendations+

---

* Data also available from spouse/partner
+ Data also available from nurse

RESULTS AND DISCUSSION

Areas in Which Problems Were Reported

Fifty-six percent of patients stated that their lives were at least moderately disrupted by their medical condition. Patients reported having problems including physical symptoms, sleep difficulties and fatigue, moodiness, sexual dysfunction and dissatisfaction, dissatisfaction with body image, fears and concerns about the future, and work and financial difficulties.

Physical symptoms were very common and all patients indicated that they were highly aware of any slight change in physical condition. Half of the patients became upset when they noticed any such change. The specific symptoms that a majority of respondents reported having frequently were bruising, fluid retention, fragile skin, headaches, hypertension, joint pain, muscle cramps, overeating, pain, poor vision, lack of strength, shakiness, and tremors. The most distressing symptoms, reported as at least moderately upsetting by a majority of recipients, were muscle cramps and lack of strength. Sleep problems also were very common among respondents. Two-thirds of patients reported frequent fatigue and 56% reported a frequent lack of sleep. Lack of sleep was rated as at least moderately upsetting by half of the patients.

In addition to these physical problems, patients reported several areas of dissatisfaction and concern. Over half of the respondents indicated that they regularly experienced mood swings (61%), irritability (56%), and tearfulness (56%). Sexual difficulties were common for both men and women, with 50% of patients reporting that their sexual activities had decreased since the surgery and only one-third reporting satisfaction with their sexual functioning. Similarly, a majority of patients reported dissatisfaction with their physical appearance. Dissatisfaction with bodily appearance was reported by 61% of respondents and dissatisfaction with facial appearance was reported by 55%. Half of the recipients believed that their physical appearance had worsened since surgery, whereas only 17% felt that their appearance had improved.

Patients indicated that they had frequent thoughts or concerns about a number of topics. The most common were fears or concerns about the family's future (72%), thoughts about the heart donor (72%), thoughts about their physical condition (56%), and uncertainty about the future (56%).

Although these thoughts were quite common, only fears
about the future of the family were associated with at
least moderate distress for most patients (67%). Perhaps
the most common and upsetting issue facing these heart
transplant recipients, however, involved the financial
problems resulting from the cost of treatment and loss of
work. Only one patient reported no financial difficulties.
Forty-seven percent stated that they were completely
unable to work.

Areas in Which Problems Were Not Reported

Despite these problems, there is clear evidence that
not all areas were associated with distress and disruption. The many physical symptoms that patients experienced did not seem to have a major impact on their overall ratings of health in that 61% considered themselves to
be in good to excellent health. Most recipients had high
levels of confidence in their treatment (72%). Almost all
patients expressed positive feelings about the treatment
and stated that they would recommend it to a friend with
similar health problems (94% in both cases).

Responses on standardized scales provided no evidence
of psychopathology or mood disturbance. Scores on the
SCL-90 indicated very low levels of psychiatric disturbance, except in the area of eating and sleeping disorders
in which slight to moderate disturbance was reported.
Consistent with the reports of physical symptomatology
described above, patients rated difficulty with early
morning wakenings, restless sleep, falling asleep, and
overeating. Although patients had reported a general
moodiness, their responses to the POMS did not reveal
either high levels of tension, depression, anger,and
confusion or low levels of vigor. On these five subscales,
patients' scores indicated more positive mood states than
were reported by the samples on which the scale was normed
(i.e., psychiatric inpatients and outpatients, adults who
did not require psychotherapy, and college students).
Moreover, patients' reponses did not differ significantly
from the responses provided by their spouses. It was only
on the Fatigue subscale that patients obtained elevated
scores.

In addition to an absence of psychiatric morbidity,
recipients reported low levels of disturbance of functional
abilities and interpersonal relationships. Half of the
respondents rated their physical capabilities as good to
excellent, with two-thirds stating that they were quite

satisfied with their abilities to perform their daily activities. With the exception of work, over 60% of patients reported at least moderate ability to perform each of a variety of activities. Improvements in functional abilities since transplantation were reported by 56% of recipients.

A majority of patients indicated that they had good to excellent relationships with their spouse/partners, children, other family members, friends, coworkers, doctors and nurses, and other patients. Sixty-one percent of recipients rated their overall level of emotional support as good to excellent, with only 11% indicating moderately low levels of support. For the vast majority, relationships had either improved or remained unchanged since surgery. The nurse rated all patients as having high levels of support. Intimate relationships also appeared to be quite strong. On the DAS, patients received a mean relationship adjustment score of 112 and their spouses/partners obtained a mean score of 109, both of which are well above the 100 point cut-off that indicates a satisfying and stable relationship.

It appears that these positive aspects were more important than the many problems reported in determining overall quality of life. When asked to assess the quality of their lives, two-thirds of patients gave ratings of good to excellent. An even higher proportion of patients (80%) reported being satisfied with the quality of their lives. Nurse's ratings of each patient's quality of life yielded very similar results, with the nurse reporting that 83% of patients had positive quality of life. Moreover, 88% of recipients rated their future outlook as positive and 75% described their lives as being improved since transplant surgery.

Table 3.   Patient and Nurse Ratings of Patients' Level of Adjustment

Patient Ratings

Response	Percent
Coping exceptionally well	29%
Coping well	41%
Coping adequately	24%
Coping poorly	6%
Coping exceptionally poorly	0%

Nurse GAIS [9] Ratings

Response	Percent
Excellent adjustment (91-100)	25%
Very good adjustment (81-90)	33%
Good adjustment (71-80)	25%
Adequate adjustment (61-70)	17%

Coping and Adjustment

These data suggest that patients somehow managed to cope with the demands of their illness in a way that limited the disruption in their lives. Indeed, when asked to rate their coping, the vast majority of recipients felt that they were doing well (see Table 3). The patients' ratings of their coping were highly correlated with the nurse's scores of patients' adjustment to their illness on the GAIS. As can be seen on Table 3, the nurse felt that all patients had made at least an adequate adjustment; all scores fell in the upper half of the GAIS rating scale.

Further evidence of successful coping can be found in the high levels of adherence to medical recommendations that were reported by both recipients and nurses. No more than 11% of patients reported nonadherence with any specific recommendation. The nurse reported that all patients had good compliance in all areas except getting adequate exercise, where only one-third of patients were rated as having good to excellent adherence. One-third of patients stated that they considered themselves to be overly cautious in avoiding health-threatening situations. The nurse, however, felt that all patients were appropriately cautious.

Table 4.   Illustrative Examples of the Coping Strategy
            Categories that Patients Reported as Common
            and Helpful on the Ways of Coping Checklist [8]

	% Using Strategy
Positive Reappraisal	
-"Rediscover what is important in life"	88%
-"Pray"	94%

	% Using Strategy
Planful Problem-solving	
-"Just concentrate on what I have to do next -- the next step"	89%
-"Draw on past experiences; I was in a similar situation before"	71%
Seeking Social Support	
-"Talk to someone to find out more about the situation"	94%
-"Talk to someone who can do something concrete about the problem"	88%
Self-controlling	
-"I try to keep my feelings to myself"	82%
-"I go over in my mind what I will say or do"	94%

What did patients do to achieve such positive coping for the most part? Table 4 contains a list of the four categories of coping responses that were most commonly reported and rated as most helpful on the Ways of Coping Checklist. Illustrative examples of specific coping responses that fall into each of these categories also are provided. For each of these examples, at least half of the respondents who had attempted the coping response stated that it had been helpful in adjusting to the demands of the illness.

It is interesting to note that patients both tried to seek social support and tried to keep their feelings to themselves. This apparent contradiction may be explained in part by the following results: Although patients over- whelmingly reported positive social support from their family and friends, they also reported some difficulty in having people understand their situation. When asked "how often do you have to put up a front and pretend that things are better than they are in order to protect others," 75% of recipients reported doing this with some frequency. Only 30% stated that people in their lives understood well what they were going through.

Table 5 provides a list of those coping stragegy categories that were found to be helpful by fewer than one-quarter of the sample. In some cases the strategies were simply not tried; whereas, in other cases, a number of individuals attempted the response, but did not con- sider it to have been helpful. Illustrations of both types of responses are listed on the Table.

Table 5. Illustrative Examples of the Coping Stragegy
          Categories that Patients Reported as Either
          Uncommon or Unhelfpul on the Ways of Coping
          Checklist [8]

	% Using strategy	% finding strategy helpful
Escape/Avoidance		
-"Hope a miracle will happen"	53%	20%
-"Try to make myself feel better by eating, drinking, smoking, using drugs or medication, etc."	0%	0%
Confrontive Coping		
-"Stand my ground and fight for what I want"	76%	24%
-"Take a big chance or do something risky"	12%	12%
Accepting Responsibility		
-"Realize I brought the problem on myself"	53%	6%
-"Criticize or lecture myself"	47%	18%

CONCLUSIONS

Clearly, these data are very preliminary and must be
interpreted cautiously. The sample size is extremely
small and the data do not allow us to draw causal conclusions to determine the extent to which reactions were due
to transplantation and ongoing treatment. Nonetheless,
these data suggest the feasibility and potential value of
assessing quality of life and coping in a comprehensive
way from multiple sources including the patient, his or
her family, and the medical staff. The data also suggest
that patients have many problems during the first two
years after successful heart transplantation, but that
most recipients learn to cope well. People working and
living with patients should neither overlook the many
problems facing recipients nor underestimate their
abilities to cope.

We have used the results of this study to design an
ongoing longitudinal study of quality of life and coping
among recipients and their families throughout pre- and

post-transplant adjustment. We hope to provide useful
descriptive and predictive data to identify which difficulties are most serious and which coping approaches may
be most fruitful.

REFERENCES

1. M. J. McAleer, J. Copeland, J. Fuller, and J. G.
   Copeland, Psychological aspects of heart transplantation, Heart Transplant. 4:232 (1985).
2. M. E. Lough, A. M. Lindsey, J. A. Shinn, and N. A.
   Stotts, Impact of symptom frequency and symptom
   distress on self-reported quality of life in heart
   transplant recipients, Heart Lung. 16:193 (1987).
3. F. M. Mai, F. N. McKenzie, W.J. Kostuk, Psychiatric
   aspects of heart transplantation: Preoperative
   evaluation and postoperative sequelae, Br. Med. J.
   292:311 (1986).
4. M. E. Lough, A. M. Lindsey, J. A. Shinn, & N. A.
   Stotts, Life satisfaction following heart
   transplantation, Heart Transplant. 4:446 (1985).
5. D. M. McNair, M. Lorr, L. F. Droppleman, "Manual:
   Profile of Mood States," Educational and Industrial
   Testing Service, San Diego (1971).
6. G. B. Spanier, Measuring dyadic adjustment: New
   scales for assessing the quality of marriage and
   similar dyads, J Marriage and Family, February: 15
   (1976).
7. L. Derogatis, "Administration, scoring and procedures
   manual for the SCL 90," Johns Hopkins University,
   Baltimore (1977).
8. S. Folkman, R. S. Lazarus, C. Dunkel-Schetter, A.
   DeLongis, and R. J. Gruen, Dynamics of a stressful
   encounter: Cognitive appraisal, coping, and
   encounter outcomes, J Person Soc Psychol. 50:992
   (1986).
9. L. R. Derogatis, "Global Adjustment to Illness Scale,"
   Johns Hopkins University, Baltimore (1975).

DEVELOPMENT OF A CONSTRUCT OF PSYCHOLOGICAL DEPENDENCY IN

PATIENTS WITH THE AUTOMATIC IMPLANTABLE CARDIOVERTER

DEFIBRILLATOR: A QUALITY OF LIFE ISSUE

Elizabeth Piasecki, Mary Gutmann,
Kathi Axtell, Patrick Tchou

University of Wisconsin Medical School
Sinai Samaritan Medical Center
Milwaukee, WI

Cardiologists involved with implantation and continuous follow-up of patients implanted with the automatic
implantable cardioverter defibrillator (AICD) have begun
to question how the patient interacts psychologically with
the device. Research to date on the psychological complications of AICD implantation has been sparse. A retrospective, descriptive study was designed to structure and
assess the numerous variables associated with AICD
implantation and psychosocial outcome.

DESCRIPTION OF DEVICE

The currently available device (Ventak-C, Cardiac
Pacemakers, Inc.) weighs approximately 290 grams and is
11.2 x 7.1 x 2.5 cm. in dimension. The device is capable
of monitoring ventricular rates via sensing electrodes
that are implanted directly on the epicardium or attached
to the endocardium through a transvenous approach. The
most common way of implanting the shocking electrodes is
by direct attachment of two patch electrodes epicardially.
These patch electrodes are also used at times to sense QRS
morphology. Implantation of the electrodes is done by
sternotomy or thoracotomy at this medical center. The
generator unit itself is implanted subcutaneously or
submuscularly over the abdomen. The electrode leads are

Impact of Cardiac Surgery on the Quality of Life
Edited by A. E. Willner and G. Rodewald
Plenum Press, New York, 1990

tunnelled to the site of the generator and plugged into
the generator. Patients may undergo concomitant coronary
artery bypass grafting, valve replacement, or other
corrective cardiac surgery at the time of implantation.

Stated succinctly, the AICD senses the presence of
an abnormal and potentially fatal cardiac arrhythmia and
delivers an internal 25-30 joule shock to the heart to
convert the abnormality to normal sinus rhythm. The
generator has the capacity to deliver 100 shocks and a
battery life of approximately two years at the current
time. Device discharge is clearly unpleasant but not
overtly painful. It has been likened to being kicked in
the chest from the inside and may be preceded by feelings
of dizziness, and occasional loss of consciousness.

PURPOSE OF THE STUDY

Clinical experience suggested that some AICD patients
seemed to respond to implantation with a renewed sense of
vigor and with a more normalized quality of life. Adjustment in others, however, has been far more problematic.
Fear of shock due to its unpredictability, emotional
reactions to the number of shocks received, body image
changes, the need for battery monitoring and the fear of
battery failure along with self-directed reductions in
physical, social, and sexual activity have contributed to
a heightened degree of implant salience. Clinical reports
from the professionals involved and the few reports of
psychological reactions of AICD patients available in the
literature [1, 2, 3] suggest that, for some patients, the
AICD may act as a stimulus which evokes dependent responses
such that it becomes a central organizing factor in
psychosocial adjustment. This kind of response could be
construed as a high dependency reaction to AICD implantation. For others, the device may function as a relatively
neutral medical intervention which is largely ego-syntonic
and which promotes a renewed sense of physical well-being.
This response can be seen as indicative of a low
dependency reaction.

This study had as its purpose the organization of
medical and psychological variables relevant to this
question of psychological dependency. Development of a
construct of AICD dependency was judged useful as a tool
to permit meaningful statistical analysis of patient
outcomes and to make identification of risk factors
associated with poor psychosocial adjustment to implantation possible in later research. This construct was

subsequently developed and then assessed in 60 patients implanted at Sinai Samaritan Medical Center. Preliminary results are offered here.

THE AICD DEPENDENCY CONSTRUCT

A review of the artificial pacemaker and AICD literature revealed no studies which have examined psychological dependency per se. Levy [4], however, has proposed that what has been learned about hemodialysis can be seen as a model for other medical modalities which evoke machine related dependency. That model was adapted to fit the specifics of AICD implantation and was utilized as the central concept in the development of the AICD-specific dependency construct.

The Levy model offers the initial assumption that stress of the disease is compounded by stress of the treatment. Construct variables include dependency and independency concerns, stress associated with chronicity of illness, the actual intervention itself, multiple losses, the expectation of others, and psychological reactions and medical complications. Stress associated with the expectation of others was judged to be better assessed in a prospective way and with input from spouses and family. Since, by design, this was a retrospective descriptive study focused on patient reaction, this component was not included in the AICD-specific dependency construct at this time. Because the central function of the AICD is delivery of shock, inclusion of another component, that of the perception of control over the number of shocks received and the correlative coping strategies utilized for that purpose were included in the AICD dependency construct. At the time of implantation, patients are instructed that they have no control over when the device will discharge. It became apparent, however, from clinical experience that some patients do not believe this and that many patients engage in behaviors directed at reduction of shock. It was hypothesized, then, for this study, that the use of coping strategies could exert a substantial impact on whether or not the device became a central organizing factor in psychosocial adjustment (high dependency).

Specifically for AICD patients, dependency and independency concerns included changes in independent functioning because of dependent/independent personality variables and change due to reality-based medical

dependency. Here the main issues for AICD patients
involved reliance on medical staff for treatment and
follow-up which could evoke a heightened degree of implant
salience. Patients are followed bimonthly and then monthy
as the device's battery approaches its normal end of life
(16-24 months post implantation). Patients must call in
every time the device discharges and must return to the
medical center if the device continues to discharge more
than several times in a short period of time. This
realistic medical dependency exists for the rest of the
patient's life. Any measure of change in the patient's
premorbid level of independence as a personality variable
could only be assessed by self-report since the sample in
this study had not undergone formal pre-implantation
psychological evaluation.

    Stress associated with the chronicity of illness was
judged very applicable for inclusion in the AICD dependency
construct since many of these patients have had long and
complicated cardiac histories with multiple cardiac diagnoses and prominent comorbidity factors. Most patients
have experienced one or more episodes of sudden cardiac
death and have failed long serial drug trials for control
of their malignant arrhythmia. All of these factors
impinge on perceived chronicity and contribute to cumulative stress. The number of pre-implant drugs failed,
number of sudden death episodes prior to implantation,
left ventricular ejection fraction, NYHA functional class,
comorbidity factors for each patient, number of cardiac
diagnoses, type of myocardial infarction if present by
history, and clinical arrhythmia type were all assessed
and included as variables in this study.

    A number of factors were singled out for assessment
relating to the stress of implantation itself. Threat of
infection of the generator pocket, worry about technological failure, the threat of battery failure, fear of
shock due to its unpredictability, body image changes,
psychological discomfort due to the number of shocks
received, fear of the pain of being shocked, concern for
repeat surgery, and concern over device effectiveness were
all included as dependent variables.

    This study also examined a number of potential losses
for AICD patients which could increase implant salience
and cause higher dependency reactions in some individuals:
loss of control, loss of physical, social, or sexual
activity, and threat of loss of life. Functional limitations were rated by responders as being due, in their

perception, to implantation with the AICD per se or as a result of general cardiac status and/or due to side effects from medication. Family changes were also assessed via patient report. Overall ratings of family change in the negative direction, that is, that a patient perceived that his/her family situation had worsened as a result of implantation, were considered to contribute to a higher dependency reaction and interpreted as loss of functional or emotional support within the family system.

Depression was considered to be a significant variable to assess independently. Other emotional reactions including discouragement, anxiety, impatience, feeling restricted, worry, hypervigilance about the implant, etc., were considered in a more generalized screening fashion with higher scores indicative of more psychological complications, creating a greater impact of implantation on psychosocial functioning.

METHOD

An AICD-specific questionnaire was developed which included items relative to all construct variables. In addition, the Beck Depression Inventory (BDI) [5] was also administered. Demographic information and medical data from chart review were also obtained.

Approximately one hundred patients constituted the potential subject pool at the time of this study. Sixty patients returned questionnaires. An overall dependency score was computed for each responder. In addition, subscores were computed for each construct variable and for the Beck Depression Inventory. Data were analyzed utilizing the SAS computer program. Descriptive statistics were developed for the sample patient profile. Pearson product moment correlations were computed for all independent variables with each other and with the overall dependency score, the subscores, and the BDI score.

RESULTS

Mean age for responders was 60.5 (SD: 13.4). Age ranged from 20 to 84 years. Twenty-two percent were female; seventy-eight percent were male. Fifteen percent were single while the remaining 85 percent were currently married. Seventy-seven percent were diagnosed with coronary artery disease. Thirty-five percent had

sustained ventricular tachycardia, while fifty-seven
percent suffered from recurrent ventricular fibrillation.
Mean number of sudden death episodes prior to implant was
1.2 (SD: 0.8).   Mean number of pre-implant drugs failed
was 2.9 (SD: 2.3).   Mean number of shocks received since
first implantation was 5.5 (SD: 9.2).   Mean number of
months since first implantation was 26 (SD: 17.9).

     Variables which were found to correlate significantly
with higher overall dependency scores were younger age
(r = 0.36, p= .005), single marital status (r = 0.39,
p= .002), and fewer cardiac diagnoses (r = 0.39,
p= .002).   Notable variables not correlated with overall
higher dependency scores were left ventricular ejection
fraction, the number of sudden death episodes prior to
implant, use of a current amiodarone drug regimen, and
frequency of shocks received.

     On the BDI, 77.6% of patients scored within normal
limits.   Mild to moderate depression was reported by
15.5%.   Moderate to severe depression was reported by 1.7%
while 5.1% reported extremely severe levels of depression.

     Although 66% of resonders believed they had no control
over the number of shocks they received, virtually all
reported the use of coping strategies to control shock to
minimize the impact of the AICD on their lives.   Approximately 5% of responders chose to center their lives around
the AICD, while 36% said they avoided emotional upset.
Fifteen percent said they depended a great deal on medical
staff as their way of coping with implantation.

     Approximately 85% of patients reported that implanta-
tion had significantly reduced their families' fear of the
patient experiencing sudden death. When asked specifically
about the impact of implantation on the quality of family
life, a disturbing 19% said that the AICD had not contributed to an improved quality of life for their families
at all.

     The results were suggestive of the following
preliminary conclusions:

     1.   The incidence of clinical depression in AICD
          patients is approximately 20 percent which is
          generally comparable to the general population.
     2.   Being married is correlated with lower dependency
          scores and better psychological adjustment.

3. Almost one out of five patients reported that the AICD did not improve the quality of their family life. This satistic is derived by patient report and may differ if family members' perceptions were sampled. Nevertheless, it is suggestive that assessment of the impact of the meaning of implantation and the demands of follow-up for the cardiac family at large may need to be specifically addressed by the AICD treatment team for optimal outcome for all patients.
4. Younger AICD patients report higher dependency and higher levels of depression.
5. Patients who have more serious disease tend to view the device in a more positive way.
6. The more traditional medical indicators of cardiac function are <u>not</u> predictive of psychological dependence on the device.
7. Functional limitations due to the device per se are reported to be minimal. Antiarrhythmic drug side effects and cardiac status are viewed as far more contributory to losses of functional status than the AICD itself.

RECOMMENDATIONS

Patient education may ameliorate some of the stress related to medical complications, fear, and management of adverse drug side effects. Care should be taken to assess the meaning and impact of AICD implantation on the entire cardiac family. Younger patients with fewer cardiac diagnoses are more at risk for negative psychological response to AICD implantation and should be targeted for follow-up intervention.

REFERENCES

1. S. Vlay, The AICD: Comprehensive clinical follow-up, economic and social impact - The Stony Brook Experience, <u>American Heart Journal</u>, 112: 189-194 (1986).
2. D. Cooper, R. Luceri, R. Thurer, R. Myerburg, The impact of the automatic implantable cardioverter defribillator on quality of life, <u>Clinical Progress in Electrophysiology and Pacing</u>, 4: 306-309 (1986).
3. A. Brodsky, AICD wearers cite fear, gratitude, and wish for smaller device, <u>Cardiovascular Disease Reports</u>, 10: 15-19 (1989)

4. N. Levy, Psychological reactions to machine
       dependency: Hemodialysis, <u>Psychiatric clinics of
       North America</u>, 4: 351-353 (1981).
5. A. Beck., R. Steer, "Beck Depression Inventory
       Manual," The Psychological Corporation: Harcourt
       Brace Jovanovich, Inc., San Antonio (1987).

QUALITY OF LIFE ISSUES AND PSYCHOLOGICAL TREATMENT

STRATEGIES AFFECTING CORONARY ARTERY DISEASE DURING

CONVALESCENCE AND REHABILITATION

M. Williams

Summit Psychological Associates
San Francisco, CA

INTRODUCTION

Over the past 20 years, researchers have shown that psychological factors influence cardiovascular health, function and disease. This paper describes identifiable dynamic phases of psychological recovery and adaptation to myocardial infarction (MI) during convalescence and rehabilitation. Psychological intervention strategies that enhance the quality of life for patients with coronary heart disease (CAD) are discussed.

Chronic emotional distress and disability can occur as secondary consequences of cardiovascular disease. The literature [1-9] on post-MI psychological recovery suggests that an understanding of psychological sequelae is important to ensure that all aspects of the disease are treated.

There are three main phases following an MI during which distinct dynamic psychological reactions can occur: prehospital phase, inpatient phase (acute stage and con-valescent stage) and rehabilitation or post-hospital phase. Table 1 describes the psychological reactions during convalescence and rehabilitation.

Impact of Cardiac Surgery on the Quality of Life
Edited by A. E. Willner and G. Rodewald
Plenum Press, New York, 1990

Table 1.   Psychological Reactions to Coronary Artery
           Disease During Convalescence and Rehabilitation

A.   Acute Phase (Days 1-3)

B.   Convalescent Phase (Day 4 - Discharge)

   1. Cardiac surgery leads to more psychological
      complications than any other major surgery [10].

   2. Psychiatric disorders occur in 25% to 50% of
      cardiac surgery cases, with open heart surgery
      having twice as many psychological complications
      as closed heart procedures.

   3. Disorders include delirium, paranoid psychosis,
      mixed affective syndrome.

   4. Denial in low to moderate levels has highest 5
      year survival rate.

        - High levels delay treatment, return to work
          prematurely, comply poorly with treatment,
          remain overactive, deny symptoms.

   5. Anxiety appears during first few days and is
      diminished by supportive care, reassurance and
      information.

   6. Depression becomes apparent around day 4 and is
      part of normal grief reaction.

   7. Behavior problems begin on Day 4.

        - Hostile or disruptive behavior lessens as
          sense of security increases.

        - Difficult patients showing preexisting
          passive, paranoid or obsessive personality
          traits are usually reverting to life-long
          patterns of coping.

        - Intolerance of medical regime is a sign of
          denial.

   8. Delirium occurs 3 to 5 days post-MI and can last
      5 to 7 days.

- Symptoms: agitation, hallucinations, impaired memory and orientation, shallow or labile affect, sleep-wake cycle disruption.

C. Rehabilitation/Outpatient Phase

1. Depression is the most frequent reaction and is a major goal of psychological rehabilitation.

   - "Homecoming depression" is evident in first 48 hours of discharge.

   - Long lasting depression, return to work problems and family turmoil persist in 25% of patients.

   - Spouses develop depression and somatic symptoms.

2. Anxiety surfaces in the form of sleep disturbances, fear of activity and fear of resuming sexual relations.

3. Denial may be mobilized in response to spouse's anxiety, leading to premature return to work and/or minimization of symptoms.

4. Sexual dysfunction is most often related to anxiety and depression.

   - 48% to 58% of patients do not return to previous levels of sexual functioning.

5. Family problems can occur even when premorbid home life is stable.

   - Problems with issues of dependence/ independence, guilt feelings and manipulations are most frequent.

   - Unmarried patients and those dissatisfied with marriage have more complications at the 1 year recovery point.

6. Chronic illness behavior or "cardiac invalidism" is shown by patients who are unwilling to abandon the sick role.

CONVALESCENT PHASE

Convalescence is the transitional period of reintegration to a previous level of functioning that begins approximately 3 to 4 days after the acute onset and treatment of a MI and continues until discharge from the hospital. Psychosocial factors such as marital status, role identity, age, cultural background, personality predisposition and availability of economic and social support influence the patient's progress through this phase. Some patients never advance past convalescence while others may reach a new level of healthy adaptation that surpasses their predisease functioning.

The course of adaptation to cardiac disease during convalescence is comparable to the process of grieving. A myocardial infarction is perceived as an unwanted or unexpected event which is a significant loss of a state of health or well-being. The resulting body changes and struggle with developmental issues raised by transition from one phase of adulthood to the next, such as from middle age to retirement age. After the initial shock and disbelief following a MI, just as with the loss experienced at the death of a loved one, the coronary patient begins the working-through process of adaptation to a major life change.

A new set of activiites, interests and renewed relationships is necessary for a sense of hope and of a future in living the new reality. As with grief, convalescence has a natural course to run. Although the rate at which this happens varies with the individual, there are predictable psychological phases of recovery which appear to be universal. The psychological reactions that most characterize the convalescent phase include denial, anxiety, depression and behavior problems.

Denial

Denial is one of the most recurring and varied psychological reactions of cardiac patients. The concept of denial includes both suppression (conscious) and classical denial (unconscious) [11]. The degree of denial determines whether there will be maladaptive or adaptive consequences. The ability to use denial as a positive coping mechanism for MI is indispensable for a good prognosis [12, 13]. Coronary patients with a low to moderate level of denial throughout their illness tend to have a

better 5-year survival rate than patients without denial
[6]. The patient who uses positive denial recognizes the
illness, but doesn't dwell upon symptoms and remains
optimistic about the future. Patients with negative
denial patterns usually delay medical attention and may
refuse to comply with medical restrictions.

Depression

In most cases, the greater the myocardial impairment,
the greater the patient's depression [7]. Anxiety and
depression occur together clinically. However, anxiety
is more apparent during the acute phases of cardiac illness, while depression is associated with chronicity [10].
Adaptation to cardiac disease during convalescence may be
compared to a grieving process, and patients described as
depressed may be having normal grief reactions. Marked
psychomotor retardation, feelings of worthlessness, and
suicidal ideation, however, are not elements of normal
grieving. Some post-MI depressions are a continuation of
an affective disorder predating the infarction. Others
are states of protracted convalescence in which the
patient is unwilling to abandon the sick role. Some
cardiac patients develop a chronic disability that is out
of proportion to their actual dysfunction and usually is
a result of anxiety over recurrrence of MI. In some
cases, especially among blue collar workers and educa-
tionally deprived patients, sick role behavior may be
reinforced if the patient receives disability compensation.
Current estimates indicate that about 1 in 6 cardiac
patients never return to work for psychological reasons
[10].

Behavioral Problems

Behavioral problems can frequently occur during the
convalescent phase. Usually the predominantly obsessive
patient will need to feel more in control, the paranoid
patient will be more guarded and suspicious, and the
passive patient will have a greater need to be cared for
[7]. Hostile or disruptive behavior usually subsides as
the sense of security increases, but patients who remain
difficult usually are reverting to a life-long pattern of
coping behavior [6]. Patients with trait anxiety and
habitual over-concern about body integrity may respond
with an overt anxiety reaction or hypochondriases.
Persons who fear passivity, dependence or enforced inactivity may not follow medical advice or rehabilitative
efforts [10].

Delirium

Delirium usually occurs 3 to 5 days after a myocardial infarction [7]. Since delirium can last 5 to 7
days, it is considered a subset of the convalescent
phase. Disruption of the sleep-wake cycle, impaired perception (hallucinations), agitation, impaired memory and
orientation, faulty judgment and shallow or labile affect
are characteristics. Delirium is especially common in
elderly patients receiving certain medications [4], or
may be due to lack of privacy, communication difficulties
and absence of windows (day-night reversal). Prompt
intervention in delirium following MI is essential as
agitation may increase demand on the cardiovascular
system and increase the chance of complications.

It is notable that cardiac surgery, especially open
heart surgery, is followed by psychological complications
more often than any other major surgery. Psychiatric
disorders range in frequency from 25% to 50% of cardiac
surgery cases, with open heart surgery having twice as
many psychiatric complications as closed heart procedures.
Besides delirum, the most commonly reported disorders
following open heart surgery include paranoid psychosis
and a mixed affective syndrome characterized by varying
degrees of anxiety, depression, apathy or elation [10].

REHABILITATION PHASE

The rehabilitation phase officially begins after
discharge from the hospital, although rehabilitative
efforts are initiated during convalescence.

Depression

The first month at home frequently is a critical
time of adjustment for the cardiac patient and family.
The joy of returning home often vanishes in the first 48
hours and is replaced by "homecoming depression" [9].
Expectations of physical recovery and a return to former
health are often contradicted by the reality of weakness,
fatigue, and dietary, sexual and recreational limits.
Anxiety begins to surface in the form of sleep disturbances, and patients often fear the recurrence of symptoms
when normal activities are resumed. Sexual dysfunction
usually is related to depression and anxiety.

Depression has been found in 15% - 20% of post-MI patients during their 1 month follow-up visit [6]. If left untreated, 75% of these patients continued to be depressed, half showing increased depressive symptoms at their 1 year follow-up examination. Long lasting depression, return to work problems and family turmoil persisted in 25% of patients [1]. Of the nearly 5 million persons in 1985 who had a history of heart attack, angina or both [14], the 25% depression rate suggests as many as 1,250,000 post-MI patients with longstanding depression.

Family Problems

The spouse's fear of recurrence of a MI can lead to overprotective behavior which includes an avoidance of sexual contact. Conflict between patient and family can occur even when the marriage and premorbid home life are stable. Long-term marital problem areas, particularly issues of dependence/independence, tend to worsen following a MI.

A negative coping pattern observed in cardiac patients involves the use of heart disease to control or manipulate family members by taking advantage of their guilt feelings or sympathy [10]. A longitudinal study of more than 600 male cardiac patients investigated the relationship of well-being to emotional intimacy in marriage [15]. Data indicated that love resources were a major determinant of long-term adjustment to cardiac illness. Married patients with a close emotional bond to their wives appeared to have significantly higher feelings of well-being and less complications at the 1 year recovery point.

PSYCHOLOGICAL TREATMENT STRATEGIES

Overall, the current literature suggests the following guidelines concerning psychological interventions for post-MI convalescence and rehabilitation: 1) intervention should be early, systematic, specific, graduated and educational; 2) specific treatment of depression should begin as early as day three; 3) social supports must be involved and mobilized; 4) continuity and follow-up are needed up to 3 years post-MI; and 5) didactic, supportive and cognitive-behavioral group therapy is desirable for general post-MI psychosocial recovery [1]. Table 2 summarizes the specific psychological treatment strategies that improve quality of life for CAD patients during convalescence and rehabilitation.

Table 2.   Psychological Treatment Strategies During
            Convalescence and Rehabilitation

Medical Phase	Psychological Treatment
A. Prehospital	
B. Cardiac Event Acute Phase (day 1-3)	Support, Information, Reassurance
C. Convalescent Phase (day 4 - discharge)	Psychological Consultation Brief Targeted Intervention Didactic Information Psychosocial Support
D. Rehabilitation	
- Early (post discharge)	Psychometric Evaluation Individual, Group, and/or Family Consultation
- Middle (2 wks. post discharge - 3 mos.)	Group for Psychosocial Support Group for Behavioral Change - Stress Management - Cognitive Strategies - Type A Behavior Change - Transition Management - Family Therapy - Sex Therapy
- Late (3 mos. - 1 yr. follow-up)	Individual Consultation Follow-up Support Group (x 1 mo. until end of 1st yr.) Follow-up Behavior Change Group (x 1 mo. until end of 1st yr.)
D. Consultation as needed	

Treatment strategies during convalescence are targeted for the specific psychological responses to CAD:
Anxiety, denial, depression and behavior problems.
Anxiety, which supportive care, information, and reassur-
ance can diminish, appears during the first days after a
MI. As the level of denial diminished and the patient
becomes more aware of the implications of cardiac injury,
signs of depression may be exhibited that indicate a need
for psychosocial intervention. Interventions are important and a patient's efforts to take responsibility and
participate in medical choices should begin while the
shock of the diagnosis is being fought and while the will
to live is being mobilized. However, for most patients,
a depressive reaction is self-limited and does not
require pharmacologic intervention [4].

Behavioral problems, such as failure to comply with
treatment or wanting to sign out against medical advice,
require individual assessment. Patients who remain difficult after the fourth day in the hospital are usually
reverting to preexisting personality characteristics and
psychiatric or psychological consultation may be
indicated.

Unlike the crisis-oriented, brief intervention
therapy that characterizes the convalescent phase, post-
hospital psychological interventions are more long-term
and may include individual, group or family consultations.
Psychometric evaluation provides baseline data for monitoring psychosocial progress as well as evaluation of
possible organic brain syndrome secondary to cardiac
surgery.

Group interventions are appealing to the majority of
MI patients who usually show enthusiastic involvement in
their recovery and who clearly seem to benefit psychologically from rehabilitation programs. In a widely
cited study of post-MI group therapy, Rahe and co-workers
[16] met with patients in 4 to 6 biweekly 90-minute group
sessions that began almost immediately after their MI.
Results 18 months post-MI showed that treated patients
had significantly fewer CAD events (coronary insufficiency, bypass surgery, reinfarction or CAD-related
death). The impact of treatment was even more evident at
3 years, which showed that combined mortality and recurrent
MI was reduced by 50%. Friedman and co-workers [17]
recently reported that modification of Type A behavior in
post-MI patients also reduced the rate of recurrent

cardiac events by 50% (from 13% to 7.2%) with the use of an intensive group counseling approach.

Family meetings and inclusion of spouse in the rehabilitation program help reduce distress and may decrease the likelihood of chronic invalidism, sexual dysfunction and marital problems [1, 2, 5].

Early psychological intervention is important, particularly when using methods of brief supportive therapy [1, 5]. Exercise programs have proven to significantly increase functional capacity and improve short-term but not long-term psychosocial outcome [1, 5, 16]. Exercise may provide the means of establishing a richer social support network for Type A patients who need structured challenges to help reorder their priorities in daily living. Type B and socially extroverted patients benefit psychologically from group exercise programs, while Type A and socially introverted patients may benefit more from solitary exercise programs which they have actively tailored to their own needs and interests [19]. Patients with severe affective disorders respond well to rehabilitation efforts that use movement in a low key, non-threatening way [20].

SUMMARY

There are predictable psychological reactions to myocardial infarction, which include denial, anxiety, depression, delirium and behavioral problems, during the convalescent phase as well as continued denial, depression, sexual dysfunction and family problems during rehabilitation. Although these psychological reactions are common, early intervention and rehabilitation can decrease long-term cardiovascular morbidity and mortality. Group treatment strategies that use a variety of methods, such as didactic information, social-emotional support and behavioral change (cognitive therapy, relaxation training, guided imagery, anger management) show the most significant results in decreasing CAD events and increasing the quality of life for cardiac patients.

REFERENCES

1. A. Razin, Coronary artery disease, Reducing the risk of illness and aiding recovery, in: "Helping Cardiac Patients," A Razin, ed., Jossey-Bass, San Francisco (1985).

2. A. Razin, Coronary artery disease, in: "Helping
    Patients and their Families Cope with Medical
    Problems," H. Roback, ed., Jossey-Bass, San
    Francisco (1984).
3. W. Gentry, R. Williams, eds., "Psychologic Aspects of
    Myocardial Infarction and Coronary Care," C. V.
    Mosby, St. Louis (1979).
4. M. Goldstein, Psychological aspects of cornary artery
    disease, The Journal of the Arkansas Medical
    Society. 83(5):205-216 (1986).
5. M. Stern, Psychosocial rehabilitation following
    myocardial infarction and coronary artery bypass
    surgery, in: "Rehabilitation of the Coronary
    Patient," N. Wenger and H. Hellerstein, eds.,
    Wiley, New York (1984).
6. M. Stern, The treatment of post-myocardial infarction
    depression, Practical Cardiology. 4:35-39 (1978).
7. R. Goldberg, Psychologic sequelae of myocardial
    infarction, American Family Physician. 25:209-121
    (1982).
8. N. Cassem, T. Hackett, Psychological aspects of
    myocardial infarction, Medical Clinics of North
    America. 61(4):711-721 (1977).
9. H. Wishnie, T. Hackett, and N. Cassem, Psychological
    hazards of convalescence following myocardial
    infarction, JAMA. 215(8):1292-1296 (1971).
10. M. Lipowski, Psychophysiological cardiovascular
    disorders, in: "Comprehensive Textbook of
    Psychiatry, 2nd Ed.," A. Freeman. H. Kaplan, and
    B. Sadock, eds., Williams, Baltimore (1975).
11. M. Freeman and D. Folks, "Psychiatric Aspects of
    Cardiovascular Disease, in: "Psychiatry, Vol. 2"
    R. Michels and J. Cavenar, eds., J. B. Lippincott,
    Philadelphia (1986).
12. J. Dimsdale and T. Hackett, Effect of denial on
    cardiac health and psychological assessment,
    American Journal of Psychiatry. 139(11):1477
    (1982).
13. W. Gentry, S. Foster, and T. Haney, Denial as a
    determinant of anxiety and perceived health status
    in the coronary care unit, Psychosomatic Medicine.
    34:39 (1972).
14. American Heart Association, 1986 Heart Facts. 1-3
    (1985).
15. W. Waltz, Marital context and post-infarction quality
    of life: Is it social support or something more?,
    Soc. Sci. Med. 22(8):791-805 (1986).
16. R. Rahe. H. Ward, and V. Hayes, Brief group therapy
    in myocardial infarction rehabilitation: Three to

four year follow-up of a controlled trial,
Psychosomatic Medicine. 41:229-242 (1979).

17. M. Friedman, C. Thoreson, J. Gill, L. Powell, L.
Ulmer, V. Thompson, A. Price, D. Rabin, W. Breall,
T. Dixon, R. Levy, and E. Boury, Alteration of
Type A behavior and reduction in cardiac
recurrences in postmyocardial infarction patients,
American Heart Jouranl. 108:237-248 (1984).

18. T. Hackett, N. Cassem, and H. Wishnie, The coronary
care unit: An appraisal of its psychologic
hazards, New England Journal of Medicine. 279:1365
(1968).

19. W. D. Gentry and M. Stewart, Psychologic effects of
exercise training in coronary-prone individuals
and in patients with symptomatic coronary heart
disease, Cardiovascular Clinics. 15(2):255-260
(1985).

20. M. Seides, Dance/movement therapy as a modality in
the treatment of the psychosocial complications of
heart disease, American Journal of Dance Therapy.
9:83-101 (1986).

APPENDIX

University of Hamburg

Federal Republic of Germany

1) **University Hospital, Hamburg-Eppendorf**

    a) Dept. of Thoracic and Cardiovascular Surgery

        P. Kalman
        H.-J. Krebber
        H.-J. Meffert
        H. Pokar
        G. Rodewald

    b) Dept. of Neurology

        Th. Emskotter
        L. Lachenmayer

    c) Dept. of Psychiatry

        P. Gotze

    d) Dept. of Psychosomatics

        U. Lamparter

Address:

    Universitats Krankenhaus Hamburg Eppendorf
    D-2000 Hamburg 20
    Martinistrasse 52
    Federal Republic of Germany

2) **Institute of Psychology**

    B. Dahme

Address:

    Psychologisches Institut III
    D-2000 Hamburg 13
    Von Park Melle 5

<u>Long Island Jewish Hospital</u>

Glen Oaks, NY

1) Department of Cardiothoracic Surgery

> John Bell-Thompson, M.D.
> Dennis Tyras, M.D.

2) Department of Neurology

> David Biddle, M.D.

3) Department of Psychiatry

> Phillip Goldberg, M.D.
> Charles J. Rabiner, M.D.
> Alice Stahl, M.D.

4) Department of Psychology

> Keneth E. Moeller, Ph.D.
> Allen E. Willner, Ph.D.

<u>Psychometricians</u>:

> Jill Bressler
> Ellen Diamond
> Gerry Hoban
> Gayle Kass
> Sharon Kaplowitz
> Sherry Kauderer
> Karen Louis
> Carol Ritter
> Janet Sendar
> Sharon Windwer

<u>Address</u>:

> Long Island Jewish Hospital
> P.O. Box 38
> Glen Oaks, NY 11004

St. Francis Hospital

Evanston, Illinois

Ralph Otto, M.D.

William Hoff, C.C.P.
Michael Quinlan, C.C.P.
Robert Tropp, C.C.P.
Susan Wener, C.C.P.

Samuel B. Kurut, M.D.
Suresh Wadhani, M.D.

Nancy Feys, Psy.D.
Joan Durlacher, M.A.
Jennifer Hoffman-Conviser, M.A.
James Schreffler, M.A.
Catherline Wilson, M.A.
Deborah Lynn Zamick, M.A.

Rita McCarthy

Address:

> St. Francis Hospital
> 355 Ridge Avenue
> Evanston, Illinois 60202

Clinica Shaio

Bogota, Columbia

Dr. Roberto Chaskel
Dr. Roberto Amador
Dr. Alberto Vejarano

Instituto do Coracao

Sao Paulo - Brazil

a) Div. of Thoracic and Cardiovascular Surgery

   Fabio Jatene
   Renato Assad
   Adib Jatene

b) Div. of Clinical Cardiology

   Ana Neri P. Miyasato

c) Services of Psychology

   Bellkiss Wilma Romano Lamosa
   Claudia Tayar
   Evani Zambon

d) Dept. of Neurology

   Renato G. Muttarelli
   Teraza Hirata
   Milberto Scaff

Address:

   Instituto do Coracao
   Av. Dr. Eneas de Carvalho Aguiar, 44
   Sao Paulo - Brazil - 05403

University of Oulu

Oulu, Finland

1) Psychologist

   Reijo Hirvenoja, M.A.

2) Neurologists

   Heikki Lidstrom, M.D.
   Matti Nikkanen, M.D.
   Merja Koivu, M.D.

3) Anaesthesiologists

   Risto Hanhela, M.D.
   Erkki Saarela, M.D.

4) Cardiologists

   Ulla Korhonen, M.D., Ph.D.
   Raimo Kettunen, M.D., Ph.D.

5) Surgeons

   Pentti Karkola, M.D., Ph.D. (Chief of the thoracic
                                    surgical ward)

   Martti Lepojarvi, M.D., Ph.D.
   Juha Nissinen, M.D.
   Risto Pokela, M.D.
   Matti Tarkka, M.D., Ph.D.

6) Special thanks for collaboration to following persons:

   Mrs. Marjatta Koivukangas, chief nurse of the
                                    thoracic surgical ward
   Mrs. Leena Sotaniemi, secretary of the thoracic
                                    surgical ward

Address:

   University of Oulu
   SF 90210 Oulu
   Finland

I° Cattedra Di Clinica Psichiatrica

Milan, Italy

1) Psychiatry

     Prof. Giordano Invernizzi
     Dr. Roberto Basile
     Dr. Nicoletta Calchi Novati
     Dr. Alberto Passerini

2) Heart Surgeons

     Prof. Paolo Biglioli
     Prof. Andrea Sala
     Dr. Pier Silvio Gerometta
     Dr. Alberto Repossini

Address:

     I° Cattredra Di Clinica Psichiatrica
     Guardia II - Ospedale Maggiore
     Via Francesco Sforza 35
     20122 Milano, Italia

Benedikt Kreutz Rehabilitationszentrum

Bad Krozingen, Federal Republic of Germany

Prof. Dr. med D. Birnbaum
Dr. Wolfgang Langosch
Dr. med D. Preis
Prof. Dr. med. G.-M. von Reutern

Address:

     Benedikt Kreutz Rehabilitationszentrum
     Sudring 15
     7812 Bad Krozingen
     Federal Republic of Germany

University of Kiel

Federal Republic of Germany

University Clinic

a) Dept. of Cardiovascular Surgery

    A. Bernhard
    D. Rogensburger

    Abteilung Kardiovasculare Chirurgic der
    Christian-Albrechts-Universitat Kiel
    Arnold-Heller-Str. 7, D-2300 Kiel 1

b) Dept. of Neurology

    H. Strenge

c) Dept. of Psychiatry

    G. Paulsen

d) Dept. of Psychotherapy and Psychosomatics

    S. Gratz
    H. Speidel
    B. Strauss

Address:

b) - d)

    Zentrum Nervenheilkunde der
    Christian-Albrechts-Universitat Kiel
    Niemannsweg 147, D-2300 Kiel 1

INDEX

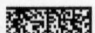